Dermoscopy Trichoscopy and Onychoscopy | In Diseases of the Pigmented Skin

AN ATLAS AND SHORT TEXT

AF067350

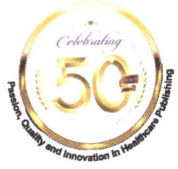

Dermoscopy Trichoscopy and Onychoscopy In Diseases of the Pigmented Skin

AN ATLAS AND SHORT TEXT

Second Edition

Editor

Uday S Khopkar MD FIDP
Consultant Dermatologist and Dermatopathologist
Emeritus Professor of Dermatology
Department of Dermatology and Venereology
Seth Gordhandas Sunderdas Medical College (GSMC) and
the King Edward Memorial (KEM) Hospital
Mumbai, Maharashtra, India

Assistant Editor

Ankit H Bharti MD FIDD
Consultant Dermatologist and Dermatopathologist
Department of Skin and Dermatopathology Referral Center
General Hospital
Vyara, Gujarat, India

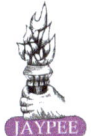

JAYPEE BROTHERS MEDICAL PUBLISHERS

The Health Sciences Publisher

New Delhi | London

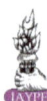

Jaypee Brothers Medical Publishers (P) Ltd.

Headquarters
Jaypee Brothers Medical Publishers (P) Ltd
4838/24, Ansari Road, Daryaganj
New Delhi 110 002, India
Phone: +91-11-43574357
Fax: +91-11-43574314
Email: jaypee@jaypeebrothers.com

Overseas Office
J.P. Medical Ltd
83 Victoria Street, London
SW1H 0HW (UK)
Phone: +44 20 3170 8910
Fax: +44 (0)20 3008 6180
Email: info@jpmedpub.com

Website: www.jaypeebrothers.com
Website: www.jaypeedigital.com

© 2020, Jaypee Brothers Medical Publishers

The views and opinions expressed in this book are solely those of the original contributor(s)/author(s) and do not necessarily represent those of editor(s) of the book.

All rights reserved. No part of this publication may be reproduced, stored or transmitted in any form or by any means, electronic, mechanical, photocopying, recording or otherwise, without the prior permission in writing of the publishers.

All brand names and product names used in this book are trade names, service marks, trademarks or registered trademarks of their respective owners. The publisher is not associated with any product or vendor mentioned in this book.

Medical knowledge and practice change constantly. This book is designed to provide accurate, authoritative information about the subject matter in question. However, readers are advised to check the most current information available on procedures included and check information from the manufacturer of each product to be administered, to verify the recommended dose, formula, method and duration of administration, adverse effects and contraindications. It is the responsibility of the practitioner to take all appropriate safety precautions. Neither the publisher nor the author(s)/editor(s) assume any liability for any injury and/or damage to persons or property arising from or related to use of material in this book.

This book is sold on the understanding that the publisher is not engaged in providing professional medical services. If such advice or services are required, the services of a competent medical professional should be sought.

Every effort has been made where necessary to contact holders of copyright to obtain permission to reproduce copyright material. If any have been inadvertently overlooked, the publisher will be pleased to make the necessary arrangements at the first opportunity. The **CD/DVD-ROM** (if any) provided in the sealed envelope with this book is complimentary and free of cost. **Not meant for sale.**

Inquiries for bulk sales may be solicited at: jaypee@jaypeebrothers.com

Dermoscopy, Trichoscopy and Onychoscopy in Diseases of the Pigmented Skin:
An Atlas and Short Text

First Edition: 2012
Second Edition: 2020
ISBN: 978-93-89034-01-1

Dedicated to

Dr SL Wadhwa
My teacher in clinical dermatology
Who has a penchant for the minutiae in clinical dermatology
and
Whose fancy for the lights and lenses caught onto me

Contributors

Anjali Pal MBBS MD (Dermatology)
Consultant Dermatologist
Rita Skin Foundation
Kolkata, West Bengal, India

Ankit H Bharti MD FIDD
Consultant Dermatologist and
Dermatopathologist
Department of Skin and
Dermatopathology
Referral Center
General Hospital Vyara
Tapi, Gujarat, India

Archana Singal
MD FAMS
Director Professor
Department of
Dermatology and Sexually
Transmitted Disease (STD)
University College of
Medical Sciences and
Guru Tegh Bahadur (GTB)
Hospital
New Delhi, India

Atul M Dongre MD Fellowship in
Diagnostic Dermatology, Fellowship
in Dermatopathology (Germany)
Associate Professor
King Edward Memorial (KEM)
Hospital and Seth Gordhandas
Sunderdas Medical
College (GSMC)
Mumbai, Maharashtra, India

Bhagyashri Abak MD
Senior Medical Officer
Department of Dermatology
Seth Gordhandas Sunderdas
Medical College (GSMC) and
the King Edward Memorial
(KEM) Hospital
Mumbai, Maharashtra, India

Deepak Jakhar MD
Senior Resident
Department of
Dermatology and STD
North Delhi Municipal
Corporation Medical College
and Hindu Rao Hospital
Delhi, India

Feroze Kaliyadan
MD DNB FRCP (London) Dip Eur Board SCE-RCP
Assistant Professor
Department of Dermatology
King Faisal University
Hofuf, Saudi Arabia

Gopalsing Rajput
MBBS MD (Derm and Ven)
Graded Specialist Dermatology
INHS Kalyani
Visakhapatnam, India

Ishmeet Kaur MD
Consultant Dermatologist
Department of Dermatology
Kaya Skin Clinic
Delhi, India

Khan Kaleem MBBS MD
Consultant
Department of Dermatology
Wockhardt Hospital
Mumbai, Maharashtra, India

KC Nischal MD
Consultant Dermatologist
Nirmal Skin and Hair Clinic
Bengaluru, Karnataka, India

Laxmisha Chandrashekhar
MD DNB
Additional Professor
Department of Dermatology
Jawaharlal Institute of Postgraduate Medical Education and Research (JIPMER)
Puducherry, India

Manas Chatterjee MD DNB
Senior Advisor
Professor and Head
Department of Dermatology
Institute of Naval Medicine
INHS Asvini
Mumbai, Maharashtra, India

Mary Thomas MD FIDD FRGUHS
Consultant Dermatologist
Department of Dermatology
Poornima Hospital
Bengaluru, Karnataka, India

Monica Bambroo DVDL DNB
Consultant Dermatologist
Anugrah Urology and Skin Clinic
Ghaziabad, Uttar Pradesh, India

Nina Madnani
MBBS DVD MD FAAD FSSVD
Department Co-ordinator
Department of Dermatology
PD Hinduja National Hospital
Mumbai, Maharashtra, India

Nirmal B MD FRGUHS
Associate Professor
Department of Dermatology
Velammal Medical College
Hospital and Research Institute
Madurai, Tamil Nadu, India

Niti Khunger MD DDV DNB
Professor and Consultant
Dermatologist
Department of
Dermatology and STD
Vardhaman Mahavir Medical
College and Safdarjung Hospital
New Delhi, India

Omprakash HM MBBS DVD
Consultant Dermatologist
Department of Dermatology
Vikram Hospital
Mysuru, Karnataka, India

Pinanky Jadhav DVDL
Consultant Dermatologist
Eternis Skin Hair and Laser Clinic
Pune, Maharashtra, India

Punit Saraogi MD
Consultant Dermatologist
Everything Skin and Hair Clinic
Mumbai, Maharashtra, India

Purva Mehta
MBBS DNB (Dermatology)
Consultant Dermatologist
Rita Skin Foundation
Kolkata, West Bengal, India
Nucleus Eye and
Skin Clinic
Mumbai, Maharashtra, India

Rachita Dhurat MD
Organizing Chairperson
Trichology Update
Professor and Head
Department of Dermatology
Lokmanya Tilak Municipal
(LTM) General Hospital and
Lokmanya Tilak Municipal
Medical College
Mumbai, Maharashtra, India

Rashmi Sharma
MBBS DDVL DNB
Dermatologist and
Aesthetic Physician
Madhukar Rainbow Children's
Hospital and BirthRight Hospital
New Delhi, India

Ruchi Hemdani MBBS
Junior Resident
Department of Dermatology
Institute of Naval Medicine
INHS Asvini
Mumbai, Maharashtra, India

Sarvesh S Thatte DVDL DNB
Consultant Dermatologist
Skin Privilege
Skin, Hair and Nail Clinic
Pune, Maharashtra, India

Shekhar S Haldar
MD Fellowship in Diagnostic Dermatology
Consultant Dermatologist
Belle Vue Clinic, Circus Avenue
Kolkata, West Bengal, India

Siddhi Chikhalkar
MD Fellowship in Diagnostic Dermatology
Associate Professor
King Edward Memorial (KEM) Hospital and Seth Gordhandas Sunderdas Medical College (GSMC)
Mumbai, Maharashtra, India

Shubhangi Mahajan
MBBS DDVL
Senior Registrar
Department of Dermatology
Seth Gordhandas Sunderdas Medical College (GSMC) and the King Edward Memorial (KEM) Hospital
Mumbai, Maharashtra, India

Subrata Malakar MBBS DCH MD
Medical Director
Rita Skin Foundation
Kolkata, West Bengal, India

Sunanda Mahajan MD DVD
Associate Professor
Department of Dermatology
Seth Gordhandas Sunderdas Medical College (GSMC) and the King Edward Memorial (KEM) Hospital
Mumbai, Maharashtra, India

Sunil N Mishra MD
Consultant Cosmetic Dermatologist and Hair Specialist
Wellness Hub, Powai
Godrej Hospital, Vikhroli
LH Hiranandani Hospital
Mumbai, Maharashtra, India

Sushil Pande MD
Associate Professor
NKP Salve Institute of Medical Sciences
Nagpur, Maharashtra, India

Tulika Yadav MD
Clinical Fellow
Department of Dermatology
Antrim Area Hospital
Northern Trust, HSC
Antrim, Northern Ireland
United Kingdom

Uday S Khopkar MD FIDP
Consultant Dermatologist and
Dermatopathologist
Emeritus Professor of
Dermatology
Department of Dermatology and
Venereology
Seth Gordhandas Sunderdas
Medical College (GSMC) and
the King Edward Memorial
(KEM) Hospital
Mumbai, Maharashtra, India

Usha Khemani MD DDV FAAD
Associate Professor
Department of Dermatology
Venereology and Leprosy
Grant Government Medical
College, Sir Jamshedjee
Jeejeebhoy Group of Hospitals
Mumbai, Maharashtra, India

Vidya Kharkar MD DVD
Professor and Head of
Department
Department of Dermatology
Seth Gordhandas Sunderdas
Medical College (GSMC) and
the King Edward Memorial
(KEM) Hospital
Mumbai, Maharashtra, India

Viral Thakkar MD
Consultant Dermatologist
Satadhar Skin and Cosmetic Clinic
Ahmedabad, Gujarat, India

Preface to the Second Edition

I am pleased to write a preface for this revised 2nd edition of *Dermoscopy, Trichoscopy and Onychoscopy in Diseases of the Pigmented Skin: An Atlas and Short Text*. Several new chapters have been added and some are completely rewritten by experts in this field like Drs Archana Singal, Laxmisha Chandrashekhar, Manas Chatterjee, Omprakash HM, Nirmal B, Feroze Kaliyadan, and Subrata Malakar among others. I am sure, this has added value to this text and made it more comprehensive.

Dermoscopy, as a technique, has rapidly evolved over the last decade and this made it necessary to replace many of the pictures in the previous edition of this book. The authors have taken efforts to introduce new dermoscopic images to cover recently described signs and conditions. This should make it instructive to go through this update. I am thankful to the contributors and my editorial assistant for delivering the goods in time and keeping the pressure on me to bring this project to completion.

I wholeheartedly thank Shri Jitendar P Vij (Group Chairman), Mr Ankit Vij (Managing Director), Ms Chetna Malhotra Vohra (Associate Director—Content Strategy) of M/s Jaypee Brothers Medical Publishers (P) Ltd, New Delhi, India, for stimulating me to bringing out this update. I am also thankful to the Jaypee desktop publication team, especially Ms Savleen Kaur, for doing job neatly in such a short time.

I appeal to my colleagues and postgraduates to send me their feedback regarding this book so that we can improve it to suit their needs. I end with expressing hope that this book stimulates interest in dermoscopy of the spectrum of pigmentary and inflammatory skin, hair, and nail diseases especially for the new entrants.

Uday S Khopkar

Preface to the First Edition

I am happy to write a preface to this short compilation of articles released on the occasion of the First National CME on Dermoscopy organized by the Department of Dermatology at Seth GS Medical College and KEM Hospital, Mumbai, Maharashtra, India. Majority of the articles are being presented as papers at the CME and we could have easily published them as an abstract book. However, I decided to do more since the most important information in any dermoscopy presentation are the images flashed, and without images, it is difficult to appreciate the findings being communicated at the presentation.

Moreover, I expect that armed with this book, my colleagues would find it easier to practice dermoscopy on their patients when they return to their clinics to cater to their patients. This should help propagating the noninvasive technique of dermoscopy in a small way. I also thank my colleagues and guest speakers at the conference for readily penning the text according to the requirement of this atlas and text on dermoscopy.

I express my deep gratitude towards our popular Dean and Director, Dr Sanjay Oak, without whose encouragement, this CME or this publication would not have been possible. I wholeheartedly thank Shri Jitendar P Vij (Group Chairman) of

M/s Jaypee Brothers Medical Publishers (P) Ltd., for agreeing to do this publication at a very short notice. I am also thankful to the Jaypee desktop publication team for doing this job neatly in such a short time. Like any publication done at short notice, there may be some shortcomings in this. If they are scientific, I am sure my colleagues will point them out and we hope to correct them in subsequent editions. If they are of technical nature, I assure you that they are due to oversight and not intentional.

I end with expressing hope that this small book stimulates interest in dermoscopy of the spectrum of pigmentary and inflammatory skin diseases observed in the brown skin and in trichoscopy.

Uday S Khopkar

Contents

SECTION 1: BASICS OF DERMOSCOPY

1. **Principles and Techniques of Dermoscopy and Videodermoscopy** 1
   KC Nischal, Uday S Khopkar

2. **Dermoscopy: Terms, Definitions, and Patterns in Diseases of the Brown Skin** 10
   Omprakash HM

3. **Choice of Dermatoscope: An End-user Perspective** 23
   Nirmal B

4. **Smartphone Dermatoscopes** 40
   Nina Madnani, Khan Kaleem

5. **Dermatoscopy of Normal Skin and Appendages** 47
   Nirmal B

6. **Vascular Patterns** 59
   Anjali Pal, Purva Mehta, Subrata Malakar

7. **Applications of Dermatoscopy** 76
   Usha Khemani, Feroze Kaliyadan

SECTION 2: DISORDERS OF HYPERPIGMENTATION

8. **Disorders of Facial Hyperpigmentation** 95
   Ankit H Bharti, Uday S Khopkar

9. **Dermoscopy in Melasma** 122
Niti Khunger, Rashmi Sharma

10. **Importance of Dermatoscopy in Diagnosing Exogenous Ochronosis** 139
Sunil N Mishra, Rachita Dhurat

11. **Pigmented Purpuric Dermatoses** 146
Siddhi Chikhalkar, Monica Bambroo, Uday S Khopkar

12. **Becker's Nevus versus Café au lait Macules: A Dermoscopic Analysis** 156
Mary Thomas, Uday S Khopkar

SECTION 3: DISORDERS OF HYPOPIGMENTATION

13. **Dermoscopy in Vitiligo: Utility for Early Diagnosis, Assessing Stability and Monitoring Therapy** 166
Laxmisha Chandreshekhar

14. **Differential Diagnosis of Hypopigmented Lesions** 175
Ankit H Bharti, Uday S Khopkar

15. **Dermoscopy in the Differentiation of Idiopathic Guttate Hypomelanosis and Guttate Vitiligo** 197
Monica Bambroo, Sushil Pande, Uday S Khopkar

SECTION 4: PAPULOSQUAMOUS DISORDERS

16. **Dermoscopy in Lichen Planus and Differential Diagnosis** 204
Sunanda Mahajan

17. **Lichen Planus Pigmentosus versus Ashy Dermatosis: Through a Dermoscope** 246
    Shekhar S Haldar, Uday S Khopkar

18. **Dermoscopy: Eczema versus Psoriasis** 259
    Manas Chatterjee, Ruchi Hemdani

SECTION 5: NAIL DISORDERS

19. **Overview of Onychoscopy** 271
    Archana Singal, Deepak Jakhar

20. **Neoplastic Nail Unit Disorders** 292
    Ishmeet Kaur, Archana Singal

21. **Nail Psoriasis versus Onychomycosis** 313
    Tulika Yadav, Uday S Khopkar

22. **Nailfold Capillaroscopy in Connective Tissue Diseases** 321
    Pinanky Jadhav, Uday S Khopkar

SECTION 6: TRICHOSCOPY

23. **An Overview of Trichoscopy** 332
    Vidya Kharkar, Bhagyashri Abak

24. **Trichoscopy of Patchy Alopecia** 369
    Viral Thakkar, Shekhar S Haldar

25. **Phototrichogram and TrichoScan®** 386
    Punit Saraogi, Rachita Dhurat

SECTION 7: MISCELLANEOUS DERMOSCOPY APPLICATION

26. **Dermoscopy of Granulomatous Skin Diseases** 396
    Shubhangi Mahajan, Uday S Khopkar

27. **Dermoscopy of Benign Skin Tumors** 410
    Manas Chatterjee, Ruchi Hemdani

28. **Dermoscopy of Malignant Cutaneous Tumors** 434
    Laxmisha Chandrashekar

29. **Dermoscopy in Keratosis Pilaris** 448
    Mary Thomas, Uday S Khopkar

30. **Porokeratosis** 457
    Sarvesh S Thatte, Uday S Khopkar

31. **Genodermatoses** 466
    Atul M Dongre, Uday S Khopkar

32. **Dermoscopy: Infections and Infestations** 473
    Manas Chatterjee, Gopalsing Rajput

Index 491

Prologue to the First Edition

The field of dermoscopy is relatively unexplored and provides exciting opportunities for original observations. Although the technique of dermoscopy was invented more than 100 years back, till recently, the instrument was used mainly on the white skin for diagnosis of skin melanoma and monitoring of melanocytic nevi.

I have been using various versions of dermoscope over the last 25 years and with help of my students and colleagues I made several observations, particularly in the field of inflammatory and pigmentary skin diseases in brown-skinned patients. While some of the observations have a diagnostic value and fill up lacunae in diagnosis (where even a biopsy is not offering reliable differentiation), and others help in clinical decision making or assessing prognosis.

Dermoscope should not be viewed as just another magnifying glass, but is a completely new way to look at the skin. It shows not only surface features but also subsurface features. The benefits of this noninvasive technique multiply as we start using it on a routine basis. Dermoscopy has its own terminologies that allow precise scientific communication. It is imperative for dermatologists to get used to the terminologies and the images that it corresponds with. This will allow them to use dermoscope on a daily basis, so as to eventually transfer its benefits to their patients. It is with this intent of creating a bank of images of applications of dermoscopy in diseases affecting the brown skin, that we have compiled this book. I am sure that many more diseases lend themselves to study with dermoscope and this compilation will stimulate my colleagues to undertake more such observations in the coming years.

Uday S Khopkar
Editor, 1st edition, January 2012

Section 1: Basics of Dermoscopy

CHAPTER 1

Principles and Techniques of Dermoscopy and Videodermoscopy

KC Nischal, Uday S Khopkar

Dermoscope synonyms: Dermatoscope, skin surface microscope, epiluminescence microscope, or episcope.

INTRODUCTION

Dermoscopy is a noninvasive, diagnostic method which requires one to visualize subtle surface and some subsurface changes in the skin using a dermoscope. It is an instrumental method to detect certain subtle changes which are not visualized even on using a magnifying lens; moreover, certain specific set of features can help in establishing a diagnosis, thus obviating need of a biopsy. With advent of the facility of connectivity to computer or other storage facility, it is also helpful in monitoring certain disease progression and treatment response as the older images are immediately available and thus, can be correlated.

Thus, dermoscope is a precise magnifying instrument, with facility of specialized illuminating systems such as visible light, polarized light and ultraviolet light; an adjustable magnification (50–500×) which helps assess structures as deep as reticular dermis, and the ability to record and save images aids documentation and monitoring. Proper knowledge and skill of dermoscopy can be a virtue in easing the process of diagnosis.

PRINCIPLES OF DERMOSCOPY

The basic principle of dermoscopy is illumination (and transillumination) of a lesion with different light sources and studying it with a high magnification lens that may or may not be connected to a camera and computer.[1,2] Any light ray incident on skin undergoes varying proportions of reflection, refraction, diffraction, and absorption dependent to physical properties of the skin (Fig. 1). Most of the light incident on dry, scaly skin is reflected, but smooth, oily skin allows most of the light to pass through it, reaching the deeper dermis and improving visibility of subsurface features.

Linkage fluids like oils applied over the lesions to be studied improve the translucency of the skin, although many modern-day videodermoscopes do not require use of linkage fluids (Fig. 2). Various linkage fluids used are oils (immersion oil, olive oil, and mineral oil), water, antiseptic solution, glycerin, and gels. A practical problem with use of oils as linkage medium is that, unless applied abundantly, they cause a lot of bubbles that may make the lesion difficult to visualize or photograph. Moreover, immersion oil is not used because it

CHAPTER 1: Principles and Techniques of Dermoscopy... 3

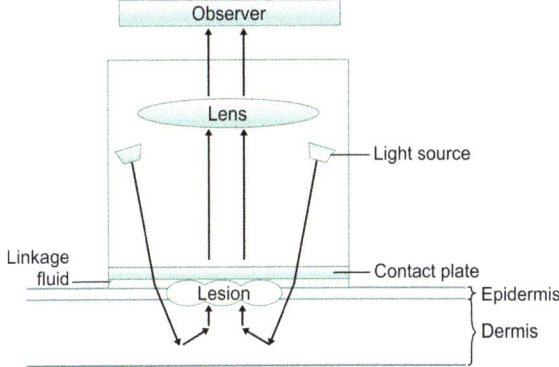

Fig. 1: Principle of a contact dermoscope.
Source: Reproduced with permission from Dr DM Thappa, Chief Editor, IJDVL; Nischal KC, Khopkar U. Dermoscope. Indian J Dermatol Venereol Leprol. 2005;71:300-3.

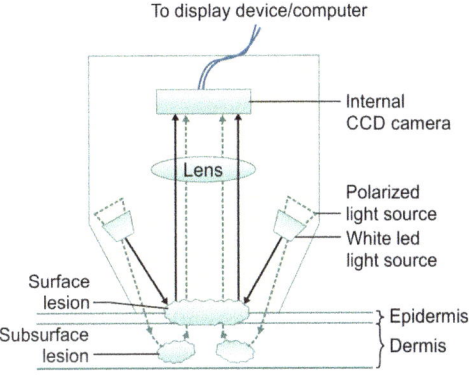

Fig. 2: Principle of a videodermoscope.

contains chlorinated paraffin and dibutyl phthalate, which have teratogenic, fetotoxic, and carcinogenic effects.[3]

Water causes fewer bubbles but evaporates quickly and hence is less preferred than oils. Besides, their refractive index is not as close to that of the skin; hence, subsurface features may not be well seen. An evidence-based study by Gewirtzman AJ et al.[4] showed that a 70% alcoholic solution gives best results in terms of image clarity, eliminating air bubbles, and better patient tolerability, as it has less strong odor. We use commercially available antiseptic solutions containing 70% alcohol. These solutions are better tolerated by patients, as they also have an additional emollient and moisturizing effect. Their use also potentially decreases the rate of transmission of infections,[5] as we deal with inflammatory dermatoses, which are likely to be excoriated and secondarily colonized with microorganisms. One can also use liquid paraffin, which is inexpensive, safe, and easily available, with good results. Air bubbles are more likely to form with paraffin oil.

Glass has a refractive index (1.52) similar to that of skin (1.55) and hence when placed over linkage fluids coated skin (as in contact plates), further enhances transillumination of the lesion. Gels (ultrasound gel) are useful, while doing dermoscopy of solid curved areas, particularly the area surrounding the nail plate.[6] By using gels, the entire curved area of the nail can be viewed as the viscous gel fills up and remains in the space between the surface to be viewed and the contact plate unlike liquids which would escape out. Another indication of using gels as linkage fluid is while doing dermoscopy around the eye region, because unlike liquids, gel would not flow into the eyes.[7]

CHAPTER 1: Principles and Techniques of Dermoscopy...

Videodermoscopes with powerful light sources do not usually use linkage fluid thereby simplifying the procedure of dermoscopy further. This also allows them to show the surface features of the skin on "as is" basis that is needed to assess dryness or oiliness of the skin.

PARTS OF A DERMOSCOPE

The essential components of a dermoscope are:
- *Achromatic lens*: Most basic instruments provide 10X magnification, but higher magnifications like 20X give better results and higher magnification or up to 1,000X can be achieved with special lenses or with CCD cameras used in modern-day videodermoscopes.
- *Inbuilt illuminating system*: Halogen lamps, which are oriented at an angle of 20°, placed within the handheld piece were the order of the day till recently. However, the color contrast of lesions gets altered by the yellow light of halogen lamps. Light-emitting diodes (LEDs) are now standard sources that provide high intensity white light and consume 70% less power than halogen lamps. Illumination can be altered by turning off a set of LEDs. They are also designed to emit lights of different colors for better visualization of the skin as penetration of the skin by light is proportional to the wavelength of light.

  Use of polarized light sources has added a new dimension to videodermoscopy by allowing them to display subsurface features of skin lesions without the use of contact plates and linkage fluids. Further, addition of ultraviolet light source allows fluorescence to be studied on a microscopic basis and its applications need more exploration. Few dermoscopes have specialized lights to enhance few dermoscopic feature viz., orange PigmentBoost™ to improve visualization of pigmented structures (DermLite DL3 and DL4, 3Gen).

- *Power supply*: Handheld instruments are usually powered by batteries and may have rechargeable handles which connect to general power supply (Heine Delta 20) or has a USB port (DermLite 4)
- *Display or viewing system*: While handheld dermoscopes have a simple see-through viewing window, the videodermoscopes have the ability to connect to a computer or another display device or have their own display screen.
- *Inbuilt photography systems*: These have become an essential component of a dermoscope (not available as standard feature with handheld dermoscopes) because of the obvious need to record and store the images. The camera may be either an attachable conventional or digital camera or an inbuilt video camera, and supporting software, for the capture, storage, retrieval, and even interpretation of images.

TECHNIQUE

Dermoscopy can be done by either the noncontact or the contact technique. In the contact technique, the glass plate of the instrument comes in contact with the surface of the linkage fluid applied to the lesion (Figs. 1 and 3). In contrast, in the

CHAPTER 1: Principles and Techniques of Dermoscopy...

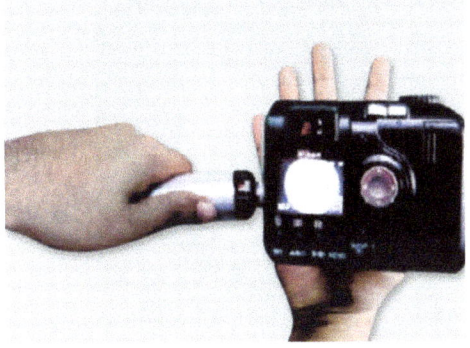

Fig. 3: Handheld dermoscope Heine Delta 20© with camera attachment.

noncontact technique, no linkage fluid is needed speeding up the procedure further. In the noncontact technique of videodermoscope, separate LEDs emit white light and polarized light and the image is captured by a CCD camera (Figs. 2 and 4). While the noncontact technique ensures that there are no nosocomial infections,[5] the ability to capture and store digital images on a computer truly puts a videodermoscope ahead of a contact dermoscope. Contact plates are made of multicoated silicone glass and are of different types. Graduated plates have inscribed scales for measuring the lesion, while nongraduated plates lack a scale. Small plates have a small contact area to facilitate use in difficult to access regions like the web spaces, flexures, and for nailfold capillaroscopy. Contact plates can be sterilized by using 2% glutaraldehyde, methylated spirit, boiling, or autoclaving.

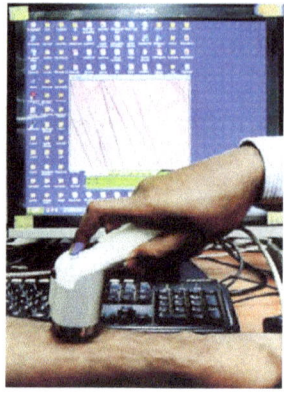

Fig. 4: Videodermoscope in use.

CONCLUSION

Dermoscopes are hand illuminated microscopes that give a lot of additional diagnostic information to clinicians. Though their major use earlier was restricted in the study of melanocytic nevi and melanoma, their importance in study of inflammatory and pigmentary dermatoses is being increasingly recognized and applied.

REFERENCES

1. Nischal KC, Khopkar U. Dermoscope. Indian J Dermatol Venereol Leprol. 2005;71:300-3.
2. Stolz W, Bilek P, Landchaer M, et al. Basis of dermatoscopy and skin-surface microscopy. In: Stolz W, Bilek P, Landchaer M (Eds). Color Atlas of Dermatoscopy, 1st edition. Germany: Blackwell Publications; 1994. pp. 7-10.

3. Binder M, Kittler H, Pehamberger H, et al. Possible hazard to patients from immersion oil used for epiluminescence microscopy. J Am Acad Dermatol. 1999;40:499.
4. Gewirtzman AJ, Saurat JH, Braun RP. An evaluation of dermoscopy fluids and application techniques. Br J Dermatol. 2003;149:59-63.
5. Stauffer F, Kittler H, Forstinger C, et al. The dermatoscope: a potential source of nosocomial infection? Melanoma Res. 2001;11:153-6.
6. Ronger S, Touzet S, Ligeron C, et al. Dermoscopic examination of nail pigmentation. Arch Dermatol. 2002;138:1327-37.
7. Melski JW. Water-soluble gels in epiluminescence microscopy. J Am Acad Dermatol. 1993;29:129-30.

CHAPTER 2

Dermoscopy: Terms, Definitions, and Patterns in Diseases of the Brown Skin

Omprakash HM

INTRODUCTION

Dermoscopy is a visible or ultraviolet light-based tool, evolving since 1655 to visualize epidermal, dermoepidermal and papillary dermal structures. The initial devices were bulkier, monocular or binocular with magnifications ranging from 10× to 172×. Some resembled a miniature telescope and others like a pathology compound microscope. Zeiss[1] idea of using oil or immersion fluid to reduce the refraction or reflection of incident light was extrapolated to dermoscopy in 1893 by Unna.[2] The initial indication for dermoscopy, not surprisingly in 1920s, was differentiating tuberculosis from syphilis.[3-6] In 1928, cretinism,[7] surprisingly entered the indications but failed. All these years dermoscopy was a predominant European science with Austria and Germany leading the way.

In 1950, Leon Goldman from USA, tried dermoscopy in pigmentary lesions including melanoma.[8] The cumbersome, bulkier dermoscope with poor illumination were later replaced with bright illumination of light-emitting diode (LED) bulbs. The need for contact plate, which again made dermoscopy messier, was improved by using polarization light technology. Now, we have handheld pocket devices with image capturing capability using smartphones or digital cameras. This evolution took place around year 2000.[9]

EVOLUTION OF TERMINOLOGY: DERMATOSCOPY TO DERMOSCOPY

In 1920, Saphier introduced the term: dermatoscopy.[3] "Vital skin histology" was used in 1958.[10] "Incident light microscopy" terminology was first used in a publication of Bernard Ackerman in 1981.[11] In 1989, Soyer et al. introduced an alternate term—"surface microscopy".[12] "Epiluminescence light microscopy" found first print in 1989, in a Journal of American Academy of Dermatology.[13] The current terminology—"dermoscopy" was coined by Freidman from USA in 1991.[14]

Is it Dermatoscopy or Dermoscopy?

The debate of terminology is torn between traditionalist and innovative group. The traditionalist argues that we have—dermatology, dermatopathology and hence the correct term is dermatoscopy.

Dr Bernard Ackerman in his article[15] beautifully argues to change for good to—"dermatoscopy".

> "I write to call attention to the fact that there is no true words "dermoscopy" and "dermoscopic": The correct words are "dermatoscopy" and "dermatoscopic"[15]
>
> —Dr Bernard Ackerman

CHROMOPHORES OF SKIN, HAIR, AND NAIL

When light is focused on skin, hair, or nail—we find various colors—black, light brown, dark brown, gray, blue or white, and red. The above colors forming different patterns helped us arrive at fewer differentials or at times final diagnosis. So, what is the basis of so many colors. These are chromophores. These include—dirt/dust on hair or skin (black/brown), keratin protein (brown), sebum in pilosebaceous orifice (yellow), melanin in—stratum corneum (black), stratum malpighii (light to dark brown), gray (papillary dermis), blue (reticular dermis), blood (black or red), and lastly collagen in dermis (white).

Chromophores to Patterns and Nomenclature—Metaphoric versus Descriptive

The different chromophores accumulate in various planes of skin, hair, and nail; and also form various morphologies. This morphology has caught the imagination of various investigators leading to different nomenclature, which may be metaphoric or descriptive. At least, we can count about 62 different metaphoric terminologies, which are well known out of nearly 128 terminologies. During the last few years, the vocabulary of dermoscopy has expanded so substantively that it has become difficult even for the authorities to remember the same.

During the last years, the vocabulary of dermoscopy has expanded so significantly that it has become difficult even for experts to remember the same.

A metaphor—"is a word or phrase used to compare two unlike objects". An example could be "brain like" (Figs. 1A and B) appearance in case of seborrheic keratosis.

Although colorful or imaginative metaphors are memorable, their sheer number—128 and the fact that some are ambiguous, make them a potential barrier to learning and research.[16] Hence, descriptive terms were framed to replace metaphors.

Descriptive terms were coined by Harald Kittler from Vienna and his other colleagues.[17,18] They coined terminologies for—pigmented lesions and cutaneous vessels. The six building blocks (basic element) for pigmented lesion description were—(1) lines, (2) dots, (3) clods, (4) circle, (5) pseudopod, and (6) structureless. A brief note on the above descriptive term is provided in the Table 1.

These above six basic elements could have patterns. A pattern of lines. The lines could be parallel (nevi in foot), curved, reticular, branched, or radial (recurrent nevi). The clods could be peripheral in lesion, central, or diffuse (compound nevi). Next in a given lesion we could have overlapping pattern of lines and clods (melanoma). Hence by using above elements and pattern along with colors, we could replace 128 metaphors.

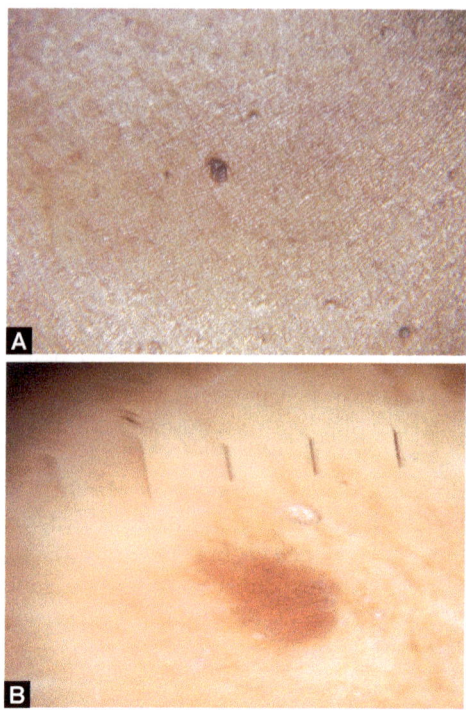

Figs. 1A and B: (A) Lesion on face—with clinical differentials—verruca plana versus seborrheic keratosis; (B) Contact dermoscopy (zoom) image showing "brain-like" appearance. Final diagnosis—seborrheic keratosis. Metaphoric terminology—"brain like".

The descriptive terms for vessels has just three terms: (1) dots, (2) clods, (3) linear vessels (Table 2). The linear

CHAPTER 2: Dermoscopy: Terms, Definitions, and Patterns in Diseases...

Table 1: Descriptive terms for pigmented structures.

Descriptive terminology	Image	Brief description
Lines		A straight, curved linear mark
Dots		A small solid pigmented spot
Clod		A larger solidly pigmented lesion of various shapes—oval, polygonal
Circle		A nonsolidly pigmented circular spot
Pseudopod		A solid line with peripheral club-shaped extension of pigmentation
Structureless		Absence of above five elements

Table 2: Descriptive terms for vessels.

Descriptive terms of vessels	Image	Brief description
Dot		A solid red dot mostly circular
Clods		An ill-defined cluster of vessels of various shapes—oval, polygonal
Linear vessels		A solid line

vessels were further subdivided into: (1) looped, (2) curved, (3) serpentine, (4) helical and (5) coiled (Table 3).

Table 3: Linear vessels.

Image	Metaphoric terms	Descriptive terms	Clinical cases
	Hairpin vessel	Looped	Squamous cell carcinoma
	Comma vessel	Curved	Dermal nevi
	Glomerular	Coiled	Bowen disease
	Arborizing	Serpentine	Basal cell carcinoma
	Corkscrew	Helical	Melanoma/metastasis

Descriptive terms were meant to be "simple and logical". But descriptive terms were self-defeating.[19] For example in Figures 2A and B, we have a metaphor "spoke wheel". This was replaced with —"central clod with radial lines". This was too cumbersome. Also some terms in descriptive terminology were themselves a minor metaphor, for example, pseudopod (false foot).

With the above controversy in background, the IV World Congress of Dermoscopy was held in Vienna from 16th to 18th April, 2015. All the experts, by hand votes favored continued usage of old metaphoric and established descriptive terms. They recommended that when creating new terminology, to use old metaphoric or descriptive terms, instead to creating new words.[16] The Vienna congress also created a dictionary of terminology used in dermoscopy incorporating both—descriptive and metaphoric terms. The abridged version of the same can be seen in Table 4.

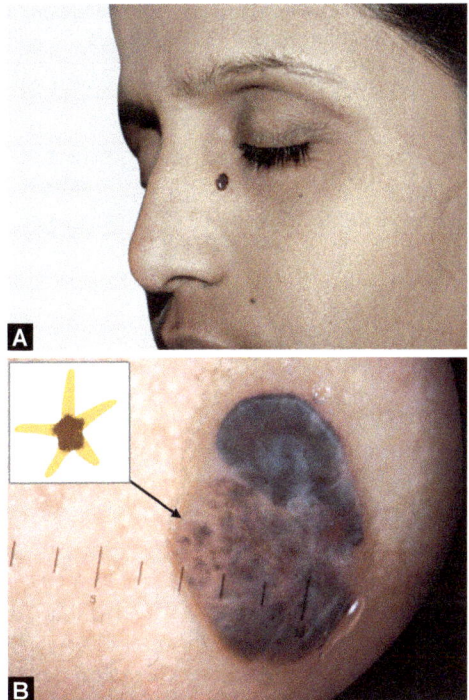

Metaphoric term—"spoke wheel". Descriptive term—"central clod with radial lines"

Figs. 2A and B: (A) Pigmented lesion on left medial canthal zone—clinical differentials—acquired melanocytic nevi versus pigmented basal cell carcinoma; (B) Contact dermoscopy image showing—"spoke wheel appearance at 9 o'clock position". Final diagnosis—pigmented basal cell carcinoma.

Table 4: Dermoscopic terms—descriptive and metaphoric used to describe common lesion findings.[16]

Descriptive	Metaphoric	Clinical significance
Lines		
Lines reticular	Pigment network	Dermatofibroma, melanocytic lesion
Lines reticular and thick	Broadened network	Melanoma
Lines radial connected to a common base	Leaf-like areas	Basal cell carcinoma
Lines radial, converging to a central clod or dot	Spoke wheel area	Basal cell carcinoma
Lines radial at periphery	Streaks	Recurrent nevi, melanoma
Clods		
Clods—yellow, brown	Comedones-like opening	Seborrheic keratosis
Clods—blue	Globules	Basal cell carcinoma
Clods—brown—large and polygonal	Cobblestone pattern	Dermal nevi
Clods—pink and small	Milky red globules	Melanoma
Clods—red or purple	Red lacunae	Hemangioma
Dots		
Dots—gray	Peppering	Melanoma
Dots—white	Milia-like cyst	Seborrheic keratosis

Contd...

CHAPTER 2: Dermoscopy: Terms, Definitions, and Patterns in Diseases...

Contd...

Descriptive	Metaphoric	Clinical significance
Circles		
Circle white		Sqamous cell carcinoma
Circle concentric	Circle within a circle	Lentigo maligna
Structureless		
Structureless zone—blue	Bluish white veil	Melanoma
Structureless zone—white	Scar-like depigmentation	Melanoma
Structureless zone—white, central	Central white patch	Dermatofibroma

Majority of time, dermoscopy is taught by teachers who have learnt in the past metaphoric terminology. Good teachers have sound knowledge of both metaphoric and descriptive terminology. But it is good to have sound knowledge of common metaphoric terminology. Aristotle believed that "it is a great thing, indeed, to make proper use of the poetic forms: but the greatest thing by far is to be a master of metaphor". So a brief summary of the classical metaphoric term is provided in the Table 5.

Table 5: Common metaphoric terms and their definition.[16]

Metaphoric term	Definition
Typical pigment network	Network with minimal variability of—color, thickness, and spacing. Symmetrically distributed
Atypical pigment network	Network with increased variability of—color, thickness, and spacing. Asymmetrically distributed. Color—gray
Cobblestone	Polygonal globules, symmetrically distributed
Radial streaming	Radial linear extensions from the lesion edge
Pseudopods	Bulbous projections seen at the lesion edge associated with network or solid tumor border
Starburst pattern	Peripheral globules or pseudopods around the perimeter of the lesion
Cerebriform pattern	Thick curved lines created by gyri and keratin-filled sulci creating a brain-like appearance
Fingerprint pattern	Light brown thin curved lines that do not interconnect and form a network
Strawberry pattern	Reddish pseudonetwork around hair follicle with white halo appearance
Blotch	Dark structureless area
Blue–whitish veil	A blue irregular blotch with overlying whitish ground–glass haze
Leaf-like areas	Brown, blue, or gray bullous structures coalescing at a common off center base, creating a leaf-like configuration
Spoke wheel area	Brown, gray, or blue radial projection from a central clod of the same color

Contd...

Contd...

Metaphoric term	Definition
Milia-like cyst	White or yellowish opalescent structure corresponding to intraepidermal cyst
Comedones-like opening	Keratin-filled clefts

CONCLUSION

Dermoscopy is an evolving science. Terminologies are created, debated, and refined with time and evidence. It is an exciting time for dermoscopists, to leave behind footprints on the sands of time.

REFERENCES

1. Diepgen P. Geschichte der Medizin. Berlin: de Gruyter; 1965. pp. 138-53.
2. Unna P. Die Diaskopie der Hautkrankheiten. Berl Klin Wochenschr. 1893;42:1016-21.
3. Saphier J. Die Dermatoskopie. I. Mitteilung. Arch Dermatol Syphiol. 1920;128:1-19.
4. Saphier J. Die Dermatoskopie. II. Mitteilung. Arch Dermatol Syphiol. 1921;132:69-86.
5. Saphier J. Die Dermatoskopie. III. Mitteilung. Arch Dermatol Syphiol. 1921;134:314-22.
6. Saphier J. Die Dermatoskopie. IV. Mitteilung. Arch Dermatol Syphiol. 1921;136:149-58.
7. Bettmann S. Felderungszeichnungen der Bauchhaut und Schwangerschaftsstreifen. Zschr Anatom Entwicklungsgesch. 1928;85:658-8.
8. Goldman L. Some investigative studies of pigmented nevi with cutaneous microscopy. J Invest Dermatol. 1951;16:407-27.

9. Stolz W, Bilek P, Landthaler M, et al. Skin surface microscopy. Lancet. 1989;2:864-5.
10. Ehring F. Geschichte und Möglichkeiteneiner Histologiean der lebenden Haut. Hautarzt. 1958;9:1-4.
11. Fritsch P, Pechlaner R. Differentiation of benign from malignant melanocytic lesions using incident light microscopy. In: Ackerman AB, Mihara I (Eds). Pathology of Malignant Melanoma. New York: Masson; 1981: pp. 301-12.
12. Soyer H, SmolleJ, Hödl S, et al. Surface microscopy. A new approach to diagnosis of cutaneous pigment tumors. J Am Acad Dermatol. 1989;11:1-10.
13. Pehamberger H, Steiner A, Wolff K. *In vivo* epiluminescence microscopy of pigmented skin lesions. I. Pattern analysis of pigmented skin lesions. J Am Acad Dermatol. 1987;17:571-83.
14. Friedman RJ, Rigel DS Silverman MK, et al. Malignant melanoma in the 1990s: the continued importance of early detection and the role of physician examination and self-examination of the skin. Cancer. 1991;41:201-26.
15. Ackerman AB. Dermatoscopy, not dermoscopy! J Am. Acad Dermatol. 2006;55:728.
16. Kittler H, Marghoob AA, Argenziano G, et al. Standardization of terminology in dermoscopy/dermatoscopy: Results of the third consensus conference of the International Society of Dermoscopy. J Am Acad Dermatol. 2016;74(6):1093-106.
17. Kittler H. Dermatoscopy: introduction of a new algorithmic method based on pattern analysis for diagnosis of pigmented skin lesions. Dermatopathology: practical & conceptual. 2007;13(1):3.
18. Kittler H, Riedl R, Rosendahl C, et al. Dermatoscopy of unpigmented lesions of the skin: A new classification of vessel morphology based on patter analysis. Dermatopathol Pract Concept. 2008;14(4):3.
19. Giacomel J, Zalaudek I, Marghoob AA. Metaphoric and descriptive terminology in dermoscopy: lessons from the cognitive sciences. Dermatol Pract Concept. 2015;5:69-74.

CHAPTER 3

Choice of Dermatoscope: An End-user Perspective

Nirmal B

INTRODUCTION

In the past few years, dermatoscopy has evolved as a useful technique to observe structures beneath the skin surface that are invisible to the naked eye. Dermatoscopy itself has various subspecialties, including inflammatory diseases (inflammoscopy), cutaneous infestations (entomodermatoscopy), nail and nailfold abnormalities (onychoscopy), and hair and scalp diseases (trichoscopy).[1] Dermatoscopes have evolved from the bulky primitive devices to extremely compact gadgets, which can easily be attached to camera for image capture.

HISTORY OF DERMATOSCOPES

The use of devices to observe skin surface dates back to the 16th century even before dermatology evolved as a science. *Pierre*

Borel, a French physician was the first to use the technique to observe capillaries of the nail bed which was published in 1656, popularly known as "capillaroscopy" today. These observations were reproduced by *Johan Christophorus Kolhaus*, 8 years later. Two centuries later, *Ernst Karl Abbe*, a German physicist and optometrist used cedar oil instead of water to increase the microscope resolution. This fact was used by German dermatopathologist *Paul Gerson Unna* to increase the epidermal translucency and called the technique as "diascopy". Beginning with works of *Maurice Raynaud*, research in second half of 19th century established direct link between capillary abnormalities and collagen vascular diseases.

Detailed descriptions of skin surface microscopy was made by *Johann Saphier* in 1920 and called the technique as "dermatoscopy" for the first time. Saphier was the first to study dermatoscopy of pigmented lesions and described pigment globules in melanocytic nevi.[2] *Leon Goldman* used a monocular microscope with a lighting source to describe nevi, melanoma, and various dermatoses. In the early 21st century, a medical device manufacturer 3Gen from California introduced the first cross-polarized dermatoscope to view subsurface features without immersion fluid.

TYPES OF DERMATOSCOPES

Nonpolarized Dermatoscopes

Nonpolarized dermatoscopes require interface fluid between the glass plate and skin to eliminate reflection from the skin surface. They are useful in the better visualization of superficial layers of skin (Figs. 1A and B). The various interface fluids used currently in dermatoscopy include alcoholic disinfectant, ethanol, isopropyl alcohol, liquid paraffin, and ultrasound gel.[3]

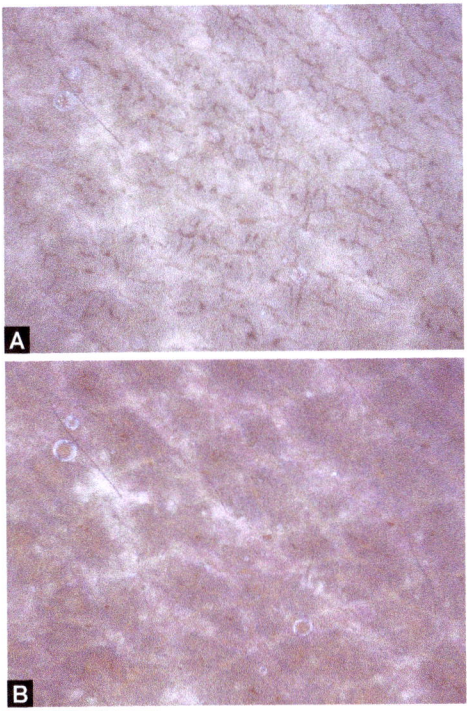

Figs. 1A and B: Dermatoscopy of acanthosis nigricans: Nonpolarized image (A) show multiple cristae and sulci clearly when compared to polarized dermatoscopy (B).

Liquid paraffin or ethanol is preferred for skin dermatoscopy while ultrasound gel is preferred for onychoscopy. Nonpolarized dermatoscopes always require contact with skin surface and interface fluid. Transparent food wraps, adhesive tapes, and disposable caps help avoid nosocomial infection while using contact dermatoscopy.

Brands: Heine Mini3000, Heine Delta20

Polarized Dermatoscopes

Polarized dermatoscopes do not require interface fluid between glass plate and skin surface. They are blind to the superficial layers of skin and are useful in viewing deeper structures (Figs. 2A and B) clearly as light penetrates deeper than nonpolarized dermatoscopes.[4] Interface fluids, however, may be used in polarized dermatoscopes to avoid color distortion

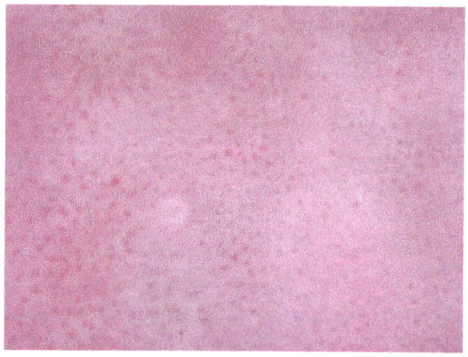

Fig. 2A

CHAPTER 3: Choice of Dermatoscope: An End-user Perspective

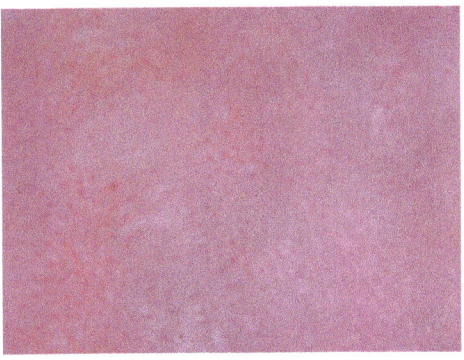

Fig. 2B

Figs. 2A and B: Dermatoscopy of psoriasis: Regular red dots and light red background are better appreciated with polarized dermatoscope (B) as opposed to nonpolarized image (A).

and to get sharper images. Later models can be used to take images by connecting with digital cameras, single-lens reflex (SLRs), and smartphones using adapters.

Brands: DermLite DL100, DermLite Carbon, DermLite DL200 HR, Heine Delta20 Plus, Canfield VEOS HD1

Hybrid Dermatoscopes

Most recent dermatoscopes allow to toggle between polarized and nonpolarized modes, which gives complementary dermatoscopic findings (Figs. 3A and B). Superficial structures like scales, milia-like cyst, comedo-like opening are seen better with nonpolarized dermatoscopy while deeper structures like

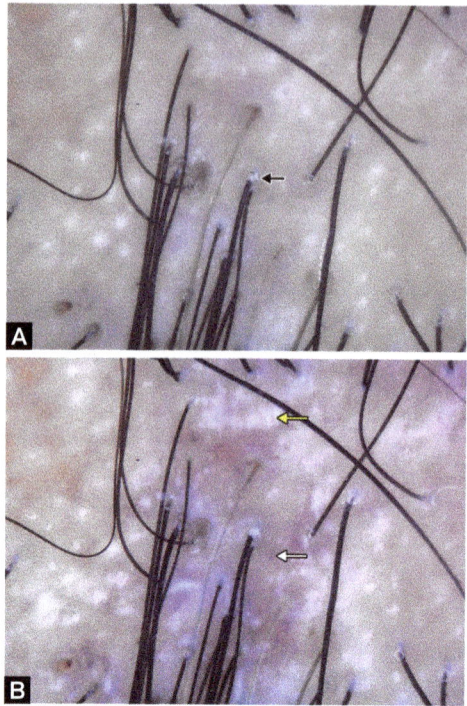

Figs. 3A and B: Dermatoscopy of lichen planopilaris: Both nonpolarized (A) and polarized modes yield complementary information. Perifollicular scales (black arrow) are better seen with nonpolarized dermatoscopy while gray globules (white arrow) and crystalline structures (yellow arrow) are better seen with polarized dermatoscopy.

dermal pigmentation, blood vessels, collagen are seen better with polarized dermatoscopy.[5] Hence, a hybrid dermatoscope switches between these two modes with the click of a button in the dermatoscope. The structures seen with one mode might not be visible with the other, so structures blink when toggled between modes.[6] Images taken with higher models of DermLite are brighter[7] and clearer while that with Heine are warmer and have a high color rendering index.[8]

Brands: DermLite DL200, DermLite DL3, DermLite DL4, Heine Delta 20T, Canfield VEOS HD2

USB Dermatoscopes

Universal serial bus (USB) dermatoscopes are used primarily in the fields of entomology, botany, and microelectronics. It has to be connected to a computer with a USB connection to view the images and stored to retrieve them later. The magnification is higher than the usual handheld dermatoscopes. The advantages of USB dermatoscopes are easy image storage with a click of a button rather than using connection kits of handheld dermatoscopes, and higher magnification.[9] On the flipside, the image quality and resolution are inferior compared to standard dermatoscopes.[10]

Brands: Ultracam TLS, Dinolite, E-scope

Smartphone Dermatoscopes

Smartphone dermatoscopes are small, compact dermatoscopes that can be used only when attached to a smartphone. The phone has software, apps for medical professionals and patients. These dermatoscopes are simple to use to monitor skin lesions and send high-quality images for review.

Brands: DermLite DL1 basic, DermLite HÜD, Heine iC1, Fotofinder Handyscope, Canfield VEOS DS3

Dermatoscopes with Analytical Capabilities

Dermatoscopes with high-resolution image capture and analytical capability are especially used to image and analyze melanomas. They are used for serial evaluation where stored dermatoscopic image of a mole is compared with recent image. Artificial intelligence helps analyze a mole and helps judge whether it is benign or malignant. It is also useful in trichoanalysis, esthetics, and psoriasis scoring. Capillaroscopy system is useful in accurate examination of morphology of capillaries, measurement, and scoring (Figs. 4A and B). These devices are expensive and are used mainly in research centers.[11]

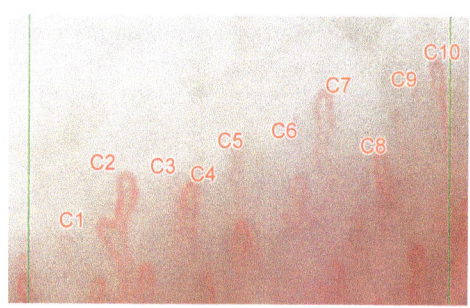

Fig. 4A

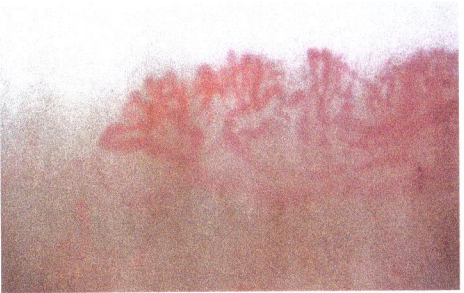

Fig. 4B

Figs. 4A and B: Images from Optilia capillaroscope. (A) Normal nailfold capillaries; (B) Bushy capillaries in systemic sclerosis.

Brands: DermoGenius MoleMap©, Fotofinder dermoscope©, Optilia Digital Capillaroscopy System

ULTRAVIOLET LIGHT IN DERMATOSCOPY

Ultraviolet (UV) light comes in-built in a few dermatoscopes along with white light and polarized light. It is useful in hypopigmented and depigmented skin lesions where it shows accentuation of hypopigmented patches and produces a white glow due to reflection back from dermal collagen in the absence or reduction of melanin in the basal layer (Figs. 5A and B). Clinically unrecognizable leukotrichia in vitiligo becomes apparent with UV mode.[12] UV light shows a "diamond necklace" appearance in superficial porokeratosis.[13] A pink glow is seen in glomus tumor under UV light dermatoscopy indicating the vascularity of glomus tumor.[14]

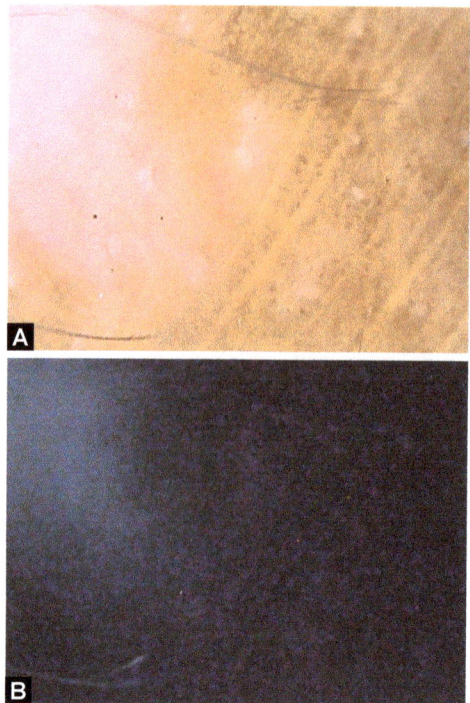

Figs. 5A and B: Dermatoscopy of vitiligo: (A) Polarized light; (B) Ultraviolet (UV) light showing white glow.

BLUE LIGHT IN DERMATOSCOPY

Lower wavelength blue light penetrates less deeper into the skin surface. Hence, it is useful in the diagnosis of alterations in the superficial layers of skin. The loss of melanin from

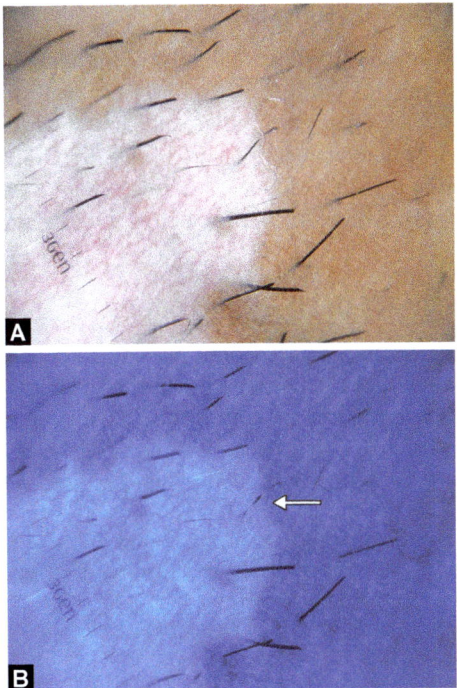

Figs. 6A and B: Dermatoscopy of vitiligo: (A) Polarized light; (B) Blue light (470 nm). Sharply defined border (white arrow) of vitiligo is better defined with blue light.

basal layer of epidermis is seen clearly as loss of pigment network continuity with 470 nm blue light (Figs. 6A and B). Blue light in dermatoscopy has found its utility in disorders of hypomelanosis like vitiligo and contact leukoderma.[15]

GREEN LIGHT IN DERMATOSCOPY

Highest absorption peak wavelengths of hemoglobin is UVA, 400 nm (blue), 541 nm (green), and 577 nm (yellow).[16] Lower wavelength colors—violet, indigo, blue, and green do not penetrate into deeper layers of skin. Hence, the utility of green light is limited to oral mucosal dermatoscopy and nailfold capillaroscopy where it offers a better contrast than white light.[17]

YELLOW LIGHT IN DERMATOSCOPY

As the wavelength increases, light penetrates deeper into the tissues. Yellow light penetrates deeper than blue and green light. Light penetrates less than 1 mm at 400 nm, up to 2 mm at 514 nm and up to 6 mm at 630 nm. Hence, yellow light is useful to delineate dermatoscopic features spikes and longitudinal

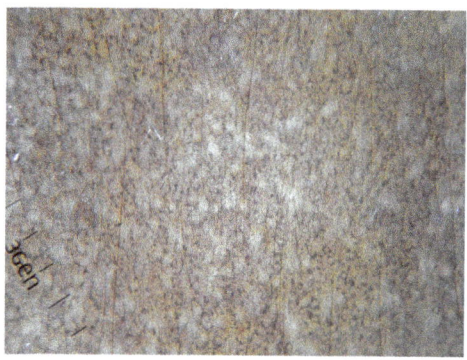

Fig. 7A

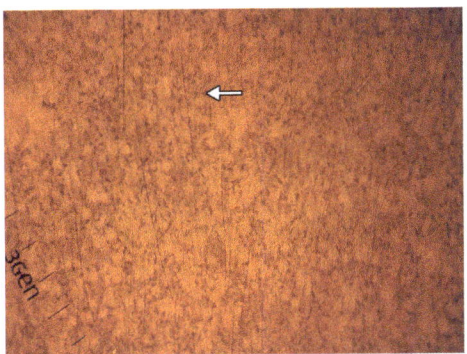

Fig. 7B

Figs. 7A and B: Dermatoscopy of lichen planopilaris: (A) Polarized light; (B) Yellow light (580 nm). Gray dots (white arrow) are visualized clearly with yellow light.

striae of onychomycosis better with yellow light at 580 nm especially in thicker nails.[18] Yellow light is also useful in defining blood vessels in the dermis and dermal pigmentation (Figs. 7A and B).[19]

FILTERS IN DERMATOSCOPY

Filters are used in photography to capture sharper images without distracters. Filters are add-ons that can be attached to the dermatoscope while capturing images (Fig. 8). Fluorescent light filters help decrease the white light reflected from nail plate while performing onychoscopy. Neutral density filters reduce the light reaching the sensor. Hence, the camera shutter

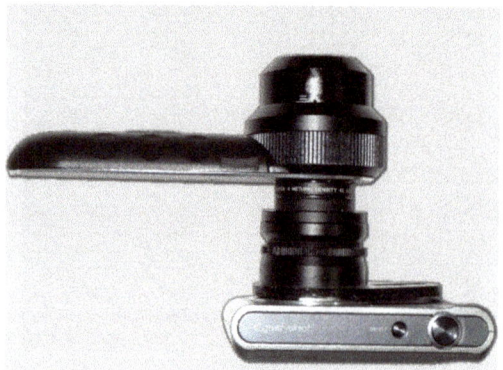

Fig. 8: Filter attached to dermatoscope and camera connection kit.

speed is decreased and maximum detail from the image is captured.[20]

USER'S CHOICE

The Dreyfus model of skill acquisition is used in education and research to demonstrate the ability of learners to acquire skills through practice. A learner goes through five stages as the skill is acquired. The stages are: (1) Novice, (2) Competence, (3) Proficiency, (4) Expertise, and (5) Mastery.[21] The choice of dermatoscopes (Fig. 9) at each stage of skill acquisition is listed in Table 1.

CHAPTER 3: Choice of Dermatoscope: An End-user Perspective

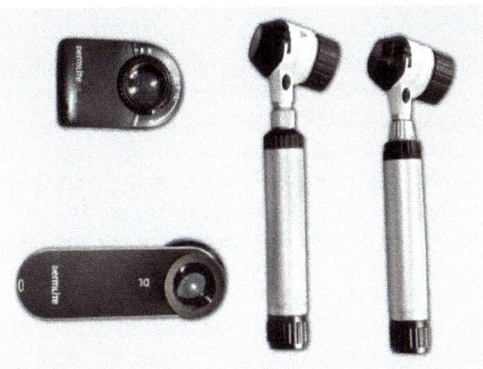

Fig. 9: Commonly used standard dermatoscopes.

Table 1: Dreyfus model of skill acquisition and choice of dermatoscope.

No.	Stage of skill acquisition	Choice of dermatoscope
1.	Novice	USB dermatoscopes, DermLite DL1, DermLite DL100
2.	Advanced beginner	Heine mini 2000, DermLite carbon
3.	Competent	DermLite DL II, Heine delta 20, iC1
4.	Proficient	DermLite DL3, DL4, Heine delta 20 plus, 20T
5.	Expert	Fotofinder, Optilia capillaroscope

(USB: universal serial bus)

REFERENCES

1. Errichetti E, Stinco G. Dermoscopy in General Dermatology: A Practical Overview. Dermatol Ther. 2016;6(4):471-507.
2. Domínguez-Espinosa AE. Historia de la dermatoscopia. Dermatol Rev Mex. 2014;58:165-72.
3. Nirmal B. Dermatoscopy: Physics and principles. Indian J Dermatopathol Diagn Dermatol. 2017;4(2):27-30.
4. Pan Y, Gareau DS, Scope A, et al. Polarized and nonpolarized dermoscopy: the explanation for the observed differences. Arch Dermatol. 2008;144(6):828-9.
5. Nirmal B, George R, Kodiatte TA. Invisible lichen planopilaris unmasked by dermatoscopy. Int J Trichol. 2017;9(2):76-8.
6. Braun RP, Scope A, Marghoob AA. The "Blink Sign" in Dermoscopy. Arch Dermatol. 2011;147:520.
7. Blum A, Jaworski S. Clear differences in hand-held dermoscopes. J Dtsch Dermatol Ges. 2006;4:1054-7.
8. Nirmal B. Dermatoscopy image characteristics and differences among commonly used standard dermatoscopes. Indian Dermatol Online J. 2017;8:233-4.
9. Kaliyadan F. The scope of the dermoscope. Indian Dermatol Online J. 2016;7:359-63.
10. Micali G, Lacarrubba F. Dermatoscopy: Instrumental Update. Dermatol Clin. 2018;36:345-8.
11. Nischal KC, Khopkar U. Dermoscope. Indian J Dermatol Venereol Leprol. 2005;71:300-3.
12. Gutte R, Khopkar US. Dermoscopy: Differentiating Evolving Vitiligo from a Hypopigmented Patch of Leprosy. In: Khopkar U (Ed). Dermoscopy and Trichoscopy in Diseases of the Brown Skin: Atlas and Short Text. New Delhi, India: Jaypee Brothers Medical Publishers (P) Ltd; 2012. pp. 108-13.

CHAPTER 3: Choice of Dermatoscope: An End-user Perspective

13. Thatte SS, Kharkar VD, Khopkar US. "Diamond necklace" appearance in superficial porokeratosis. J Am Acad Dermatol. 2014;70:e125-6.
14. Thatte SS, Chikhalkar SB, Khopkar US. "Pink glow": A new sign for the diagnosis of glomus tumor on ultraviolet light dermoscopy. Indian Dermatol Online J. 2015;6 Suppl S1:21-3.
15. Nirmal B, Santhikiran B, Mukhopadhyay S. Multispectral dermatoscopic features of chemical leucoderma with pigmented contact dermatitis. Indian Dermatol Online J. 2018;9:107-9.
16. Barolet D. Light-emitting diodes (LEDs) in dermatology. Semin Cutan Med Surg. 2008;27:227-38.
17. Weekenstroo HH, Cornelissen BM, Bernelot Moens HJ. Green light may improve diagnostic accuracy of nailfold capillaroscopy with a simple digital videomicroscope. Rheumatol Int. 2015;35:1069-71.
18. Nirmal B. Utility of a multispectral dermatoscope in onychomycosis. Indian J Dermatol. 2018;63:87-8.
19. Nirmal B. Yellow light in dermatoscopy and its utility in dermatological disorders. Indian Dermatol Online J. 2017;8:384-5.
20. Nirmal B. Use of filters in dermatoscopy to capture better images. Indian Dermatol Online J. 2018;9:137-8.
21. Wikipedia. (2018). Dreyfus model of skill acquisition. [online] Available from https://en.wikipedia.org/wiki/Dreyfus_model_of_skill_acquisition. [Accessed December, 2018].

CHAPTER 4

Smartphone Dermatoscopes

Nina Madnani, Khan Kaleem

Traditional dermatoscopes were usually "stand-alone", relatively bulky, with no facility for photographing, storing or emailing images. Also, many required a contact medium for improved clarity. For a dermatoscope to be of significant benefit over a magnifying device, it should provide polarized light capabilities necessary for visualizing the dermis. This facility was often missing in the older models.

Modern day dermatoscopes have evolved to support the ever-growing need of a clinician. Good clinical practice requires maintaining a data base of clinical images of suspect lesions for review on subsequent follow-up, for publication/presentation in journals and discussion at various forums. Since smartphones are an integral part of our lives today, it would seem logical to incorporate the necessary optics of a dermatoscope with the camera/imaging power of the smartphone and hand us "smartphone dermoscopy". These newer devices are efficient and portable enough to fit in a pocket or ladies purse for easy availability.

The smartphone dermatoscopes usually attach to the smartphone with the help of a template, which aligns the optics with the phone camera. The template may enclose the entire phone, or more likely serve as a back-plate to mount the device. These templates are designed to be easy-to-use and are usually "slip-on" or "clip-on" types and can be formatted for any smartphone.

All dermatoscopes, which attach on to a smartphone, have these basic features:
- Optics and light source
- Battery to power the light source
- A software optimized for the specific hardware.

The major players for these smartphone devices are as follows:
- Canfield VEOS DS3
- DermLite 3Gen DL1
- HEINE iC1
- FotoFinder Handyscope
- MoleScope 1 and 2.

These devices vary in their external esthetics, mode of connecting, magnification, facility of polarizing/nonpolarizing, and option of use of a contact medium.

All smartphone dermatoscope devices are recommended to be used along with the software provided by the manufacturer. These are available as free download apps from the app store.

The software shares similar functionality in that they are able to log images into a patient's profile and maintain a reference (Fig. 1). It also allows for rapid review of the lesion in question on subsequent follow-ups. The images are stored locally on the phone, can be downloaded to a computer, or can be emailed to any specified person. The applications are renewed on a regular basis to increase functionality thus making them future proof.

The Canfield VEOS DS3 (Fig. 2) is designed for use with the iPod touch (which is included in the cost of the device). Its unique touch screen has a zoom option and a millimeter scale for measuring the size of the lesion. It offers up to 10× magnification with both polarized and nonpolarized options achieved with a tap on the screen. A removable magnetic cap, protects the delicate optics, and can be sterilized/cleaned after every use. The battery pack provides 3.5 hours and is rechargeable with a

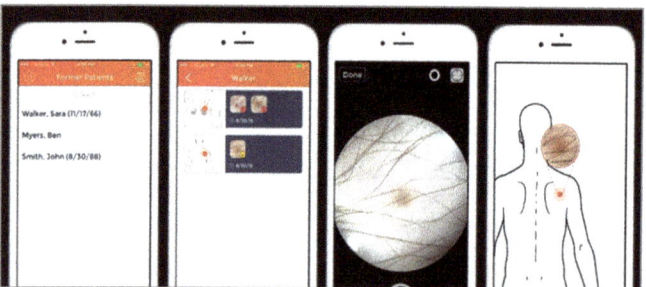

Fig. 1: App-based software allows for storing and cataloging dermoscopy images.

CHAPTER 4: Smartphone Dermatoscopes

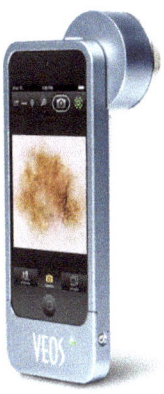

Fig. 2: Canfield VEOS DS3.

standard USB (universal serial bus) mini charger. A moveable lens design allows for taking standard photograph of the area of interest. It is also available as an attachment to an iPhone or Intelli Studio, or android smartphone by means of a clip and plate. When used with the Canfield Dermagraphic body mapping software and the Canfield Intelli Studio, images are wirelessly captured and rapidly mapped to body sites on the computer screen.

The DermLite DL1 (Fig. 3) on the other hand can be used with iPhones, iPads, and even Samsung Galaxy phones when used with a compatible adaptor. The device itself is very compact and can also be used as a "stand-alone" dermatoscope. It too offers up to 10× magnification with both polarized and nonpolarized options. This device can be used by patients

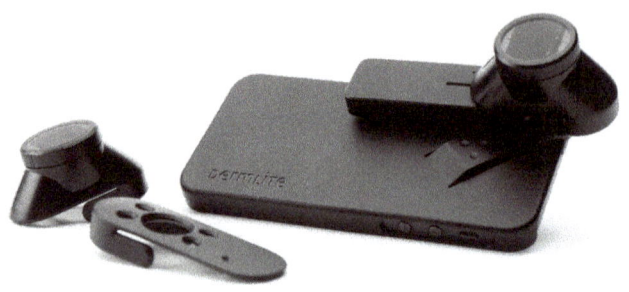

Fig. 3: DermLite DL1.

at home to track their moles and upload the images for the physician to see. The DermLite series have been upgraded to more sophisticated versions, which do not require smartphones for their use.

The HEINE iC1 (Fig. 4) has an edge over the others as it offers up to 40× magnification with up to 12 MP image quality. It has optics for both, polarized and nonpolarized light but can only be used as a contact dermatoscope. It is compatible with recently released iPhones using suitable templates.

The FotoFinder Handyscope (Fig. 5) is another dermatoscope, which is available for use with the iPhone and iPod touch. It uses a slide-in design for ease of use. The advantage it offers over other smartphone dermatoscopes is its long battery life (8 hours), reducing the need to charge the device often.

MoleScope (Fig. 6) is a smartphone dermatoscope attachment for capturing and storing images. It is compatible with both IOS and android devices providing both polarizing/

CHAPTER 4: Smartphone Dermatoscopes

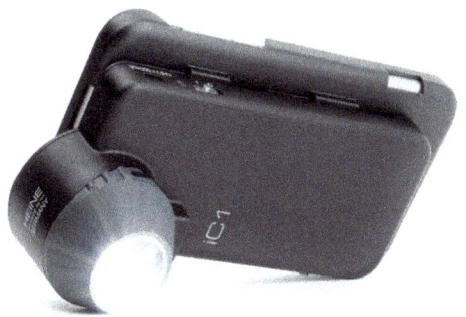

Fig. 4: HEINE iC1.

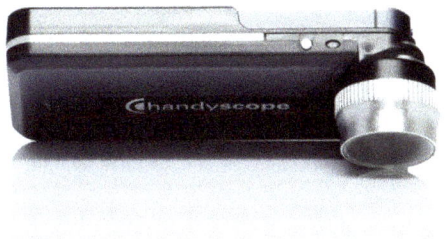

Fig. 5: FotoFinder Handyscope.

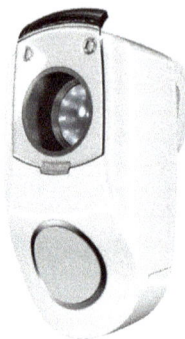

Fig. 6: MoleScope.

nonpolarizing options (depending on the model) with a rechargeable lithium battery (only in MoleScope II).

Over the last decade, a dermatoscope has become an essential diagnostic tool in clinical dermatology akin to a stethoscope for medical personnel. The ease of use and the significant impact a dermatoscope with imaging capabilities can make to one's clinic practice includes it in "must have" for every clinician. The choice of model purchased is regulated mostly with the convenience of use and the cost of the device.

CHAPTER 5

Dermatoscopy of Normal Skin and Appendages

Nirmal B

INTRODUCTION

Dermatoscopy, also known as epiluminescence microscopy or dermoscopy, is widely used for the examination of pigmented and nonpigmented lesions of the skin, scalp, nails, palms, and soles. It increases the clinician's diagnostic accuracy allowing the recognition of malignant skin tumors at an early, curable stage and multitude of nonmalignant lesions including inflammatory disorders and infections.[1] It is imperative to know and be familiar with the dermatoscopy of normal skin and its appendages with variations with respect to site before recognition of its abnormalities.

NORMAL SKIN

Dermatoscopy of normal skin shows brown lines in a reticular pattern resembling a honeycomb called the pigment network, with white circles in-between (Figs. 1 A and B). Typical pigment

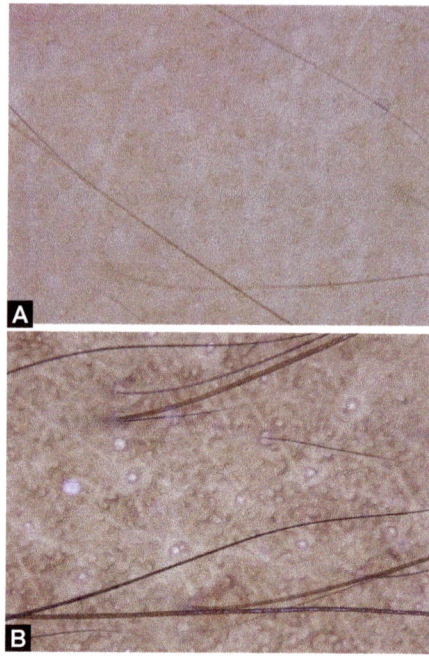

Figs. 1A and B: Dermatoscopy of normal skin: Homogeneous pigment network in light (A) and dark (B) skin.

network is homogeneous in color, meshed regularly, and relatively uniform.[2] The brown lines in the pigment network in the normal skin correspond to melanin in the epidermis arranged along the rete ridges where the tips of the rete ridges appear as white or light brown circles. This is because the concentration of melanin in the slope of the rete ridges in a unit area is higher than that at the tips.

FACE

True pigment network which is a hallmark of pigmented lesions of the body, it is rarely found on facial skin. Facial skin exhibits the following histological characteristics being the reason for the unique dermatoscopic findings: flat dermoepidermal junction and presence of pilosebaceous units at a higher density, larger than those present in truncal skin[3] (Figs. 2A and B). The distinctive dermatoscopic findings of facial skin include:

- *Pseudonetwork*—constituted by diffuse brown pigmentation interrupted by numerous light brown circles or holes of variable sizes. Pigmentation is diffuse brown structureless due to the melanin along the flat rete ridges of epidermis. Holes correspond to the numerous pilosebaceous and sweat gland openings.
- *Yellow clods*—correspond to keratin plugs over follicular ostia.
- *Gray circles* are located around the hair follicle and they denote melanocytes in the hair follicle.

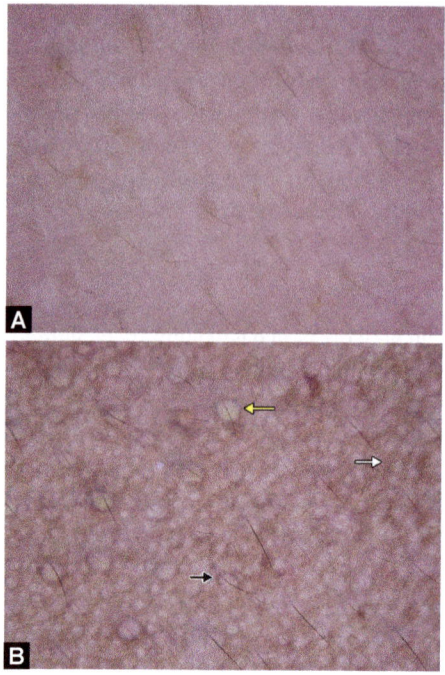

Figs. 2A and B: Dermatoscopy of facial skin in light (A) and dark (B) skin showing pseudonetwork (white arrow), yellow clods (yellow arrow), and gray circles (black arrow).

MUCOSA

Dermatoscopy of mucosa is less investigated and the literature on the topic is scarce.[4] The reticular pigment network is rarely seen in mucous membranes due to nearly flat rete ridges.[5] The various pigment patterns (Fig. 3) seen in normal oral mucosa include:

- *Ring*-like pattern—distinguished by the presence of brown circles
- *Fish scale*-like pattern—characterized by semilunar curved lines, which form either a U-pattern or V-pattern
- *Hyphal* pattern—characterized by irregularly curved lines of varying length similar to fungal hyphae[6]
- *Parallel* pattern—distinguished by the presence of brown straight lines
- *Fingerprint*-like pattern—characterized by thin curved parallel lines.

Blood vessels located in the connective tissue papillae assume a *loop* pattern or a *dot* pattern depending on the direction from which they are observed. They are located superficial

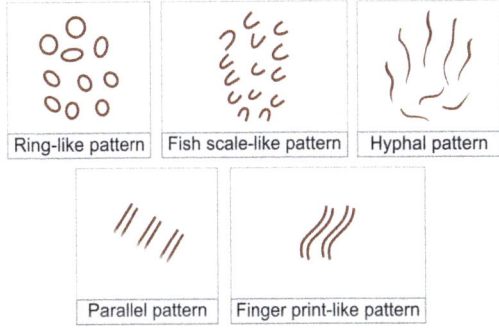

Fig. 3: Normal mucosal pigment patterns.

directly under the mucosa and are called intrapapillary capillary loops (IPCL).[7] These pigment and vascular patterns are due to changes in the angle while capturing images and curvature of the surface mucosa (Figs. 4A and B).

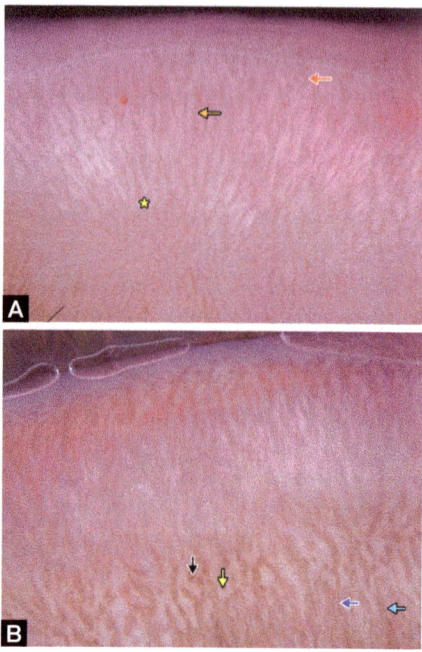

Figs. 4A and B: Dermatoscopy of lip mucosa in light (A) and dark (B) skin showing blood vessels in dot (red arrow), loop (orange arrow) patterns, and pigment in hyphal (yellow star), ring-like (yellow arrow), fish scale-like (black arrow), parallel (light blue arrow), fingerprint-like (dark blue arrow) patterns.

ACRAL SKIN

The skin over palms and soles has a distinct anatomy compared with skin of nonglabrous skin with the presence of furrows and ridges giving rise to unique dermatoglyphic pattern for that individual. It is characterized by epidermis comprising of compact cornified layer and two types of epidermal rete ridges—crista profunda intermedia under the surface ridge and crista profunda limitans under the furrow. Eccrine sweat glands open into the ridges (Fig. 5). Pilosebaceous units are absent in palmoplantar skin.

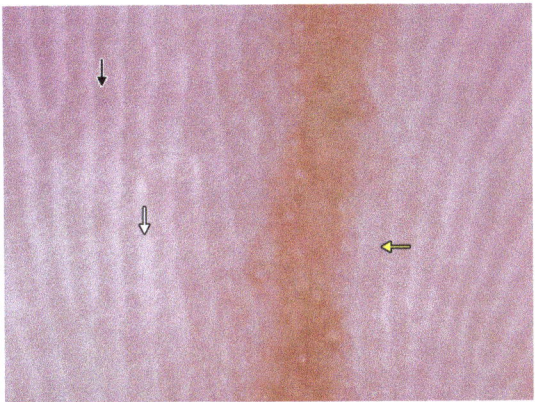

Fig. 5: Dermatoscopy of palmar skin showing ridges (black arrow) and furrows (white arrow) with eccrine sweat glands (yellow arrow) opening into ridges.

NAIL

Nonpolarized contact dermatoscopy of the nail plate requires the use of ultrasound gel as an interface medium, as it allows a better contact with the convex nail surface. Areas to be examined include the nail plate, the nail plate-free edge, the hyponychium, and the nail folds.

- *Proximal nail fold (PNF)*: PNF is characterized by the presence of looped vessels resembling a hairpin bend arranged parallel to the skin surface (Fig. 6). Normal density of capillaries is 30 linear capillaries per 5 mm. The following characteristics should be looked for in normal capillaries in PNF designated by the acronym "A–H without F in-between" (ABCDEGH)[8]:
    - *Architecture*—looped vessels formed by two arms making a convex loop distally

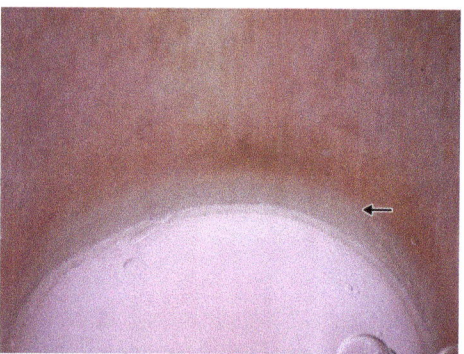

Fig. 6: Dermatoscopy of proximal nail fold showing looped vessels (black arrow) resembling hairpin bend.

- *Background*—clear
 - *Capillary distribution*—organized arranged parallel to each other
 - *Dropouts*—absent
 - *Enlarged/Giant vessels*—absent
 - *Hemorrhage*—absent.
- *Nail plate*: Normal nail plate is translucent and has a smooth surface.
- *Cuticle*: Cuticle attaches the PNF to the nail plate and appears as transparent transverse band.
- *Nail bed*: Nail bed appears pink in color visible through the nail plate and distally shows linearly arranged capillaries along the dermal ridges (Fig. 7).
- *Hyponychium*: Blood vessels in the hyponychium show red dot pattern as they are arranged perpendicular to the skin surface. Red dots correspond to top of each capillary loop.[9]

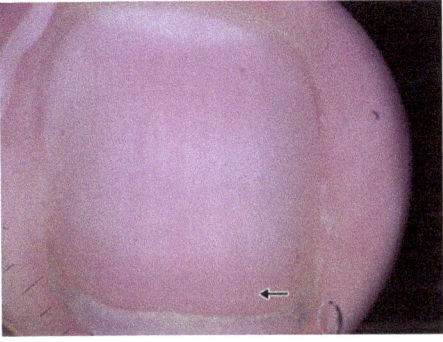

Fig. 7: Dermatoscopy of nail plate and nail bed showing capillaries arranged linearly (black arrow) along the dermal ridges.

HAIR AND SCALP

Hair and scalp dermatoscopy or trichoscopy, as it is popularly called, includes visualization of the following structures:

- *Hair shafts*—comprise terminal and vellus hairs. Normal terminal hairs have a consistent diameter and color along the length of the hairs. Vellus hairs are shorter (less than 3 mm) and narrower (less than 30 μm) than terminal hairs. Vellus hairs constitute less than 20% of all the hairs in normal scalp[10] (Fig. 8).
- *Follicular ostia*—appear as circular small structures that are regularly spaced referred to as white dots.[11] Normally 2–3 hair follicles emerge from single follicular ostium. The temporal scalp has mostly single, double follicular units, and the occipital scalp largely has triple follicular units.

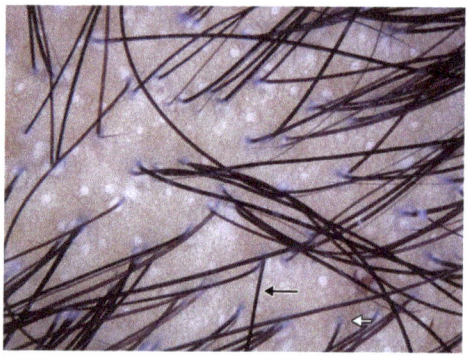

Fig. 8: Dermatoscopy of scalp showing predominantly terminal hairs (black arrow) and vellus hairs (white arrow) constituting less than 20%.

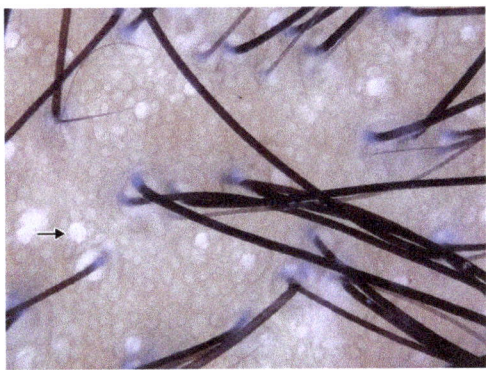

Fig. 9: Dermatoscopy of scalp showing white dots (black arrow).

- *Perifollicular and interfollicular skin*—is characterized by honeycomb-like reticular pigment network especially in darker skin types and small regular pinpoint white dots. These dots correspond to the opening of eccrine sweat ducts and empty follicular ostia (Fig. 9). Bigger irregularly distributed white dots correspond to areas of perifollicular fibrosis seen in scarring alopecia.[12]
- *Blood vessels*—appear as simple red loops and thin arborizing red lines, corresponding to vessels of the dermal papilla and subpapillary vascular plexus, respectively. Blood vessels of scalp are visible at more than 50× magnification. Thin arborizing vessels are commonly found in temporal and occipital scalp. Simple red loops are seen normally in frontal scalp.[13]

REFERENCES

1. Kittler H, Marghoob AA, Argenziano G, et al. Standardization of terminology in dermoscopy/dermatoscopy: Results of the third consensus conference of the International Society of Dermoscopy. J Am Acad Dermatol. 2016;74:1093-106.
2. Nirmal B. Dermatoscopy: Physics and principles. Indian J Dermatopathol Diagn Dermatol. 2017;4:27-30.
3. Thomas L, Phan A, Pralong P, et al. Special locations dermoscopy: facial, acral, and nail. Dermatol Clin. 2013;31: 615.
4. Olszewska M, Banka A, Gorska R, et al. Dermoscopy of pigmented oral lesions. J Dermatol Case Rep. 2008;2:43-8.
5. Mannone F, De Giorgi V, Cattaneo A, et al. Dermoscopic features of mucosal melanosis. Dermatol Surg. 2004;30:1118-23.
6. Lin J, Koga H, Takata M, et al. Dermoscopy of pigmented lesions on mucocutaneous junction and mucous membrane. Br J Dermatol. 2009;161:1255-61.
7. Okamoto T, Sasaki R, Kataoka T, et al. Dermoscopy imaging findings in the normal oral mucosa. Oral Oncol. 2015;51:e69-70.
8. Nirmal B. Checklist for Nailfold Capillaroscopy findings in systemic sclerosis: ABCDEGH. Int J Dermoscop. 2017;1:54-5.
9. Lencastre A, Lamas A, Sá D, et al. Onychoscopy. Clin Dermatol. 2013;31:587.
10. Mubki T, Rudnicka L, Olszewska M, et al. Evaluation and diagnosis of the hair loss patient: part II. Trichoscopic and laboratory evaluations. J Am Acad Dermatol. 2014;71:431.e1.
11. Abraham LS, Piñeiro-Maceira J, Duque-Estrada B, et al. Pinpoint white dots in the scalp: dermoscopic and histopathologic correlation. J Am Acad Dermatol. 2010;63:721-2.
12. Miteva M, Tosti A. Hair and scalp dermatoscopy. J Am Acad Dermatol. 2012;67:1040-8.
13. Pirmez R, Tosti A. Trichoscopy Tips. Dermatol Clin. 2018;36:413-20.

CHAPTER 6

Vascular Patterns

Anjali Pal, Purva Mehta, Subrata Malakar

INTRODUCTION

Dermoscopic diagnosis involves a step-by-step approach. The first step is to determine whether the lesion is melanocytic or nonmelanocytic. In a melanocytic lesion, the identification of the melanocytic pattern helps in diagnosis. In a nonmelanocytic lesion, the vascular pattern often gives clues to the diagnosis.

To recognize the vascular pattern in a lesion, we need to consider two main characteristics—the shape of the vessels and its structural arrangement. In addition to these, some associated features may help in narrowing down the diagnosis.

ANATOMY OF THE DERMAL VASCULAR PLEXUSES[1]

The dermal vasculature consists of a subpapillary plexus and a deep plexus of arterioles and venules.

The subpapillary plexus is situated in the upper part of the reticular dermis. It runs parallel to the skin surface, and from it, capillaries loop into each dermal papilla forming arcades. These loops are perpendicular to the skin surface. The deep plexus is located in the lower part of the reticular dermis.

PRELIMINARY NOTE

Lines: These are vessels of the subpapillary dermal plexus, and run parallel to the skin surface. Hence, they are seen as lines on dermoscopy (Fig. 1).

Dots: They are vessels in the dermal papillae that arise from the subpapillary vascular plexus and are oriented perpendicular to the skin surface.[2] Thus, they are seen as dots on dermoscopy, or hairpin loops, when they are oriented obliquely to the skin surface (Fig. 2).

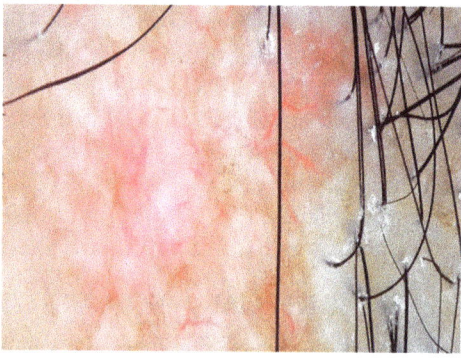

Fig. 1: Vessels parallel to the skin surface are linearly oriented.

CHAPTER 6: Vascular Patterns

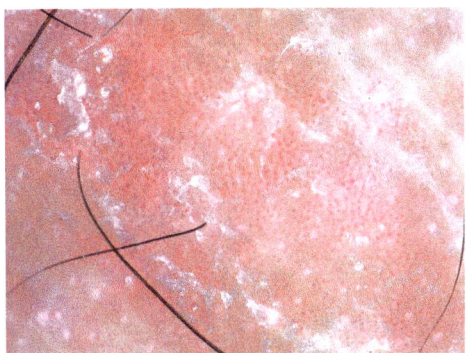

Fig. 2: Vessels perpendicular to the skin surface appear as dots or loops.

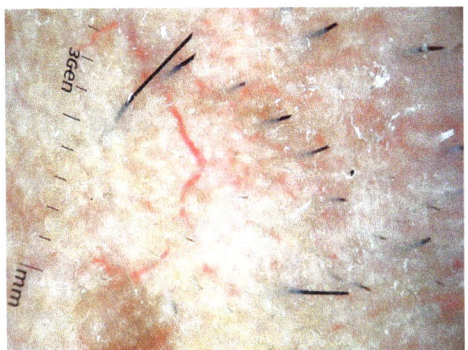

Fig. 3: Superficial vessels appear bright red and in focus.

Superficial dermal vessels (just below the epidermis) appear bright red, prominent and in-focus (Fig. 3). In contrast,

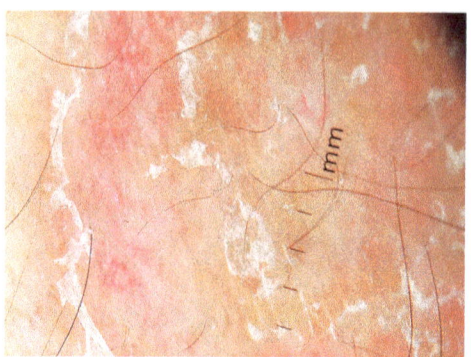

Fig. 4: Deep vessels appear pink and out of focus.

deeper dermal vessels appear pink, less prominent and out of focus due to dispersion of light through the dermal connective tissue (Fig. 4).

Shortlist of dermoscopic vascular patterns (Table 1).[3-5]

1. Dotted Vessels

Dotted vessels correspond histopathologically to capillaries in the dermal papillae.

- When seen in a regular distribution, it is the dermoscopic hallmark for psoriasis (Fig. 5). They serve as a therapeutic marker, as their density decreases on clinical improvement.[6]
- Dotted vessels in a patchy distribution are seen in eczematous conditions.
- Dotted vessels arranged in a linear "string of pearls" distribution is highly characteristic of clear cell acanthoma.[7]

Table 1: Dermoscopic vascular patterns.

Pattern of the vessels	Description	Arrangement of the vessels			
1. Dotted vessels	Rounded, small diameter vessels resembling a pinhead	Regular arrangement, e.g. psoriasis	Patchy arrangement, e.g. eczema	Dotted vessels arranged linearly resembling a "string of pearls", e.g. clear cell acanthoma	
2. Comma vessels	Curved vessels with one end being thicker than the other	Isolated arrangement, e.g. dermal nevi			
3. Hairpin vessels	Loop vessels with a U-shaped bend	Peripheral, irregular arrangement, e.g. keratoacanthoma squamous cell carcinoma	Coursing throughout the lesion: seborrheic keratosis		
4. Crown vessels	Branching vessels along the periphery that never cross the midline	Radial arrangement, e.g. sebaceous hyperplasia, molluscum contagiosum			

Contd...

Contd...

Pattern of the vessels	Description	Arrangement of the vessels			
5. Arborizing vessels	Prominent large-bore vessels dividing into finer vessels	Branching throughout the lesion, e.g. basal cell carcinoma, adnexal tumors			
6. Glomerular vessels	Vessels curling up on each other in a tortuous manner	Clustered arrangement, e.g. Bowen's disease, stasis dermatitis			
7. Corkscrew vessels	Linear vessels arranged spirally/helically	Irregular arrangement, e.g. melanoma, melanoma metastasis			
8. Linear irregular vessels	Straight vessels	Irregular arrangement, e.g. melanoma, squamous cell carcinoma			

Contd...

Contd...

Pattern of the vessels	Description	Arrangement of the vessels
9. Coral vessels	Vessels in a flowery arrangement resembling the tentacles of a coral	Superficial arrangement, e.g. secondary milia
10. Lacunae	Well demarcated, round to oval, reddish blue structures	Solitary/clustered arrangement, e.g. angiokeratoma, hemangioma
11. Polymorphous vessels	Various patterns coexisting in the same lesion	Irregular arrangement, e.g. melanoma, carcinomas

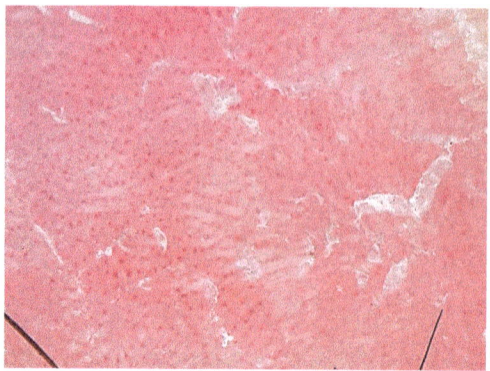

Fig. 5: Regularly distributed red dots in a case of scalp psoriasis.

- Dotted vessels are also commonly seen in nevi. In benign nevi such as dermal melanocytic nevi or Spitz nevus, their arrangement is regular whereas in dysplastic nevi, their arrangement varies from regular to irregular.
- In malignant melanoma (thin lesions), the distribution is completely irregular.[4,8,9]

2. Comma Vessels

These vessels are the key dermoscopic feature for the diagnosis of mature melanocytic nevi (Fig. 6).

Comma vessels are also found in other conditions such as dysplastic nevi, dermatofibroma, etc.

The presence of comma vessels in a melanoma, however, is a negative predictive factor, almost ruling out its possibility.[4,9]

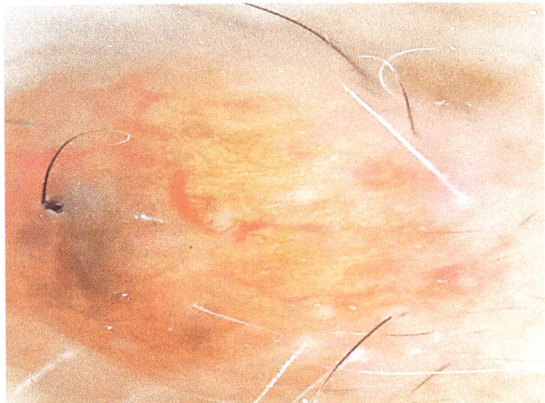

Fig. 6: Comma vessels in a case of compound nevus.

3. Hairpin Vessels

Hairpin vessels on dermoscopy are characteristic of keratinizing tumors such as seborrheic keratosis, keratoacanthoma, squamous cell carcinoma, etc. In these lesions, there is a whitish halo seen surrounding the hairpin vessels, a dermoscopic marker for keratinization. The presence of this halo helps to differentiate them from hairpin vessels in melanoma, which lack this halo (Fig. 7).[2,4]

The hairpin vessels have a characteristic peripheral arrangement in keratoacanthoma and this helps to distinguish it from hairpin vessels in seborrheic keratosis, where they are dispersed throughout the lesion.[3]

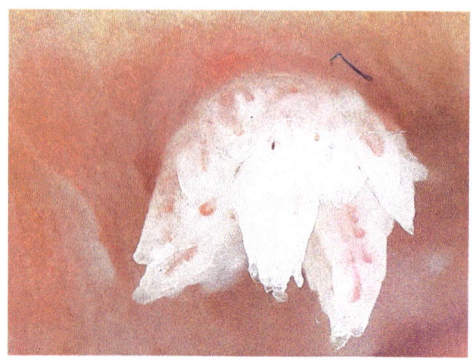

Fig. 7: Hairpin vessels visible in a filiform wart.

4. Crown Vessels

These are characteristically branching vessels, distributed radially at the periphery of the lesion and do not cross the midline.[10,11]

Crown vessels on dermoscopy are seen in sebaceous hyperplasia and molluscum contagiosum (Fig. 8).

- In sebaceous hyperplasia, crown vessels surround a central whitish yellow lobulated or crateriform area, which corresponds to sebaceous lobules.
- In molluscum contagiosum, they surround lobules of squamous epithelium filled with molluscum bodies. As the central lobulated mass expands, the dermis is displaced and hence the dermal vessels are pushed to the periphery, resulting in crown vessels.[2]

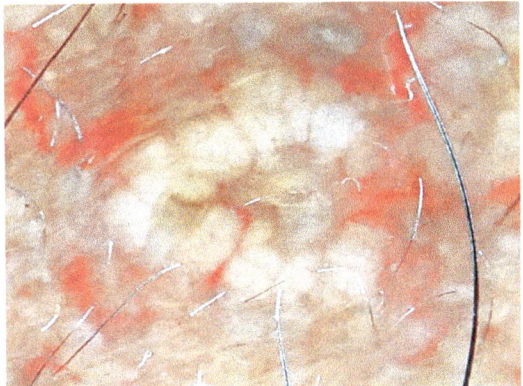

Fig. 8: Crown vessels in a radial distribution in sebaceous hyperplasia.

5. Arborizing Vessels

These are large-bore vessels, which branch at abrupt irregular intervals into finer vessels. They are the feeding vessels of a tumor, essential for its growth, and appear bright red in color, prominent and "in focus" on dermoscopy, indicating their superficial location in the dermis. They correlate to dilated vessels in the superficial dermis histopathologically.[2]

- Arborizing vessels are a vascular dermoscopic hallmark for basal cell carcinoma—especially nodular basal cell carcinoma, and adnexal tumors (Fig. 9).[2,4,12]
- Arborizing vessels are also seen in other malignancies such as squamous cell carcinoma, melanoma.

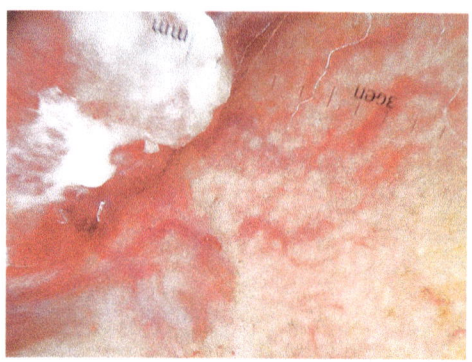

Fig. 9: Arborizing vessels.

6. Glomerular Vessels

They are tortuous vessels, curling upon each other and are named after the glomerular apparatus of the kidney owing to their resemblance to it (Fig. 10).
- Glomerular vessels are seen most commonly in Bowen's disease in a clustered distribution. They are commonly associated with surface scaling in Bowen's.
- Glomerular vessels are also seen on dermoscopy of stasis eczema over the legs.[13,14]

7. Corkscrew Vessels

They are helically designed vessels and are distributed irregularly throughout the lesion.[15]

Corkscrew vessels are a dermoscopic indicator of melanoma, and more commonly, melanoma metastasis.

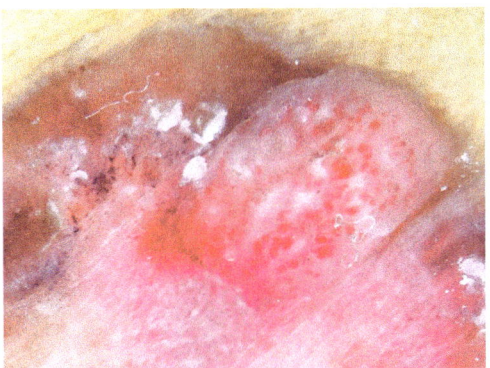

Fig. 10: Glomerular vessels, in a clustered distribution.

8. Linear Irregular Vessels

Linear but irregularly arranged vessels on dermoscopy are seen in premalignant conditions such as actinic keratotis, Bowen's disease and in frankly malignant conditions such as squamous cell carcinoma, melanoma, etc.[3]

9. Coral Vessels

These are vessels that loop peculiarly, resembling the tentacles of oceanic corals.

They have been identified on dermoscopy in secondary milia. Stretching of the skin over the surface of secondary milia, as a part of the postinflammatory process, causes dermal vessels to branch and loop extensively, resulting in a coral pattern (author's observation) (Fig. 11).

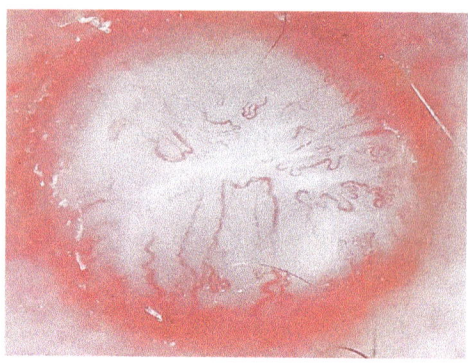

Fig. 11: Coral pattern of vessels seen on the surface of secondary milia.

10. Lacunae

Lacunae are round to oval, well defined, reddish, or reddish-blue structures on dermoscopy, corresponding to dilated vascular spaces in the superficial dermis on histopathology.

- They are characteristically seen on dermoscopy in solitary angiokeratomas, hemangiomas, angioma serpiginosum, and lymphangioma circumscripta.[5,16,17]

  They are either singularly placed or arranged in clusters and vary in color depending on the underlying condition.[16] Thrombosed hemangiomas tend to have dark lacunae, whereas regressing hemangiomas have a whitish scar like appearance.[5]

- The lacunae in angioma serpiginosum are bright red in color, whereas those in lymphangioma circumscripta are yellow to brown, surrounded by a pale septa (Fig. 12).[2,17]

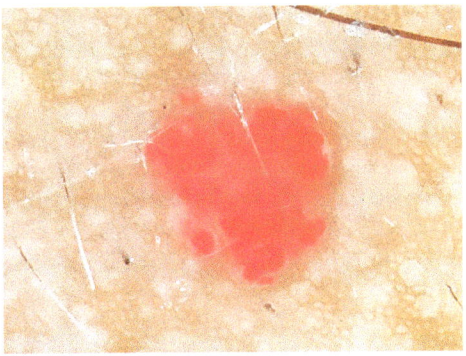

Fig. 12: Well demarcated round to oval red lacunae in a cherry angioma.

11. Polymorphous Vessels

Polymorphous vessels on dermoscopy indicate that more than one vascular pattern coexists in the same lesion. Vascular polymorphism is not restricted to malignancies but has been documented in adnexal tumors, dermatofibroma, irritated seborrheic keratosis, etc.[2]

Recognition of these vascular patterns on dermoscopy is of utmost importance as they highlight features invisible to the naked eye, and thus give vital clues in establishing clinical diagnoses.

REFERENCES

1. Murphy GF. Histology of the skin, In: Elder DE, Elenitsas R, Johnson Jr BL, Murphy GF (Eds). Lever's Histopathology of the

skin. 9th edition. Philadelphia: Lippincott Williams & Wilkins; 2005. pp 9-58.
2. Martin JM, Bella-Navarro R, Jorda E. Vascular patterns in dermoscopy. Actas Dermosifiliogr. 2012;103(5):357-75.
3. Zalaudek I, Kreusch J, Giacomel J, et al. How to diagnose nonpigmented skin tumors: a review of vascular structures seen with dermoscopy: part I. Melanocytic skin tumors. J Am Acad Dermatol. 2010;63:361-74.
4. Argenziano G, Zalaudek I, Corona R, et al. Vascular structures in skin tumors: a dermoscopy study. Arch Dermatol. 2004;140: 1485-9.
5. Wolf IH. Dermoscopic diagnosis of vascular lesions. Clin Dermatol. 2002;20:273-5.
6. Micali G, Lacarrubba F, Musumeci ML, et al. Cutaneous vascular patterns in psoriasis. Int J Derm. 2010;49:249-56.
7. Bugatti L, Filosa G, Broganelli P, et al. Psoriasis-like dermoscopic pattern of clear cell acanthoma. J Eur Acad Dermatol Venereol. 2003;17:452-5.
8. Ferrara G, Argenziano G, Soyer HP, et al. The spectrum of Spitz nevi: a clinicopathologic study of 83 cases. Arch Dermatol. 2005;41:1381-7.
9. Menzies SW, Kreusch J, Byth K, et al. Dermoscopic evaluation of amelanotic and hypomelanotic melanoma. Arch Dermatol. 2008;144:1120-7.
10. Zaballos P, Ara M, Puig S, et al. Dermoscopy of sebaceous hyperplasia. Arch Dermatol. 2005;141:808.
11. Zalaudek I, Kreusch J, Giacomel J, et al. How to diagnose nonpigmented skin tumors: a review of vascular structures seen with dermoscopy: part II. Nonmelanocytic skin tumors. J Am Acad Dermatol. 2010;63:377-86.

12. Menzies SW, Westerhoff K, Rabinovitz H, et al. Surface microscopy of pigmented basal cell carcinoma. Arch Dermatol. 2000;136:1012-6.
13. Zalaudek I, Leinweber B, Citarella L, et al. Dermoscopy of Bowen's disease. Br J Dermatol. 2004;150:1112-6.
14. Zaballos P, Salsench E, Puig S, et al. Dermoscopy of venous stasis dermatitis. Arch Dermatol. 2006;142:1526.
15. Minagawa A, Koga H, Sakaizawa K, et al. Dermoscopic and histopathological findings of polymorphous vessels in amelanotic cutaneous metastasis of pigmented cutaneous melanoma. Br J Dermatol. 2009;160:1134-6.
16. Zaballos P, Daufi C, Puig S, et al. Dermoscopy of solitary angiokeratomas: a morphological study. Arch Dermatol. 2007;143:318-25.
17. Kalisiak MS, Haber RM. Angioma serpiginosum with linear distribution: case report and review of the literature. J Cutan Med Surg. 2008;12:180-3.

CHAPTER 7

Applications of Dermatoscopy

Usha Khemani, Feroze Kaliyadan

INTRODUCTION

Dermatoscopy is a noninvasive examination technique that upsurges the dermatologist's diagnostic capacity in numerous cutaneous diseases. Its application in the evaluation of pigmented skin lesions and prompt recognition of skin cancer is well known. In comparison to the hand lens that has been used over the decades, the dermatoscope has the ability to not just magnify but also to look at the subsurface structures, especially the pigment network and vascular patterns.

Dermatoscopy has significantly increased the sensitivity and specificity of diagnosing melanoma in the hands of the experienced users and is now recognized as a good screening test for melanoma, leading to better triage and decreased morbidity and mortality caused by this condition.[1]

CHAPTER 7: Applications of Dermatoscopy

In the context of evaluation of pigment, color and patterns are two parameters to be appreciated in dermatoscopy. The color is largely dependent on location of pigment in the epidermis or dermis—for example, the color is black when melanin is in the stratum corneum and the color changes to brown as the pigment is found deeper in the epidermis. Blue color is seen, if melanin is present in papillary dermis due to the Tyndall effect. Being a technology-dependent investigation, dermatoscopy findings are subject to the lighting and resolution of the instrument and camera being used. Variation in the features also occurs with the type of dermoscope used (polarized vs nonpolarized).[1]

Dermatoscopy may obviate the need of a skin biopsy thus reducing healthcare cost. Data shows that the ratio of benign/malignant pigmented lesions of the skin is reduced on application of dermatoscopy as compared to diagnoses made on naked eye examination.

A basic dermoscope is quite affordable instrument as compared to other state-of-art equipment, e.g. reflectance confocal microscopy. Handheld dermoscopes are relatively inexpensive, thus making such an advanced diagnostic technology affordable for most practitioners.

There has been enough research data including meta-analysis, which has demonstrated the advantage and the expediency of dermatoscopy in diagnosing cutaneous diseases. With the beginning of polarized light dermatoscopy, the necessity of using a liquid interface or direct skin contact fluid has been eliminated.

Several helpful algorithms have been created to aid in classifying lesions of the skin.

Dermatoscopy permits a dermatologist to re-examine the lesion microscopically and thus offers another chance to rethink the naked-eye diagnosis and to make the correct diagnosis. Dermatoscopy helps to isolate suspicious foci within larger lesions. Identifying such foci can be useful for directing pathology sectioning (or dermatoscopy-guided biopsies) of such suspicious sites within a lesion. Dermatoscopy can aid in more precisely defining borders of some lesions for improved presurgical margin mapping. An example of this is the ability to recognize subclinical extensions of facial lentigo maligna melanomas using dermatoscopy.

APPLICATIONS

Dermatoscopy may result in confirmation of clinical diagnosis, often avoiding the need for a skin biopsy. Although a skin biopsy and clinicopathological correlation (CPC) remain the gold standard for cutaneous diagnosis, but with dermatoscopy around, we are gradually moving from CPC clinical pathological correlation to clinico-dermoscopic-pathological correlation (CDPC).

The main application of dermatoscopy in the initial stages has been for differentiation between melanoma and the various benign lesions of the skin including seborrheic keratoses (Fig. 1), solar lentigo, simple lentigo, melanocytic nevi, and basal cell carcinoma. Some of the other conditions for which dermatoscopy was used commonly at the initial stages included—vascular lesions (like hemangiomas) (Fig. 2),

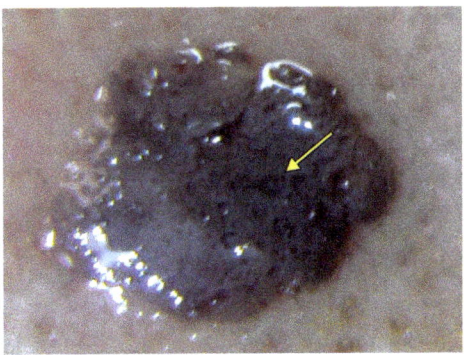

Fig. 1: Dermatoscopy of a seborrheic keratosis showing brain-like cerebriform appearance of the surface (E-SCOPE nonpolarized magnification 10×) with comedo like openings (yellow arrow).

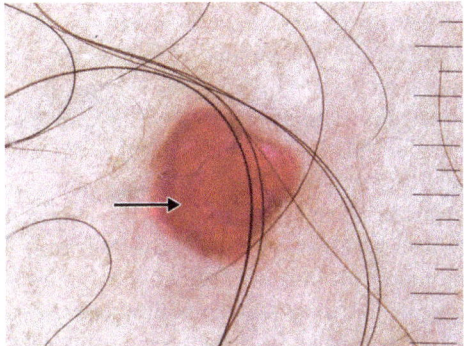

Fig. 2: Cherry angioma–Vascular lacunae (black arrow) seen in cherry angioma (Foto ii pro, Dermlite, 10x polarized).

actinic keratosis, squamous cell carcinoma, Bowen's disease, clear cell acanthoma, and dermatofibromas.

Infectious diseases have recently received increasing attention from clinicians practicing dermatoscopy. Simple antiseptic precautions should be observed in case a contact plate is being used in the dermoscope. Use of ethanol-based antiseptic solution as a linkage fluid acts as self-sterilizer. Transparent adhesive tape can also be used to prevent transmission of infectious disease through dermatoscopy. Some of the common infectious diseases, which have characteristic diagnostic patterns on dermatoscopy, include—molluscum contagiosum and viral warts. Early lesions of molluscum contagiosum, where the central umbilication is difficult to visualize, are easily picked up using dermatoscopy. They are seen as multilobular white–yellow amorphous structures surrounded by a crown of vessels (Fig. 3A). The central crater is seen well even with the white light. Viral warts on dermatoscopy show the characteristics brown, red, or black dots on the hyperkeratotic surface clearly (Fig. 3B). Entomodermoscopy—in the context of conditions like scabies has helped to improve diagnosis in parasitic infestation (Fig. 3C). Dermatoscopy can also help in the diagnosis of less common cutaneous infections like cutaneous leishmaniasis and deep fungal infections.[2-4]

Hair and scalp diseases lend themselves readily to dermoscopic examination and show distinct patterns in most cases narrowing down the clinical differential diagnoses. Dermatoscopy of hair and scalp diseases is now termed as trichoscopy and is currently the most practiced area of dermatoscopy in India. In addition, dermatoscopy has also been used to calculate the

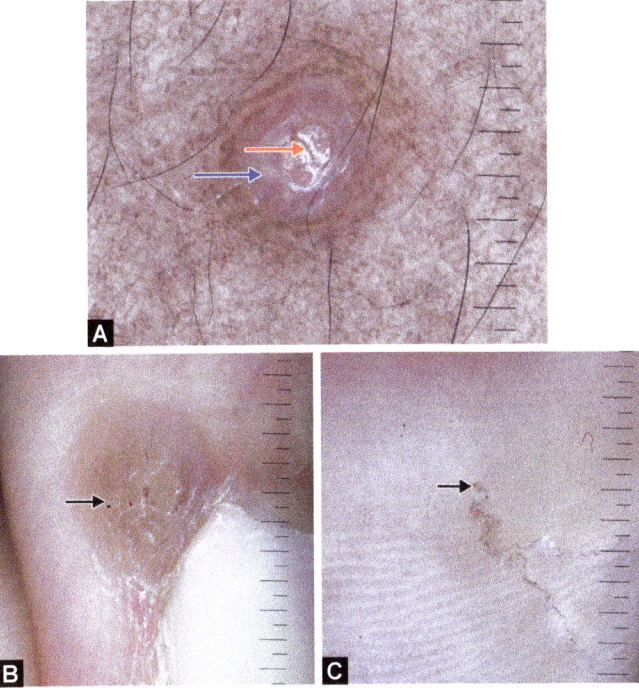

Figs. 3A to C: Entomodermoscopy improves the diagnosis of skin infestations and infections. (A) Molluscum contagiosum is typified by central opaque yellowish or whitish globules (red arrow), which are surrounded by blurred vessels (blue arrow) (Foto ii pro, Dermlite, 10x polarized); (B) Viral wart—polarized dermatoscopy showing the black dots which are often missed on naked eye examination (black arrow) (Foto ii pro, Dermlite, 10x polarized); (C) Dermatoscopy of scabies showing the classical dermoscopic image of triangle or delta wing jet sign (black arrow showing head of the delta). (Foto ii pro, Dermlite, 10x polarized)

follicular density in general and especially in the donor area before follicular unit hair transplantation. Combined with appropriate software, this can make pre- and postevaluation of hair transplant less cumbersome.[5]

Dermatoscopy of androgenetic alopecia, alopecia areata, trichotillomania, discoid lupus erythematosus (Fig. 4A), lichen planopilaris (Fig. 4B), and hair shaft diseases (Fig. 4C) shows patterns characteristic of those diseases, for example monilethrix shows uniform elliptical nodes with intermittent constrictions and bent regularly at multiple locations with a majority of broken hair and are discussed in detail in separate sections in this handbook.[6-9]

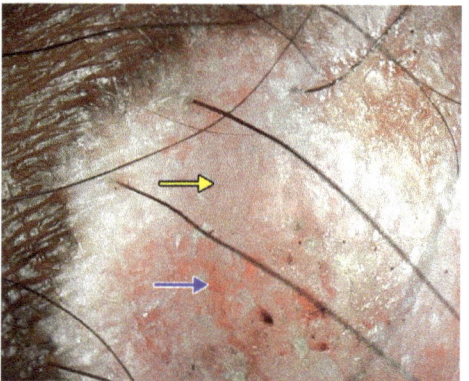

Fig. 4A: Trichoscopy (E-SCOPE nonpolarized magnification 10×). (A) Trichoscopy—showing scarring alopecia due to discoid lupus erythematosus. There is a marked reduction of the hair follicles with pinkish–white areas and loss of follicular openings (yellow arrow). Some linear vessels (blue arrow) indicate telangiectasia.

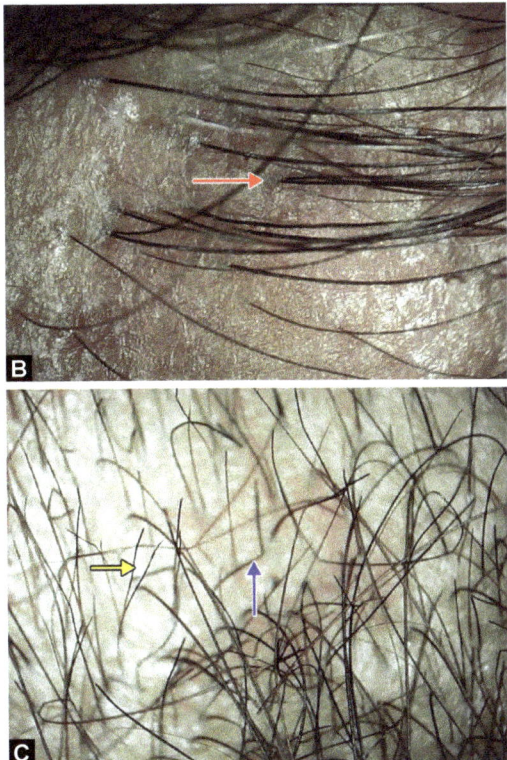

Figs. 4B and C: (B) Trichoscopy of lichen planopilaris is characterized by keratotic scales within and around the hair shaft (red arrow) and reduced number of follicular openings; (C) Trichoscopy of monilethrix hair shaft defect showing uniform elliptical nodes with intermittent constrictions (yellow arrow) and bent regularly (blue arrow) at multiple locations with a majority of broken hair.

Disorders of the nails are also amenable to dermoscopic examination and this may, at times, obviate the need for a nail biopsy. Tosti found specific patterns for many nail disorders including pigmentation of nail plate. The term onychoscopy is used to denote dermatoscopy of the nail and related structures. Handheld dermatoscopy can also be a useful tool in screening nail fold capillaries in the context of connective tissue diseases like scleroderma (Figs. 5A and B) and dermatomyositis (Fig. 5C).[10,11]

Dermatoscopy patterns in primary pigmentary disorders have been described—including vitiligo, melasma, and ochronosis. Pigmentary purpuric dermatosis also has characteristic dermatoscopy patterns. In the case of vitiligo, dermatoscopy has been suggested as a possible tool to assess stability and prognosis.[4]

The use of dermatoscopy in cutaneous inflammatory diseases (inflammascopy) is growing and studies around the world, especially in skin of color patients is helping to build a database of dermatoscopy patterns under this group. Mucosal lesions are also amenable to dermoscopic examination (mucoscopy) and can help in the diagnosis of conditions like oral lichen planus.

A proposed "algorithm" for the dermoscopic examination of inflammatory diseases suggested four categories of criteria to be evaluated, namely vessel morphology and distribution, background color, surface scales or keratin and follicular disturbances, while additional clues that typify a specific diagnosis do also exist. Dermatoscopy in common inflammatory dermatoses, e.g. psoriasis vulgaris, usually

CHAPTER 7: Applications of Dermatoscopy

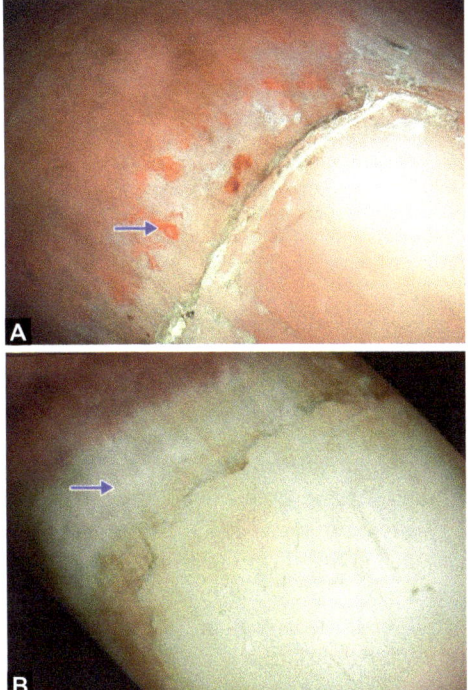

Figs. 5A and B: Nail fold capillaroscopy (E-SCOPE nonpolarized magnification 10×). (A) Capillaroscopy of the nail fold of a patient with systemic scleroderma active stage reveals twisted and elongated nail fold capillaries (blue arrow) as well as microhemorrhages in the cuticle; (B) Another nail fold in systemic scleroderma showing avascular areas in late scleroderma (blue arrow).

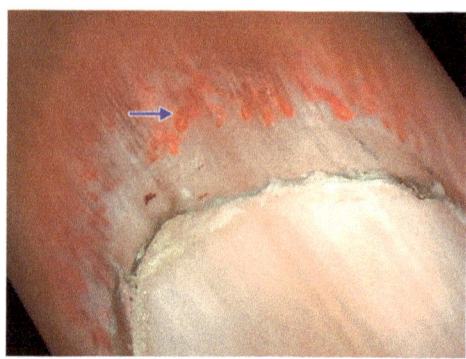

Fig. 5C: Tortuous and ramified capillaries in dermatomyositis (blue arrow).

presents with regularly distributed dotted vessels on a light or dull background. Whenever due to presence of hyperkeratosis, the underlying features are veiled and removal of scale can be done thus exposing the above-mentioned vascular pattern as well as possible tiny red blood drops (dermoscopic "Auspitz sign") (Fig. 6A). In lichen planus (Fig. 6B), presence of characteristic whitish striae on dermatoscopy can be observed, whereas pityriasis rosea shows peripheral whitish scaling (collarette sign or curtain sign) (Fig. 6C) as well as dotted vessels, which, differently from psoriasis, are distributed in an irregular or focal pattern.[12,13] Reactive perforating collagenosis shows a three-zone area yellowish–brown hyperkeratotic plug in the center, elevated rim, and pinkish halo at periphery (Fig. 6D).

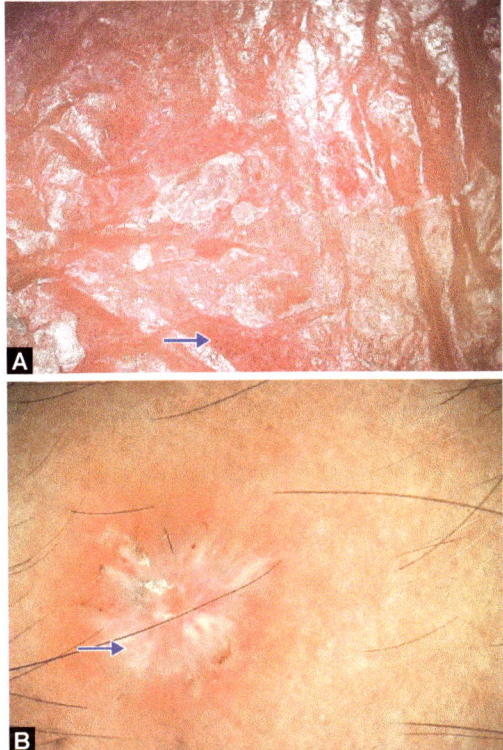

Figs. 6A and B: Inflammoscopy improves the differential diagnosis of inflammatory skin disorders (E-SCOPE magnification 10×). (A) Dermatoscopy of psoriasis shows regularly arranged dotted vessels (blue arrow) and white scales over a pink or red background; (B) Lichen planus shows white streaks (Wickham striae – blue arrow) of various morphologies.

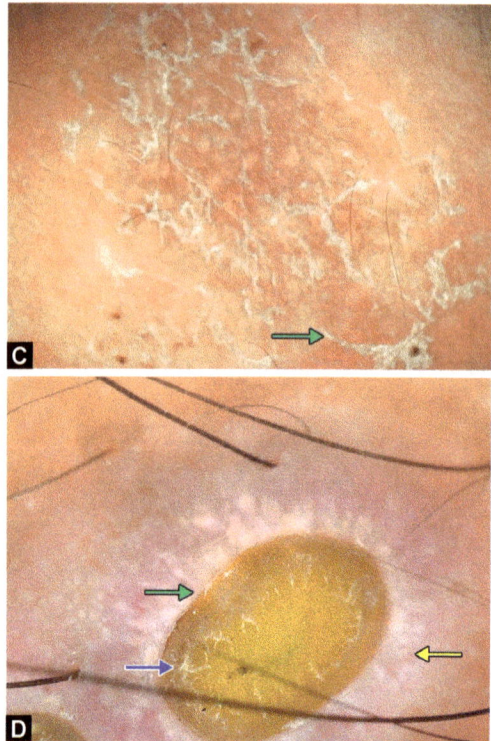

Figs. 6C and D: (C) Pityriasis rosea is characterized by a red-brown structureless color and fine white translucent scales that "hang" from the periphery toward the center like a curtain (green arrow); (D) Three zone area in a lesion of reactive perforating collagenosis showing yellowish-brown hyperkeratotic plug in the center (blue arrow), whitish elevated rim (green arrow) and pinkish halo at periphery (yellow arrow) (Dinolite polarized 10X).

For general dermatological condition, Errichetti and Stinco have suggested classifying conditions based on gross morphological patterns—dermatoses presenting with erythematous—desquamative patches plaques (like psoriasis), papulosquamous—papulokeratotic dermatoses (like lichen planus), facial inflammatory skin diseases (like rosacea, lupus vulgaris, sarcoidosis, discoid lupus, etc.), acquired keratodermas, sclero-atrophic dermatosis (like morphea), hypopigmented macular dermatosis, hyperpigmented maculopapular diseases, itchy papulonodular lesions, erythrodermas, noninfectious balanitis, scaling scalp disorders, inflammatory cicatricial alopecia, and nonscarring alopecia.[14] However, there may be more conditions outside this list that may be amenable to dermoscopic diagnosis.

Dermatoscopy for Treatment Decision and Monitoring

Dermatoscopy has also been used for monitoring adverse effects of topical treatment (for example, the evaluation of potent topical corticosteroids in psoriasis and to monitor response of lentigo maligna to treatment with topical imiquimod).[1] Dermatoscopy can be used in assessing treatment response in various conditions including hair disorders and pigmentary disorder. It can also help in follow-up of treated cases of skin cancers. This application gains importance, especially in the light of the steadily increasing availability and use of topical treatment options for nonmelanoma skin cancer like photodynamic therapy for basal cell carcinoma (Figs. 7A to D). Also certain dermoscopic criteria, namely pigmented structures, ulceration and arborizing vessels, predict the presence of residual disease (residual disease-associated dermoscopic criteria) in skin tumors such as basal cell carcinoma.[15-17]

A miscellaneous use of dermatoscopy described recently is in recognition and extraction of foreign bodies in the skin.

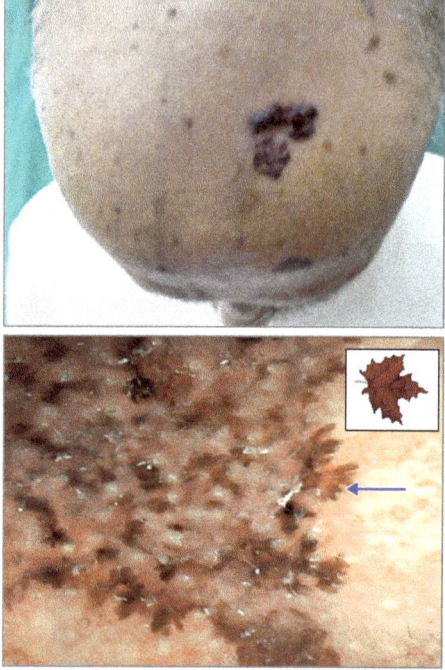

Fig. 7A: Malignancy-basal cell carcinoma (Dino-Lite polarized magnification 10X). (A) Nodular pigmented BCC.

CHAPTER 7: Applications of Dermatoscopy

Dermatoscopy has also been found to help patients understand their skin condition better by using the dermatoscopy images as a patient education tool.[18,19]

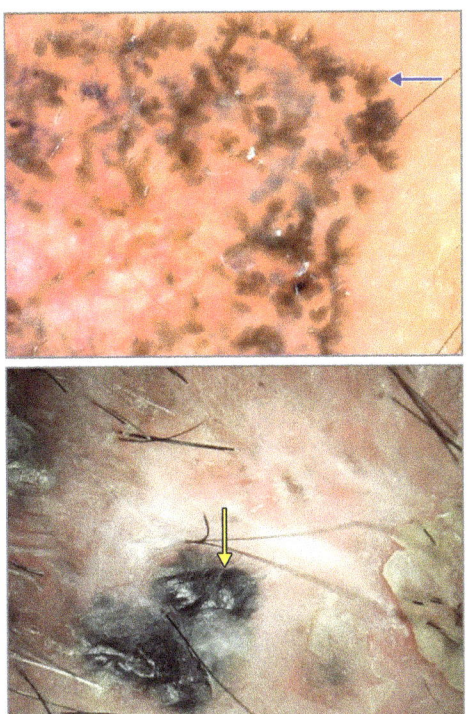

Fig. 7B: Dermatoscopy of basal cell carcinoma at baseline showing maple leaf like structures (blue arrow) and brownish pigmented structures with blue-gray globules (yellow arrow) prephotodynamic therapy.

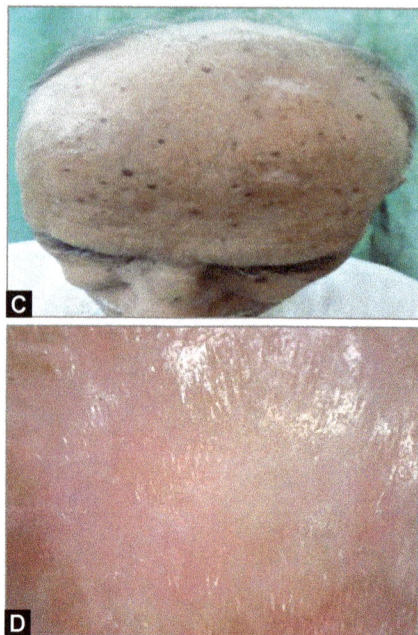

Figs. 7C and D: (C) Post-PDT scar and postinflammatory hypopigmentation; (D) Dermatoscopy after successful topical PDT treatment, there is absence of criteria suggestive of persistence. Only white scar-like areas are visible showing post two months after two cycles of photodynamic therapy.

CONCLUSION

To conclude, while dermatoscopy continues to be used extensively for the primary indications it was initially used for the diagnosis of pigmented skin tumors, its indications in general dermatology are growing rapidly. Evidence-based development of guidelines is the need of the hour in the context of dermatoscopy in general dermatology, especially in patients with skin of color. The future might see an increased correlation of dermoscopic findings to newer tools like confocal reflectance microscopy, further improving the diagnostic capabilities of a dermatologist. It is important that dermoscopic patterns always need to take into account the clinical context—clinical examination and history, and not be interpreted in isolation.

REFERENCES

1. Marghoob A, Malvehy J, Braun R. Chapter 1: Introduction. In: Marghoob A, Malvehy J, Braun RP (Eds). Atlas of Dermoscopy, 2nd edition. London, UK: Informa Healthcare; 2012. pp. 1-2.
2. Zalaudek I, Lallas A, Moscarella E, et al. The dermatologist's stethoscope—traditional and new application of dermoscopy. Dermatol Pract Conc. 2013;3(2):11.
3. Zalaudek I, Giacomel J, Cabo H, et al. Entodermoscopy: A new tool for diagnosing skin infections and infestations. Clinical and Laboratory investigations. Dermatology. 2008;216:14-23.
4. Zalaudek I, Argenziano G, Di Stefani A, et al. Dermoscopy in general dermatology. Dermatology. 2006;212(1):7-18.
5. Haldar SS, Nischal KC, Khopkar U. Chapter 2: Dermoscopy: Applications and patterns in Diseases of the Brown skin. Dermoscopy and Trichoscopy in Diseases of the Brown Skin. Atlas and short Text. New Delhi: Jaypee Brothers Medical Publisher (Pvt) Ltd; 2012. pp. 10-37.
6. Lallas A, Apalla Z, Lefaki I, et al. Dermoscopy of discoid lupus erythematosus. Br J Dermatol. 2012;168(2):282-8.
7. Olszewska M, Rudnicka L, Rakowska A, et al. Trichoscopy. Arch Dermatol. 2008;144(8):1007.

8. Rudnicka L, Olszewska M, Rakowska A, et al. Trichoscopy Update, 2011. J Dermatol Case Rep. 2011;5(4):82-8.
9. Miteva M, Tosti A. Hair and scalp dermatoscopy. J Am Acad Dermatol. 2012;67(5):1040-8.
10. Bergman R, Sharony L, Schapira D, et al. The handheld dermatoscope as a nail-fold capillaroscopic instrument. Arch Dermatol. 2003;139(8):1027-30.
11. Hasegawa M. Dermoscopy findings of nail fold capillaries in connective tissue diseases. J Dermatol. 2011;38(1):66-70.
12. Ankad BS, Beergouder SL. Dermoscopy of Inflammatory Conditions: The journey so far. Eur J Dermatol. 2017;5(1):98-105.
13. Lallas A, Kyrgidis A, Tzellos TG, et al. Accuracy of dermoscopic criteria for the diagnosis of psoriasis, dermatitis, lichen planus and pityriasis rosea. Br J Dermatol. 2012;166(6):1198-205.
14. Errichetti E, Stinco G. Dermoscopy in General Dermatology: A Practical Overview. Dermatol Ther (Heidelb). 2016;6(4):471-507.
15. Christensen E, Mork C. High and sustained efficacy after two sessions of topical 5-aminolevulinic acid photodynamic therapy for basal cell carcinoma: a prospective, clinical and histological 10-year follow-up study. Br J Dermatol. 2012;166:1342-8.
16. Thissen MR, Schroeter CA. Photodynamic therapy with delta-aminolevulinic acid for nodular basal cell carcinomas using a prior debulking technique. Br J Dermatol. 2000;142:338-9.
17. Soler AM, Warloe T. A follow-up study of recurrence and cosmesis in completely responding superficial and nodular basal cell carcinomas treated with methyl 5-aminolevulinate-based photodynamic therapy alone and with prior curettage. Br J Dermatol. 2001;145:467-71.
18. Sonthalia S, Jha AK, Kaliyadan F. Dermoscopy for the detection and safe extraction of an intracutaneous foreign body. J Am Acad Dermatol. 2018;79:e19-e20.
19. Kaliyadan F, Kuruvilla J, Al Ojail HY, et al. Clinical and Dermoscopic study of pseudofolliculitis of the beard area. Int J Trichology. 2016;8(1):40-2.

Section 2: Disorders of Hyperpigmentation

CHAPTER 8

Disorders of Facial Hyperpigmentation

Ankit H Bharti, Uday S Khopkar

INTRODUCTION

Facial hyperpigmentation is a major cosmetic concern in the current era. With increased predisposition of the brown skin to tan, there has also been observed an increased tendency for postinflammatory hyperpigmentation (PIH). Thus, the two major sources of melanin in facial skin are the follicular melanocytes and epidermal melanocytes. The normal pigment network, which is typically seen at other sites is interrupted by numerous appendages on the face.[1] This results in a reticuloglobular pattern that is normal on face.

Differentials for facial hyperpigmentation vary widely from generalized tanning to vitamin B_{12} deficiency, acanthosis nigricans, periorbital hyperpigmentation, PIH, to patchy pigmentation due to melasma, exogenous ochronosis, lichen planus pigmentosus (LPP), erythema dyschromicum perstans (EDP), fixed drug eruption (FDE), pigmentary demarcation lines, freckles, lentigines, or even the less common causes like drug-induced (cyclophosphamide or bleomycin) pigmentation, dyskeratosis congenita, morphea, discoid lupus erythematosus, argyriasis, arsenic pigmentation, porphyria cutanea tarda, and Becker's nevus among others.

Dermoscopy assists in judging the depth of pigmentation. Hyperpigmentation can be epidermal or dermal, the dermoscopic color varies according to the depth of melanin deposition. The melanin located in the stratum corneum and the upper epidermis appears black on dermoscopy. The melanin in the epidermis appears light to dark brown on dermoscopy, when in papillary dermis, it appears gray to bluish gray and steel blue when located in the reticular dermis. The melanin located in the deeper parts of the skin appears blue because portions of visible light with the shorter wavelengths (blue–violet end of the spectrum) are dispersed more than those with longer wavelength (red end of visible spectrum).[2]

The dermoscopic findings of some of the common disorders of facial hyperpigmentation are as follows.

MELASMA (FIGS. 1 AND 2)

Discussed in Chapter 7.

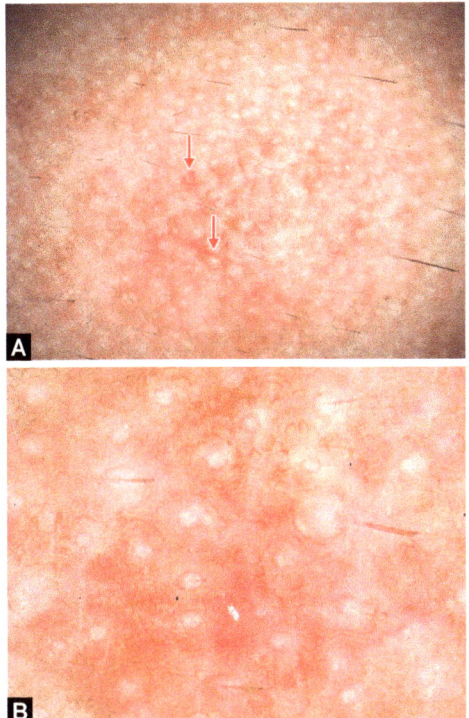

Figs. 1A and B: (A) Epidermal melasma displaying patchy accentuation of the reticuloglobular pigmentary pattern with cluster of fine brown granules can be seen on higher magnification (B) in pigmented areas encircling the white globules representing appendages.

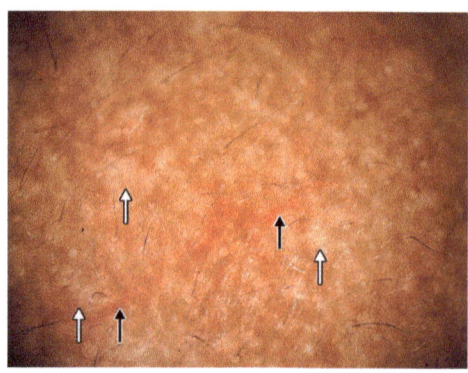

Fig. 2: Mixed melasma with dark-brown fine granular pigment in reticuloglobular pattern. Patchy loss of pattern (white arrow) indicating confetti-like macules within the area of hyperpigmentation. Black arrow shows marked linear telangiectasia suggesting topical steroid abuse.

EXOGENOUS OCHRONOSIS

Discussed in Chapter 8.

LICHEN PLANUS PIGMENTOSUS (FIGS. 3A AND B)

Discussed in Chapter 15.

ERYTHEMA DYSCHROMICUM PERSTANS OR ASHY DERMATOSIS OF RAMIREZ

Erythema dyschromicum perstans was recognized as a distinct entity in 1957 by Ramirez; thus, it is also known as ashy dermatosis of Ramirez. It is clinically characterized by

CHAPTER 8: Disorders of Facial Hyperpigmentation

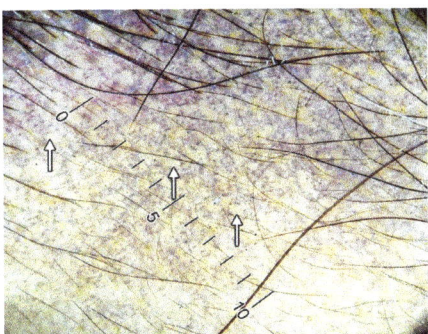

Fig. 3A: An established lesion of lichen planus pigmentosus (Heine Delta 20) shows speckled distribution of blue-gray and violet granules and globules with acrosyrigeal sparing (white arrow).

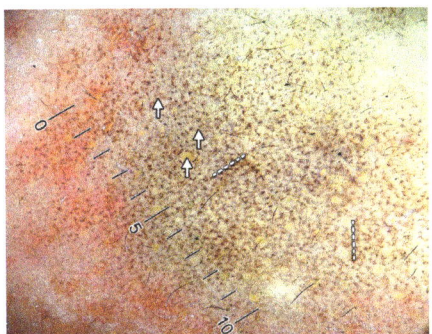

Fig. 3B: An established lesion of lichen planus pigmentosus (Polarized light microscopy—Heine Delta 20) shows speckled distribution of blue-gray and violet granules and globules forming acrosyrigeal arciform structures. The erythema on the left side and bottom of the image suggests active disease process.

numerous rounded or oval macules and circumscribed patches of varying shades of gray usually found over trunk and limbs; there may initially be signs of inflammation with a red, slightly raised, and palpably infiltrated margin.[3]

On dermoscopic evaluation, it shows a uniformly accentuated reticular pigment network over the face. The reticular pigment network shows more thickened lines and granules superimposed on the pigment network. The clusters of melanophages in the papillary dermis appear as brown, black, or gray-black granules. The reticular pattern of pigment network is complete at places, though sometimes it is disintegrated into discrete speckled, granular, linear, angulated, bluish-gray dots and a few globules. The reticular pigment network appears blunted around the acrosyringium on the extremities.

The granules of pigment clusters seen in EDP are limited by the skin surface marking and do not tend to cross them. Unlike LPP, they do not encircle the follicular openings. Thus, dermoscopy can be helpful in differentiating EDP from LPP.

ACANTHOSIS NIGRICANS

White light surface dermoscopy in a case of early acanthosis nigricans (AN) with dark band over neck shows linear crista cutis and sulcus cutis; focal hyperpigmented dots and globules that represent follicular plugging and white dots representing follicular openings and eccrine pores along with hyperpigmented globules and follicular plugging.[4]

Mild AN (Figs. 4A and B) shows follicular plugging and subtle sulci pattern with irregular brown globules and

CHAPTER 8: Disorders of Facial Hyperpigmentation

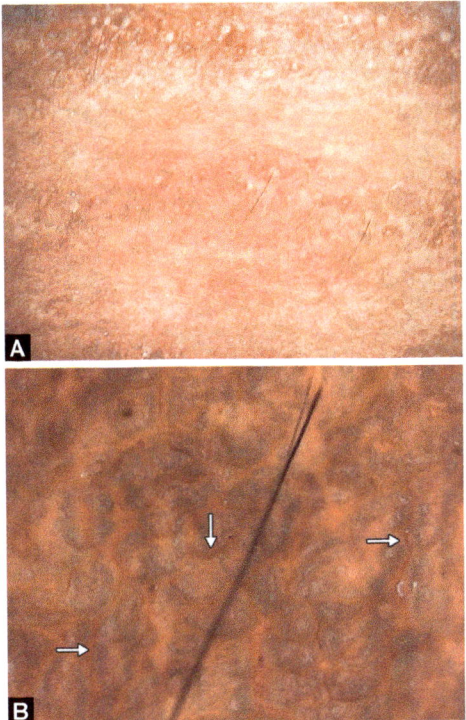

Figs. 4A and B: (A) Mild acanthosis nigricans (50X)—showing follicular plugging and subtle sulci pattern (white arrows) that is brought out clearly in the higher magnification (B) (200X). The red glow along the sulci pattern is because of the warmth produced due to the dermoscopy light.

perifollicular pigmentation along with occasional white and yellow dots.

Moderate AN (Figs. 5A and B) shows sulci that tend to connect with each other as AN progresses and the subtle cristae pattern of folding becomes visible along with larger brown globules and perifollicular hyperpigmentation.

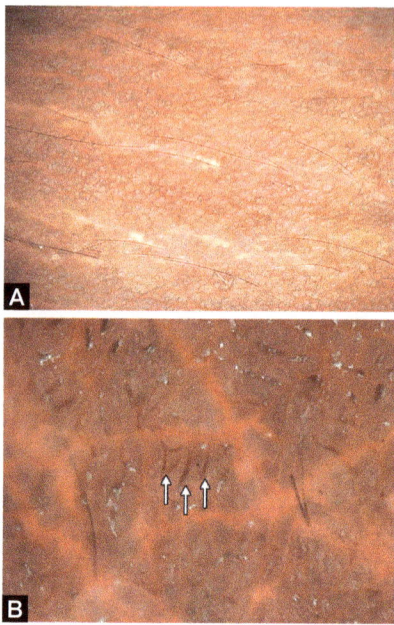

Figs. 5A and B: (A) Moderate acanthosis nigricans (50×) sulci tend to connect with each other as acanthosis nigricans progresses and the subtle cristae pattern (white arrow) (B) of folding becomes visible between the sulci resembling folds within mitochondria on higher magnification (200×). The red glow along the ridges pattern is because of the warmth produced due to the dermoscopy light.

The red glow along the ridges pattern is because of the warmth produced due to the dermoscopy light.

Severe AN (Figs. 6A and B) shows rhomboid (diamond)- shaped islands typical of the condition which at higher

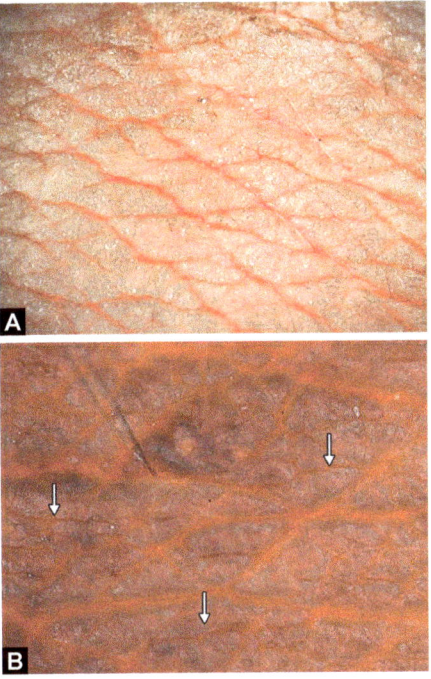

Figs. 6A and B: (A) Severe acanthosis nigricans (50×) shows rhomboid (diamond)-shaped islands typical of the condition which at the higher magnification (200×) shows markedly depressed sulci and prominent cristae (white arrows) (B).

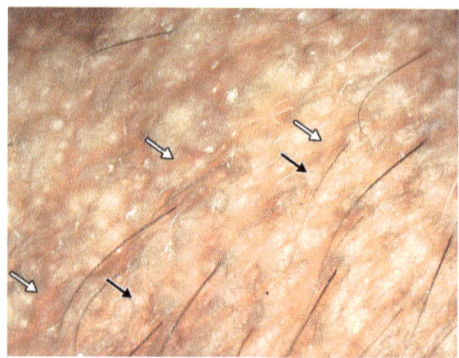

Fig. 7: Early facial acanthosis nigricans shows on higher magnification (200×) curvilinear depressions (white arrows) (over forehead) around follicular globules forming sulci pattern. Black arrows show a few follicular plugs.

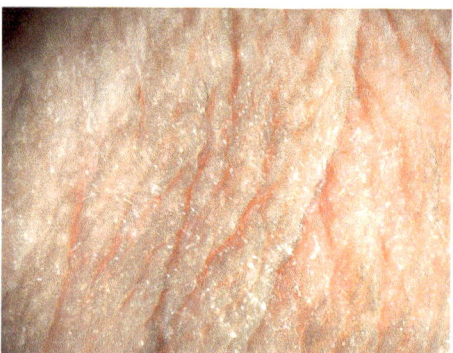

Fig. 8: White light image showing sulci pattern of acanthosis nigricans accentuated with background edema, erythema, and microscales in a patient with acanthosis nigricans with underlying atopic dermatitis.

magnification (200×) shows markedly depressed sulci and prominent cristae with large brown globules and irregular multiple white and yellow dots.

Facial AN (Fig. 7) shows curvilinear depressions around follicular globules forming sulci pattern with few follicular plugs. Infraorbital AN (Fig. 8) on higher magnification displays curvilinear depressions around follicular globules forming sulci pattern along with a few follicular plugs.

PERIORBITAL HYPERPIGMENTATION

Periorbital melanosis develops due to multiple components such as vascular congestion, reduced epidermal thickness, deposition of melanin in the dermis, and hereditary factors affecting pigmentation.[5]

Periorbital hyperpigmentation can have following components: vascular, pigmented, and mixed. The most common patterns of pigmentation observed include: (1) blotchy pattern (2) pseudonetwork pattern, and (3) multicomponent pattern.[6]

In the vascular type of pigmentation pattern, there is presence of diffuse erythema or thin blood vessels, sometimes diffuse vascular networks are observed.

Dermoscopic evaluation of periorbital melanosis/hyperpigmentation is valuable in classifying and the etiologic determination of the degree and pattern of pigmentation.

POSTINFLAMMATORY HYPERPIGMENTATION

Postinflammatory hyperpigmentation is characterized by irregular patchy accentuation of the normal pigment network and pseudoreticular pattern (Honeycomb like) that exists over the face with or without whitish irregular blotches. Blotches ranging from black to brown color, of variable intensity, are observed, based on the underlying condition and the level of melanophages in the epidermis. There is presence of perifollicular sparing of pigment network giving it a targetoid appearance with multiple islands of sparing, which correspond histologically to the dermal papillae.[3]

Polarized light dermoscopy in PIH postacne vulgaris displays perifollicular hyperpigmentation with brown granules spreading centrifugally from the follicles with ice pick scars and rolling scars (Figs. 9A and B). PIH following atopic

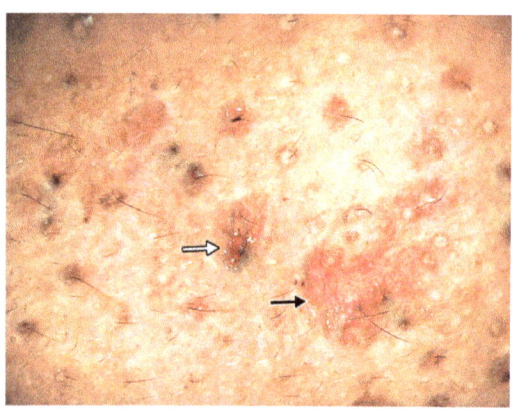

Fig. 9A

CHAPTER 8: Disorders of Facial Hyperpigmentation

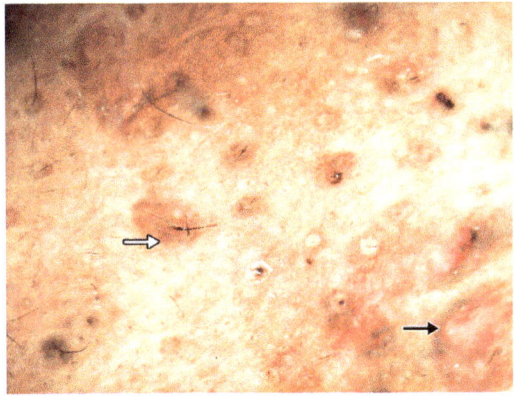

Fig. 9B

Figs. 9A and B: Postinflammatory hyperpigmentation (polarized light dermoscopy) following acne vulgaris displays perifollicular hyperpigmentation with brown granules spreading centrifugally from the follicles with ice pick scar (white arrow) and rolling scar (black arrow).

dermatitis (Fig. 10A) displaying clusters of speckled brown and black granules and globules with sparing of acrosyringeal openings and background blotchy erythema. On higher magnification (Fig. 10B), it displays disturbed reticuloglobular pattern. The specks are made up of fine granules of varying shades of brown while some brown dots have coalesced to form globules.

SECTION 2: Disorders of Hyperpigmentation

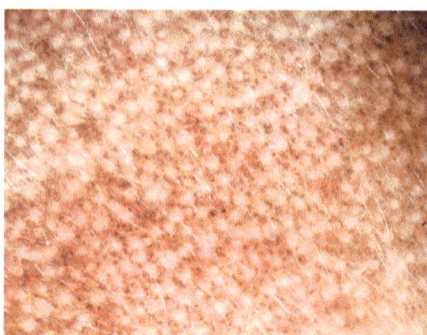

Fig. 10A: Polarized light dermoscopy of postinflammatory hyperpigmentation following atopic dermatitis displaying clusters of speckled brown and black granules and globules with sparing of acrosyringeal openings and background blotchy erythema.

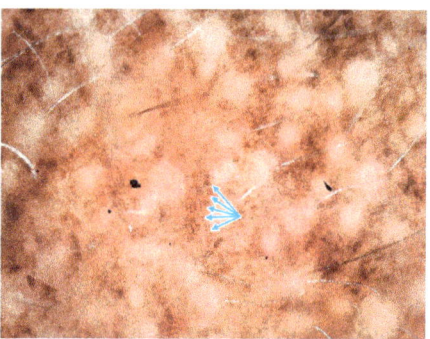

Fig. 10B: Higher magnification of the same showing disturbed reticuloglobular pattern. The specks are made up of fine granules of varying shades of brown while some brown dots have coalesced to form globules (blue arrows). The two black specks toward the center are artifacts due to dust.

PIGMENTED CONTACT DERMATITIS

Pigmented contact dermatitis is a disorder of cutaneous melanosis attributed to a complex series of interaction to specific kind of allergen, which requires recurrent exposure, at a very low dose in a specific manner to elicit a noneczematous phototoxic reaction to skin, in predisposed individuals, resulting into bizarre pigmentation pattern.[7] It has also been labeled as Riehl's melanosis, melanodermatitis toxica, or pigmented cosmetic dermatitis when on face.

In pigmented contact dermatitis, the dermoscopic findings (Fig. 11) include irregular accentuation of reticuloglobular network with speckling and bluish-gray globules along

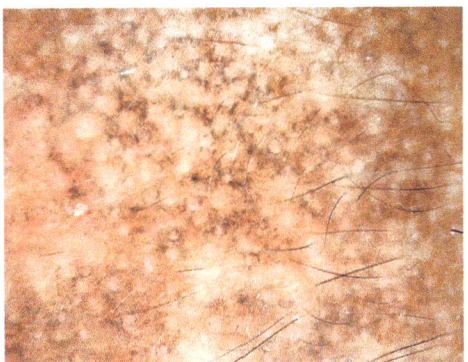

Fig. 11: Pigmented contact dermatitis shows patchy accentuation of pigment network with speckling of brown and gray globules and diffuse blotchy erythema. Suggesting an overlap between pigmentation observed in postinflammatory hyperpigmentation and lichen planus pigmentosus.

presence of microscaling, brown granules, follicular plugs, and curvilinear pattern around the acrosyringeal openings. The less commonly observed features also include brown granules, perifollicular halo diffuse telangiectasia, linear telangiectasias, and pigment cluster limited by skin markings. The histopathology of pigmented contact dermatitis seems similar to LPP, but presence of epidermal and follicular spongiosis along with superficial perivascular and periappendageal infiltrate help to diagnose pigmented contact dermatitis along with patch testing and an elaborate history. Pigmented contact dermatitis due to kumkum has been documented in India, which shows diffuse brown gray pigment granules in interfollicular region (Fig. 12). The follicles are seen as variably sized red globules

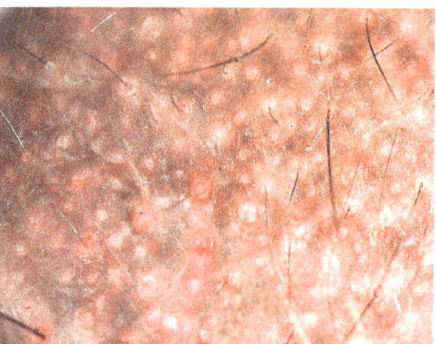

Fig. 12: Pigmented contact dermatitis due to kumkum displays diffuse brown-gray pigment granules between follicles. The follicles are seen as variably sized red globules due to inflammation. At higher magnification, the red globules show dark-red granules of kumkum pigment trapped within follicular infundibulum.

due to inflammation. At higher magnification, the red globules show dark red granules of kumkum pigment trapped within follicular infundibulum.

FIXED DRUG ERUPTION

The dermoscopy of a circumscribed patch of fixed drug eruption (FDE) displays multiple black, brown, or bluish–gray-colored dots and globules depending on the depth of the melanophages in the epidermis or dermis, secondary to pigment incontinence and damaged dermoepidermal junction.[8]

Dermoscopy of PIH post-FDE (Fig. 13) displays multiple brown dots and elongated globules ranging from brown to gray color without sparing of perifollicular region. Involvement of

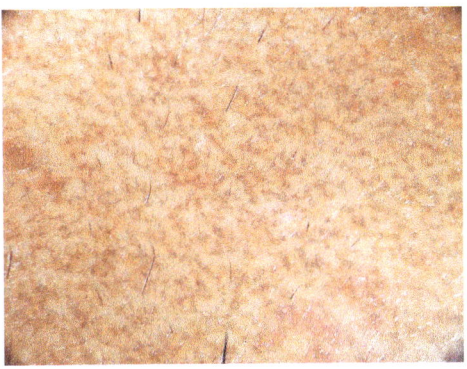

Fig. 13: Dermoscopy of postinflammatory hyperpigmentation (PIH) following fixed drug eruption (FDE) displays multiple brown dots coalescing haphazardly with globules broad pigmented lines with globular ends ranging in color from brown to gray.

perifollicular areas is observed in FDE unlike LPP, PIH, or ashy dermatosis. Thus, dermoscopy in a case of FDE, though not well described, could prove to be a valuable tool for a dermatologist, particularly to determine the depth of melanin pigment and thus verify the lesion and decide the prognosis of it.

DISCOID LUPUS ERYTHEMATOSUS

Dermoscopy in a depigmented patch of DLE with hyperpigmented margin has been described to display loss of pigment network with linear as well as branching vessels, keratin plugs, perifollicular whitish halo, rosettes, and structureless white and brown areas.[9]

Supplementing the above finding, Lallas et al. also described loss of follicular ostia, honeycomb-pigmented networks, dyschromia, and variable scaling. He described follicular red dots as a specific dermoscopic finding of DLE, which was not detected in other cases of alopecia. The morphologic distribution of the red dots corresponds to follicular openings was assumed to be resulting from dilated vessels and red blood cell extravasation in perifollicular distributions around the isthmus.[10]

An early lesion of DLE is characterized by presence of erythema, microscaling, follicular plugging and (a) typical perifollicular halo (duration 2 months), (b) with evolution of disease, fibrosis becomes more diffuse yet, perifollicular whitish halo can still be detected. There is presence of follicular plugging and short telangiectasias are also present (duration 5 months). (c) The advanced stages are characterized by more prominent pigmentation structure such as honeycomb network or an unspecified pattern. Follicular plugging and telangiectasias are present (duration 12 months). (d) End-stage plaques exhibit whitish structureless areas, which correspond to diffuse fibrosis in dermis, whereas the pigmentary changes and telangiectasias represent a common additional finding (duration 3 years).[11]

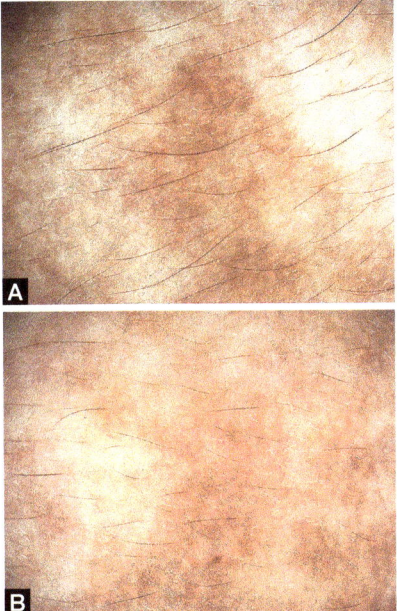

Figs. 14A and B: Dermoscopy of nevus of Ota displays patchy areas of accentuated reticuloglobular pattern varying from brown to gray color along with a few blotches of erythema which may be normal to facial skin.

NEVUS OF OTA

Dermoscopy of nevus of Ota (Figs. 14A and B) displays patchy areas of accentuated reticuloglobular pattern varying from brown to gray color along with a few blotches of erythema. It is characterized by accentuation of the reticular areas with bluish–gray blotches along with brown and bluish-gray globules with some normal areas and few dark brown areas.

NEVUS SPILUS

Dermoscopy of Nevus Spilus (Figs. 15A and B)

Dermoscopy of nevus spilus (NS) displays dark brown patchy areas with accentuated reticuloglobular pattern on a background of lighter reticuloglobular pattern.[12] In typical cases of NS, dermoscopy shows a reticular pattern without atypia. In suspected cases of atypical NS, dermoscopy displays irregular patches with hypopigmentation. The most characteristic pattern observed consists of reticular pattern, occasionally admixed with homogeneous globular components, located focally in the form of numerous patchy macules of varying colors, ranging from light brown to gray-black. On dermoscopy, the frequency of occurrence of reticular pattern and mixed pattern is similar. The homogeneous reticular and homogeneous globular pattern occur together sometimes which is also labeled as mixed pattern. The dermoscopic pattern of the lesions resembles the "Sparkle pattern".

CHAPTER 8: Disorders of Facial Hyperpigmentation

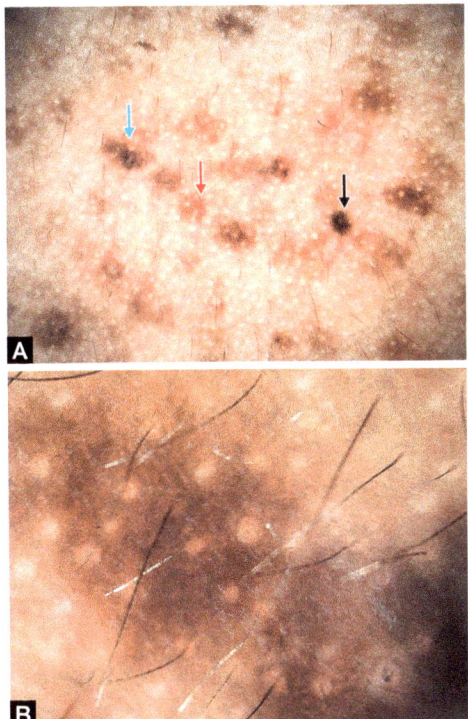

Figs. 15A and B: Nevus spilus in lower magnification shows islands ranging from brown (red arrow) to gray (blue arrow) and black (black arrow) areas with white dots (acrosyringeal openings).

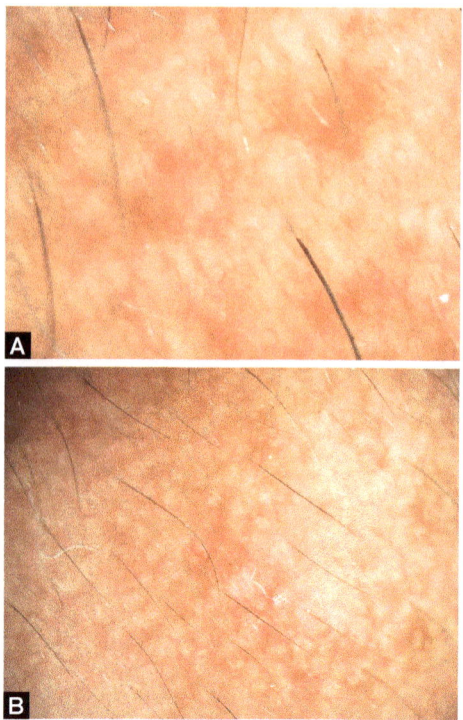

Figs. 16A and B: (A) Pigmentary demarcation lines (W type): At 50× displays cluster of brown granules which become confluent to form leaf-like pattern in some places and accentuation of reticuloglobular pattern to display a darker brown shade visualized on the left side of the image. (B) (50X): Diffuse blotchy telangiectasia and few linear vessels are visualized, which are probably normal on malar area or may be attributed to steroid application.

PIGMENTARY DEMARCATION LINES

Pigmentary demarcation lines (W type) on dermoscopy displays cluster of brown granules and globules (Figs. 16A and B), which become confluent to form leaf-like pattern in some places along with accentuation of the reticuloglobular pattern to display shades of dark brown. There is presence of diffuse blotchy telangiectasia and few linear vessels, which can be normal on malar area or secondary to steroid application.

LENTIGO SIMPLEX

The dermoscopy of lentigo simplex displays a typical brown–black pigment network, consisting of thin and uniformly arranged stitches. This is probably due to elongated and hyperpigmented rete ridges. On dermoscopy, one may observe a typical delicate pigment network with regularly sized mesh pattern, which is evenly distributed throughout the lesion. The pattern is caused by elongated rete ridges housing increased number of regularly spaced melanocytes. Dermoscopy of lentigo simplex displays at low-magnification confluence of accentuated dark-brown pigment network with white dots which at 200× displays (Figs. 17A and B) brown granules, which fuse at places to form globules and thus form a confluent pattern with white dots without perifollicular sparing.[13]

ACTINIC/SOLAR LENTIGO

On dermoscopy, actinic lentigo appears with a homogeneous pattern and uniform coloration. Commonly they display a "moth-eaten" or "jelly-like" edge. On the face, the dermoscopic

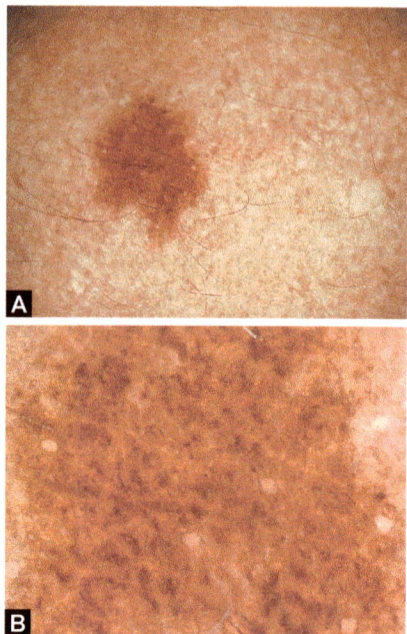

Figs. 17A and B: Dermoscopy of lentigo simplex displays at low-magnification confluence of accentuated dark brown pigment network with white dots. The lesion at 200X displays brown granules, which fuse at places to form globules and thus form a confluent pattern with white dots without perifollicular sparing.

features need to satisfy specific criteria according to the specific histological architecture, shown by the sun-damaged skin. The pigmentation displays a diffuse discoloration with circular hypopigmented follicular openings, known as pseudonetwork (similar to seborrheic keratosis).[14]

CUTANEOUS MASTOCYTOSIS

Two dermoscopic patterns have been described in cutaneous mastocytosis predominantly, i.e. microvessels in linear and/or reticular pattern in telangiectasia macularis eruptiva perstans (TMEP) and accentuated pigment network in urticaria pigmentosa. This was followed by identification of four dermatoscopic patterns by Vano-Galvan,[15] they were:

- Light-brown blot
- Pigment network
- Reticular telangiectasias
- Yellow–orange blot.

It was emphasized by the authors that the light brown blot and accentuated pigment pattern is more commonly observed in patients with maculopapular mastocytosis, while reticular vessels are mostly observed in TMEP, whereas the yellow-orange blots are more prevalent in mastocytoma.

CONCLUSION

Thus, dermoscopy of facial hyperpigmentation can be an essential tool for rapid diagnosis and may obviate the need for a skin biopsy. Though facial pigmentation can be a distressing symptom to patient, the pigmentation patterns, if assessed carefully using dermoscopy, can prove to be an important investigation to diagnose the common disorders and it can also be helpful in diagnosis of uncommon disorders.

REFERENCES

1. Haldar SS, Khopkar U, Nischal KC. Dermoscopy: Applications and Patterns in Diseases of the Brown Skin. In: Khopkar US (Ed). Dermoscopy and Trichoscopy in Diseases of the Brown Skin: Atlas and Short Text. New Delhi: Jaypee Brothers Medical Publishers (P) Ltd.; 2012. pp. 10-37.
2. Braun RP, Rabinovitz HS, Oliviero M, et al. Dermoscopy of pigmented skin lesions. JAAD. 2005;52(1):109-21.
3. Griffiths C, Barker J, Bleiker T, Chalmers R, et al. Acquired Pigmentary Disorders, 9th edition. New York: Wiley blackwell; 2016. pp. 32-3.
4. Phiske MM. An approach to acanthosis nigricans. Ind derm online. 2014;5(3):239-49.
5. Ga NQ, Romero W. Dermoscopy in periorbital hyperpigmentation: an aid in the clinical type diagnosis. Surg Cosm Dermatolo. 2014;6(2):171-2.
6. Mostafa WZ, Kadry DM, Mohamed EF. Clinical and dermoscopic evaluation of patients with periorbital darkening. J Egypt Women's Dermatol Soc. 2014;11(3):191-6.
7. Shenoi SD, Rao R. Pigmented contact dermatitis. Indian J Dermatol Venereol Leprol 2007;73:285-7.
8. Valdebran M, Salinas RI, Ramirez N, Velásquez CF, Thomas A, Domingo S, et al. Fixed Drug Eruption of the Eyelids. A Dermoscopic Evaluation Alba Rodriguez, Leyla Guzman, Silvia Marte, Max Suazo; 2013;344-6.
9. Tsai TM, Yang KC TT. Dermoscopic features of discoid lupus erythematosus. Dermoscopic Featur discoid lupus erythematosus. 2012;30(2):78-80.
10. Juan S. Dermatologica Sinica Dermoscopic features of discoid lupus erythematosus. 2012;30:78-80.

CHAPTER 8: Disorders of Facial Hyperpigmentation

11. Lallas A, Apalla Z, Lefaki I, Sotiriou E, Lazaridou E, Ioannides D, et al. Dermoscopy of discoid lupus erythematosus; 2013;284-8.
12. Kaminska-Winciorek G. Dermoscopy of nevus spilus. Dermatologic Surgery. 2013;39(10):1550-4.
13. Carli P, Salvini C. Lentigines Including Lentigo Simplex, Reticulated Lentigo and Actinic Lentigo.
14. Tanaka M, Sawada M, Kobayashi K. Key points in dermoscopic differentiation between lentigo maligna and solar lentigo. 2011;(October 2010):53-8.
15. Vano-Galvan S, án Álvarez-Twose I, De las Heras E, Morgado JM, Matito A, Plana MN, Orfao A, Escribano L. Dermoscopic features of skin lesions in patients with mastocytosis. Archives of dermatology. 2011;147(8):932-40.

CHAPTER 9

Dermoscopy in Melasma

Niti Khunger, Rashmi Sharma

INTRODUCTION

Melasma is a common skin condition with various shades of pigmentation ranging from light-brown to dark-brown to grayish-brown, presenting frequently on the face in a bilateral symmetrical manner. It affects globally, more commonly seen in women with darker skin tones. There are various factors contributing to the pathogenesis such as ultraviolet radiation, visible light, family history, genetics, thyroid diseases, drugs, and hormonal disturbances.[1] Increased cutaneous vasculature, through vascular endothelial growth factor (VEGF), may also play a role in increased pigmentation seen in melasma.[2]

Though more common in females, it is said to be more resistant to treatment in males.

CLASSIFICATION

Melasma can be classified by various methods:
- Clinical classification
- Histopathological classification
- Instrument based:
  - Wood's lamp
  - Dermoscopy.

Clinical Classification of Melasma

This classification is based on the predominant site of involvement (Figs. 1A to C).
- *Centrofacial*—predominant symmetrical involvement of the center of the face around glabella, forehead, nose, zygoma, upper lip, and chin areas (Fig. 1A).
- *Malar*—predominant involvement of the cheeks (Fig. 1B).
- *Mandibular*—predominant involvement of the lower half of the face over the mandibular area (Fig. 1C). It is a rare type and considered as a variant of poikiloderma of Civatte, present in postmenopausal women mainly after extensive sun exposure. It is most resistant to treatment.
- *Nonfacial*—involvement of the neck and extensors of the forearms.

The most common type in Asians is malar type, whereas the centrofacial type is most common worldwide.

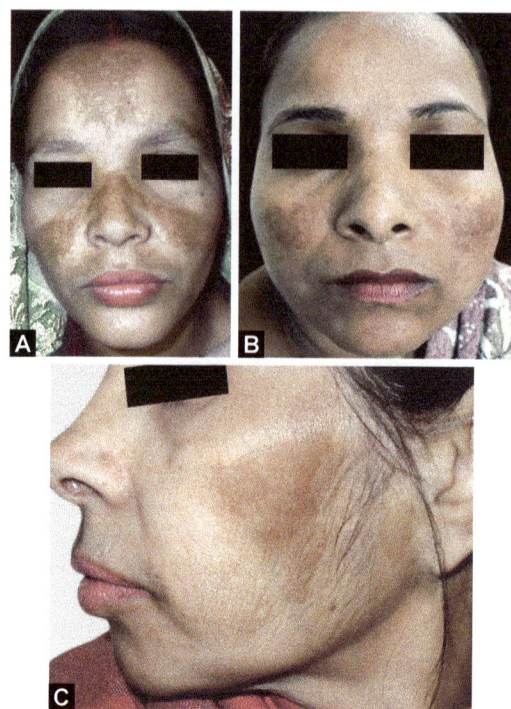

Figs. 1A to C: Clinical classification of melasma. (A) Centrofacial; (B) Malar; (C) Mandibular.

Histopathological Classification

Melasma can be epidermal, dermal, or mixed type, mixed being the most common (Table 1). In melasma, melanin is increased

Table 1: Histopathological classification of melasma.

Type	Histology
Epidermal	Melanin is increased in epidermal layer with increase in melanosomes in melanocytes and keratinocytes
Dermal	Melanophages in dermis with increase in vascularity and elastosis in affected skin
Mixed	Increase in melanin in epidermal layer with increased mature melanosomes, with increase in vascularity and elastosis in the dermis and presence of melanophages

in the epidermal layers. Mature melanosomes are increased in number and also increased in keratinocytes in the affected area. There is an increase in free melanin and melanophages in the dermis. The number of melanocytes is not increased but they are hypertrophied with increased number of dendrites and cytoplasmic organelles, depicting higher metabolism. In the dermis, there is increased vascularity and elastosis.[3,4] Pure dermal melasma is not observed and most melasma is epidermal or mixed.

Instrument-based Classification

Wood's Lamp

In Wood's lamp examination, the epidermal and dermal type can be differentiated depending upon the enhancement of pigmentation, which is enhanced in epidermal type and shows no change in dermal type (Table 2). However, in mixed type, there is enhancement of pigmentation in spotty areas.[5]

Table 2: Classification of melasma based on Wood's lamp.

Type	Wood's lamp
Epidermal	Increase in pigmentation
Dermal	No change
Mixed	Increase noticed in few areas

Dermoscopy-based Classification

Dermoscopic features of normal skin in cases of melasma: In normal skin, pigmentation is seen due to melanin present in keratinocytes and melanocytes. The typical pigment pattern observed in normal skin is seen as a honeycomb pattern composed of intersecting lines with hypopigmented holes present in-between which is denoted by tips of dermal papillae. Also brown dot on the pigment network is a melanocytic nest at tip of the rete ridges. However, in facial lesions, pseudonetwork is formed by interruption of pigmentation by adnexal openings. In melasma, the normal skin may show patchy accentuation of the normal pseudonetwork pattern even in clinically normal skin (Fig. 2).

Dermoscopic features of melasma: The dermoscope is a very important assessment tool in melasma. It helps in diagnosing the type of melasma as well as in assessing the response to treatment and assists in early detection of adverse effects to treatment. It also helps in differentiating melasma from other hyperpigmentary skin conditions. It holds special importance in prognosis to treatment. It is noninvasive, quick, and an important hand-held instrument which is very easy to operate.

CHAPTER 9: Dermoscopy in Melasma

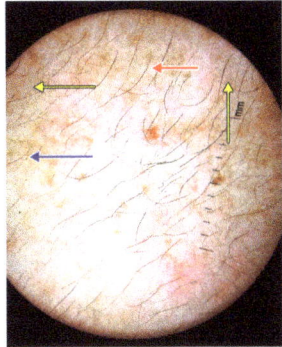

Fig. 2: Dermoscopy of normal skin in melasma. Normal pseudonetwork pattern (red arrow), patchy accentuation of the pattern (yellow arrow), increased vascularity seen as faint erythema (blue arrow).

Global and local dermoscopic features: Dermoscopic features can be described on the basis of color, pattern, vascularity, and special features[6-9] (Table 3). The global feature is the reticular network pattern which is consistently present along with the pigmented background (Fig. 3). The local features are details along with other features like vascular pattern. The reticular network is regular in epidermal melasma and irregular and blotchy in dermal melasma. The color varies depending on the level of involvement, being dark brown in the stratum corneum, becoming progressively lighter brown in the deeper epidermis to blue or bluish gray, when present in the dermis. A characteristic feature of melasma is the "jelly sign" which is aggravated pigmentation with concave borders with characteristic sparing of adnexal openings[6] (Fig. 4).

Table 3: Dermoscopic characteristics of melasma.

Dermoscopy	Epidermal	Dermal	Mixed
Color	Dark brown to light brown	Blue to bluish gray	Dark brown
Pattern	Regular pigment network	Irregular pigment network	Diffuse reticular pigmentation or blotches of irregular varying shades of brownish pigmentation of varying sizes
Vascular	Diffuse erythema may be present with widened vessels	Diffuse erythema may be present with widened vessels	Diffuse erythema may be present with widened vessels

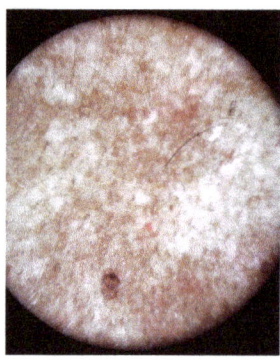

Fig. 3: Global feature of melasma—reticular network pattern with pigmented background.

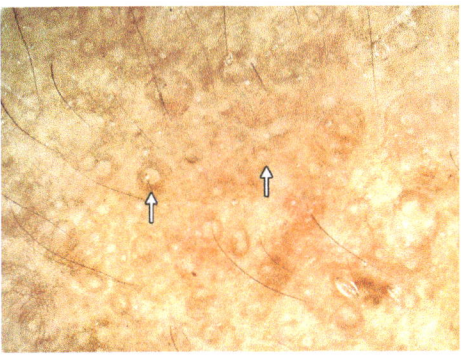

Fig. 4: Denser distribution of brown granules around follicular globules lead to their concave or circular coalescence (jelly sign).

There are also dark brown granules and globules noticed with sparing of perifollicular openings. The color intensity and arrangement of network pattern reveal the level of involvement. The presence of dark brown color and well-defined network is noticed in involvement of upper layer of epidermis, light brown pigmentation with irregular network seen in lower level of epidermal involvement (Figs. 5A to C). If there is involvement of dermis, then the shades of blue color are seen (Figs. 6A and B).

Increased vascularity has also been observed in patches of melasma even in untreated patients. It has been reported that VEGF receptors are present on melanocytes and this contributes to increased pigmentation in melasma.[10]

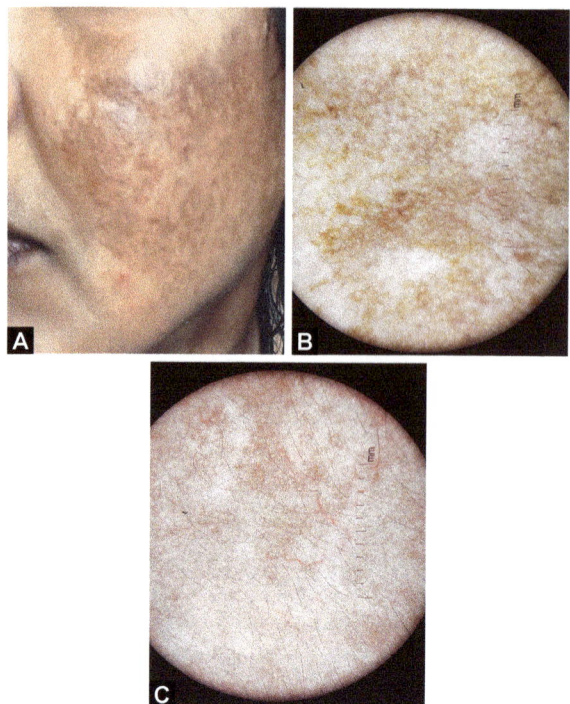

Figs. 5A to C: Epidermal melasma. (A) Clinical appearance with dark brown pigmentation; (B) Dermoscopy showing light brown pigmentation with irregular network; (C) Increased vascularity.

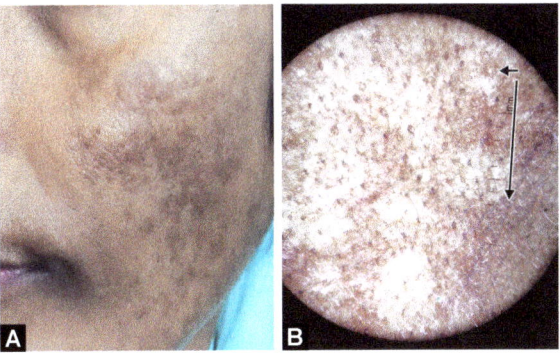

Figs. 6A and B: Dermal melasma. (A) Clinical appearance showing irregular patchy bluish gray pigmentation; (B) Irregular patchy bluish gray pigmentation (black arrow).

DIFFERENTIAL DIAGNOSIS

Dermoscopy can help in differentiating from other facial pigmentary disorders like lichen planus pigmentosus,[11,12] Riehl's melanosis, ochronosis, pigmentary demarcation lines, lentigines, freckles, and nevus of Ota[6] (Table 4).

TREATMENT ASSESSMENT OF STEROID ABUSE AND OCHRONOSIS

Dermoscopy can be used as an assessment tool for selection of treatment and assessing response to treatment. Patients showing increased vascularity on dermoscopy may respond better with the pulsed dye laser, which targets vascular lesions

Table 4: Differential diagnosis of common facial melanosis based on dermoscopy.

	Reticular network	Pigment deposition	Color	Vascular pattern	Other features
Melasma	Accentuation of regular pseudonetwork pattern in epidermal melasma, irregular network in dermal and combination in mixed melasma	Dots and globules, blotchy in dermal, sparing follicular, and adnexal openings	Dark to light brown in epidermal and bluish gray in dermal	Telangiectasia Localized	Jelly sign
Ochronosis	Irregular network	Deposition of blue gray to blackish pigment in arcuate, curvilinear, worm-like pattern with obliteration of follicular openings	Blue gray amorphous areas in a background of brown color White confetti-like dots interspersed	Telangiectasia	

Contd...

Contd...

	Reticular network	Pigment deposition	Color	Vascular pattern	Other features
Lichen planus pigmentosus	Accentuated network, which may be uniform or irregular	Pigment deposition in the form of grayish blue dots and globules in a perifollicular, perieccrine, annular, arcuate, cobblestone, reticular or linear pattern	Erythematous background in active cases and diffuse brown background in older cases	Classic peripheral red dots and globules of lichen planus are rare	Hem-like, interrupted linear pigment pattern
Riehl melanosis		Uneven pigment dots	Regular distribution of brown-to-gray-colored dots and globules		
Pigmentary demarcation lines	Accentuated normal pigment network		Occasional brown dots and globules		
Hori nevus			Dark brown areas with bluish gray dots in a reticular pattern		

combined with low-fluence Q-switched neodymium-doped yttrium aluminum garnet (Nd:YAG) laser as compared with Q-switched Nd:YAG laser alone.[13] Tranexamic acid, which targets vascularity may also be more useful in such patients.

It has been observed that following treatment blotchy pattern changes to globules and globular pattern changes to dots progressively with treatment. The pattern becomes irregular with clearing of lesions and fading of pigment. Vascularity also reduces with response to treatment.[14,15]

Dermoscopy can also pick up early signs of topical steroid side effects seen as presence of telangiectasia and hypertrichosis (Fig. 7). The detection of exogenous ochronosis following use of hydroquinone is also easier seen as the presence of depigmented confetti-like areas, globular,

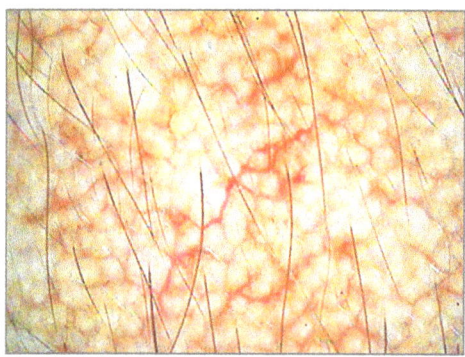

Fig. 7: Topical steroid abuse showing presence of telangiectasia and hypertrichosis.

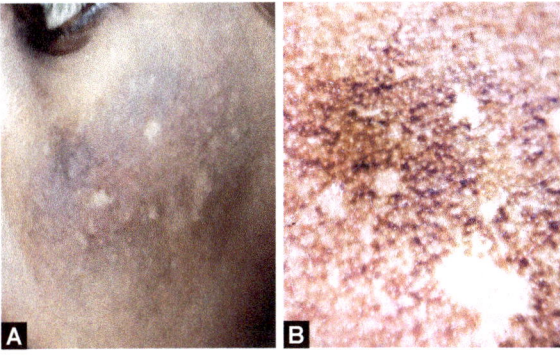

Fig. 8A and B: Exogenous ochronosis. (A) Clinical appearance of bluish gray pigmented papules with areas of confetti-like depigmentation; (B) Globular, arcuate, and worm-like pattern of bluish gray pigmentation, with obliteration of follicular openings.

arcuate, and worm-like pattern of bluish gray pigmentation, with obliteration of follicular openings (Figs. 8A and B). It can also help in selecting the right site of biopsy in suspected cases.[11]

EXOGENOUS OCHRONOSIS

There has been increase in the incidence of exogenous ochronosis due to unsupervised application of skin lightening agents. Hence, it is an important differential diagnosis and dermoscopy is helpful in differentiating them at an early stage. It is important to rule out ochronosis in a resistant case of melasma as early as possible as further treatment with hydroquinone will increase the pigmentation and make the patient worse. Clinically, there are areas of hyperpigmented macules with "confetti"-like hypopigmented to depigmented macules, with pinpoint papules present in-between them, better appreciated on palpation (caviar-like papules). There can also be erythema and telangiectasia with mild atrophy. Though the gold standard for diagnosis of exogenous ochronosis remains biopsy, the dermoscope aids in selecting the biopsy site. The typical histopathology reveals stout, curvilinear, "banana-shaped", and ochre-colored fibers of varying thicknesses in the papillary dermis.

PROGNOSIS

The presence of features suggestive of epidermal melasma signifies a better prognosis as compared with dermal melasma.

CONCLUSION

To conclude, the dermoscope is an important assessment tool in diagnosis, treatment, and prognosis of melasma. It can also aid in differentiating it from other facial pigmentary disorders. On dermoscopy, melasma can be classified as epidermal, presenting with a regular pigmentary network and dark brown to light brown hue, which has better prognosis as compared with dermal melasma, seen as an irregular pigmentary network with bluish-gray hue, and mixed melasma with areas compatible with both categories. It can also assist in early detection of adverse effects to treatment such as increasing telangiectasia and hypertrichosis due to topical steroids and exogenous ochronosis, with distinct dermoscopic features.

Thus dermoscopy in melasma should be routinely done for assessment and follow-up of patients.

REFERENCES

1. Grimes PE. Melasma. Etiologic and therapeutic considerations. Arch Dermatol. 1995;131:1453-7.
2. Kim EH, Kim YC, Lee ES, et al. The vascular characteristics of melasma. J Dermatol Sci. 2007;46:111-6.
3. Kwon SH, Hwang YJ, Lee SK, et al. Heterogeneous Pathology of Melasma and Its Clinical Implications. Sugumaran M, ed. Int J Molecul Sci. 2016;17(6):824.
4. Kang WH, Yoon KH, Lee ES, et al. Melasma: histopathological characteristics in 56 Korean patients. Br J Dermatol. 2002;146(2):228-37.
5. Tamler C. Classification of melasma by dermoscopy: comparative study with Wood's lamp. Surgical Cosmetic Dermatol. 2009; 1(3):115-9.
6. Khopkar US. Dermoscopy and trichoscopy in diseases of the brown skin—atlas and short text, Volume 1. New Delhi: Jaypee Brothers Medical Publishers; 2014: pp. 50-62.
7. Nanjundaswamy BL, Joseph JM, Raghavendra KR. A clinico-dermoscopic study of melasma in a tertiary care center. Pigment Int. 2017;4:98-103.
8. Manjunath KG, Kiran C, Sonakshi S, et al. Melasma: Through the eye of a dermoscope. Int J Res Dermatol. 2016;2(4):113-7.
9. Neema S, Chatterjee M. Dermoscopic characteristics of melasma in Indians: A cross-sectional study. Int J Dermoscope. 2017;1:6-10.
10. Cho SB, Kim JS, Kim MJ. Melasma treatment in Korean women using a 1064-nm Q-switched Nd:YAG laser with low pulse energy. Clin Exp Dermatol. 2009;34:e847-50.

11. Sharma VK, Gupta V, Pahadiya P, et al. Dermoscopy and patch testing in patients with lichen planus pigmentosus on face: A cross-sectional observational study in fifty Indian patients. Indian J Dermatol Venereol Leprol. 2017;83:656-62.
12. Güngör S, Topal IO, Göncü EK. Dermoscopic patterns in active and regressive lichen planus and lichen planus variants: a morphological study. Dermatol Pract Concept. 2015;5(2):6.
13. Kong SH, Suh HS, Choi YS. Treatment of melasma with pulsed-dye laser and 1,064-nm Q-Switched Nd:YAG Laser: A Split-Face Study. Ann Dermatol. 2018;30(1):1-7.
14. Passeron T. Long-lasting effect of vascular targeted therapy of melasma. J Am Acad Dermatol. 2013;69:e141-2.
15. Khunger N, Khandari R. Dermoscopic criteria for differentiating exogenous ochronosis from melasma. Indian J Dermatol Venereol Leprol. 2013;79:819-21.

CHAPTER 10

Importance of Dermatoscopy in Diagnosing Exogenous Ochronosis

Sunil N Mishra, Rachita Dhurat

INTRODUCTION

In 1866, Virchow coined the term exogenous "ochronosis" for brownish yellow or ochre-colored accumulation of pigment in dermis.[1] Ochronosis can be divided into two types on the basis of origin, i.e. endogenous or exogenous.[2] Exogenous ochronosis is an acquired deposition of polymerized homogentisic acid in collagen due to prolonged application of hydroquinone. Exogenous ochronosis is usually limited to dermis and presents in form of asymptomatic blue or slate gray cutaneous pigmentation which develops usually over malar area including temples, inferior part of cheeks, neck, back, and over the extensor parts of extremities in form of hyperchromatic, pinpoint, and caviar-like papules (Figs. 1 to 3).[2] Exogenous ochronosis can be divided into three clinical

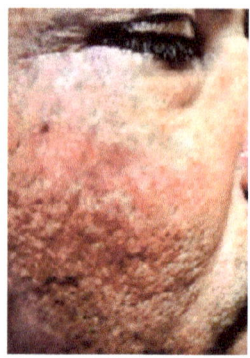

Fig. 1: Exogenous ochronosis over malar area: Hyperchromatic, brown caviar-like papules, with presence of confetti-like depigmentation within the melasma patches.

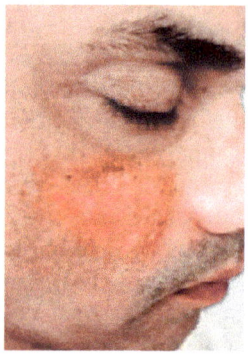

Fig. 2: Exogenous ochronosis over the zygomatic process: Black-colored (caviar-like) pinpoint-sized papules which is admixed with confetti-like depigmentation.

CHAPTER 10: Importance of Dermatoscopy in Diagnosing Exogenous...

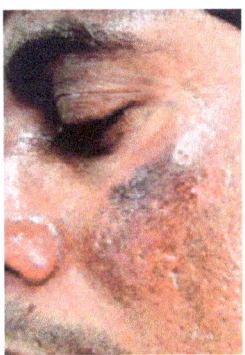

Fig. 3: Initial stage of exogenous ochronosis: Caviar-like pinpoint papules in the zygomatic region with surrounding zone of erythema.

stages as described by Dogliotti: (1) Initial erythema and mild pigmentary change, followed by hyperpigmentation, (2) Black colloid milia, and atrophy, and (3) Finally papulonodules.[3]

DERMOSCOPY

The dermoscopic features in ochronosis are unique though they have received little attention till now. Some of the common features described are presence of blue, gray annular and granular structures in perifollicular region.[4] In 2008, Charlin et al. described blue-gray amorphous areas occasionally surrounding follicular regions as one of the important dermoscopic features. In 2009, Berman et al. reported dark brown globular structures on a diffuse brown background as another dermoscopic features. In 2009, Berman et al. reported the presence of globular dark brown colored structures. Gil et al. reported the presence of thin annular and arciform structures around follicular openings.[5]

Dermoscopy of melasma displays accentuation of the normal pseudoreticular pattern over face. There is also presence of caviar-like hyperchromic papules suspected of exogenous ochronosis shows:

- Brown amorphous structures which can be seen obliterating the follicular structures and sometimes even surrounding them (Fig. 4).
- Numerous brown pigment globules can be observed over the melasma patch (Fig. 5).
- Numerous thin, short arciform structures (Fig. 6).

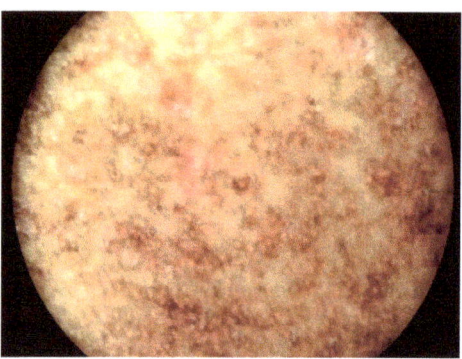

Fig. 4: Dermoscopy of the patches shown in Figure 2: Accentuation of the normal pseudonetwork pattern over face with hyperpigmented brown amorphous structures with some obliterating the follicular openings and confetti-like depigmentation.

CHAPTER 10: Importance of Dermatoscopy in Diagnosing Exogenous...

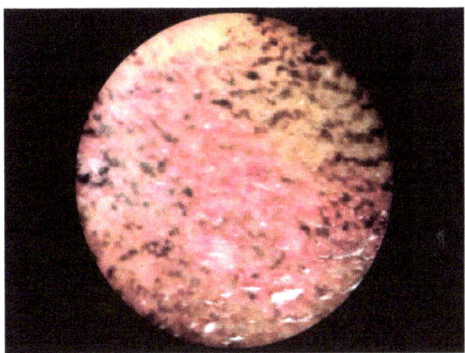

Fig. 5: Dermoscopy from a darker area of the same patch from Figure 2: Multiple thick globular structures.

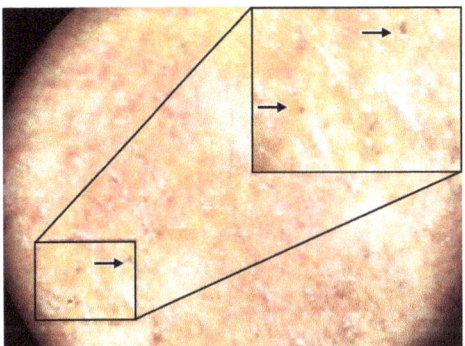

Fig. 6: Dermoscopy from a different foci of the same patch from Figure 2: Multiple thin, short arciform structures with few hyperpigmented grayish-brown amorphous areas obliterating some follicle.

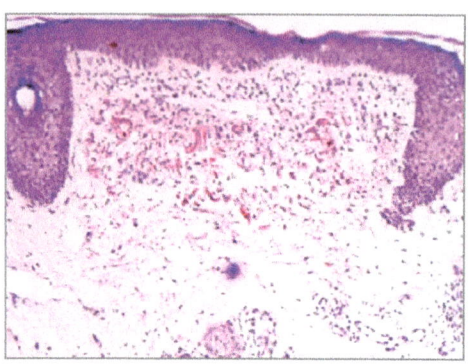

Fig. 7: Histopathology of the patch seen in Figure 2: Numerous "ochre colored-banana-shaped" curvilinear structures in the dermis observed on hematoxylin and eosin (H&E) stain that represent deposition of hydroquinone on collagen.

- Confetti-like depigmented dots (Figs. 4 and 6) and red dots (Fig. 6).

A diagnosis of ochronosis can be confirmed by histopathology which is characterized by: there is effacement of the rete ridges, with presence of melanophages in the dermis, with numerous "ochre colored-banana-shaped" curvilinear structures in the dermis observed on hematoxylin and eosin (H&E) stain (Fig. 7).

CONCLUSION

Exogenous ochronosis is probably more common than diagnosed. Reluctance to undertake a biopsy for a cosmetic facial problem complicates this situation. Dermatologists should be aware of the value of dermoscopy in early diagnosis of exogenous ochronosis complicating melasma. An early diagnosis necessitates immediate discontinuation of hydroquinone, rather than increasing the concentration in an attempt to clear the hyperpigmentation. Exogenous ochronosis has been largely refractory to topical agents, oral medications, dermabrasion, and CO_2 laser irradiation.[2] Dermoscopy shows different patterns for lesions of melasma, exogenous ochronosis, and confetti like depigmentation due to hydroquinone and it should be employed more frequently to differentiate between them.

REFERENCES

1. Charlín R, Barcaui CB, Kac BK, et al. Hydroquinone-induced exogenous ochronosis: a report of four cases and usefulness of dermatoscopy. Int J Dermatol. 2008;47:19-23.
2. Levin CY, Maibach H. Exogenous ochronosis: an update on the clinical features, causative agents, and treatment options. Am J Clin Dermatol. 2001;2:213-7.
3. Dogliotti M, Leibowitz M. Granulomatous ochronosis—a cosmetic-induced skin disorder in Blacks. S Afr Med J. 1979;56:757-60.
4. Penneys NS. Ochronosis-like pigmentation from bleaching creams. Arch Dermatol. 1985;121:1239-40.
5. Gil I, Segura S, Escala EM, et al. Dermoscopic and reflectance confocal microscopic features of exogenous ochronosis. Arch Dermatol. 2010;146:1021-5.

CHAPTER 11

Pigmented Purpuric Dermatoses

Siddhi Chikhalkar, Monica Bambroo, Uday S Khopkar

INTRODUCTION

Pigmented purpuric dermatoses (PPD), also called purpura simplex or chronic capillaritis,[1-3] is a group of chronic and relapsing disorders characterized by petechiae and pigmentation. These conditions result from minimal inflammation and hemorrhage of superficial papillary dermal vessels, usually capillaries. The exact etiology of the inflammation is unknown. PPD have traditionally been divided into five clinical entities: (1) progressive pigmented purpuric dermatosis or Schamberg´s disease (Fig. 1); (2) purpura annularis telangiectodes Majocchi or Majocchi´s disease (Fig. 2); pigmented purpuric, lichenoid dermatosis of Gougerot and Blum; eczematoid-like purpura of Doucas and Kapetanakis (Fig. 3); and lichen aureus.[1-3]

CHAPTER 11: Pigmented Purpuric Dermatoses

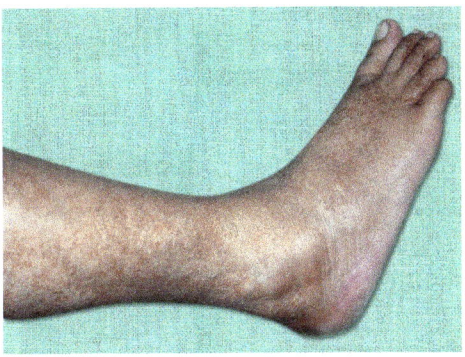

Fig. 1: Progressive pigmentary dermatosis or Schamberg's disease: Multiple, discrete and confluent nonpalpable and nonblanching lesions of long duration.

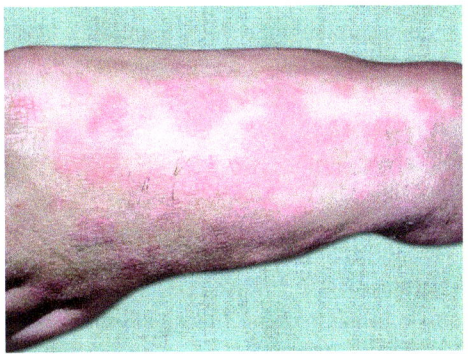

Fig. 2: Purpura annularis telangiectodes or Majocchi purpura: Multiple discrete to confluent nonpalpable and nonblanching purpuric lesions arranged in an annular pattern.

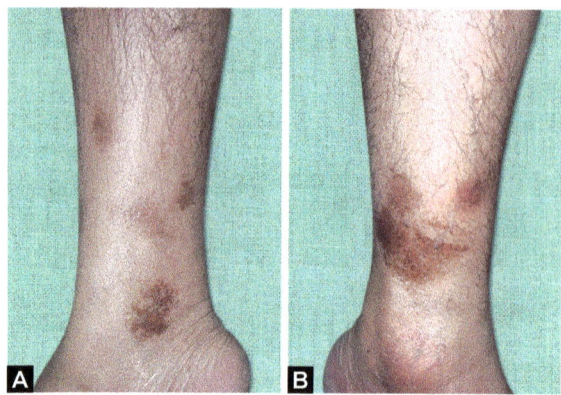

Fig. 3: Eczematoid-like purpura of Doucas and Kapetanakis: Mild scaling over typical patches of pigmented purpuric dermatosis lesions.

The most common subtype is Schamberg's disease. This group of disorders is often neglected by patients due to their asymptomatic nature and patients seek medical attention only for cosmetic reasons.

There is paucity of reports in literature regarding use of dermatoscopy in PPD. Only one Spanish case series has been reported in lichen aureus, which mentioned findings in only three cases.[4] Role of dermatoscopy in PPD has not been mentioned in any of the textbooks. There are no dermatoscopic studies done in Indian patients having PPD.

CLINICAL NEED OF DERMOSCOPY

In PPD, differentiation from stasis pigmentation, post-inflammatory hyperpigmentation, purpuric clothing dermatitis

CHAPTER 11: Pigmented Purpuric Dermatoses

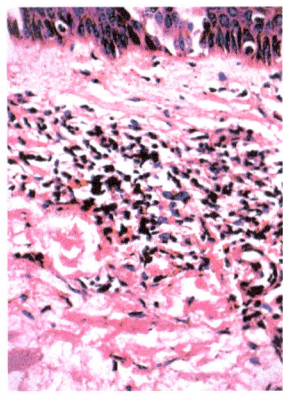

Fig. 4: Histopathological features in Schamberg's disease: Lichenoid superficial perivascular infiltrate with extravasation of red blood cells and hemosiderin deposit.

(khaki), leukocytoclastic vasculitis (LCV), and senile or steroid-induced purpura may be difficult clinically and hence a biopsy is needed. Some patients may not be ready for biopsy, and it is risky to do a biopsy in patients receiving anticoagulants like warfarin. Dermatoscopy being a noninvasive tool may come handy in such situations for aiding clinical diagnosis. However, diagnosis should not be solely dependent on dermoscopic findings, which must be interpreted in the light of clinical features, and if needed, histopathology (Fig. 4).

COMMON DERMOSCOPIC OBSERVATIONS IN PPD[4]

- Round to oval globules
- Red dots, and patches

- Brownish or coppery-red, diffuse, homogeneous background
- Gray dots, network of brownish to gray interconnected lines.

DERMOSCOPIC FINDINGS AND HISTOPATHOLOGIC CORRELATION WITH EVOLUTION OF LESIONS OF PPD[4]

The dermoscopic findings with evolution of lesions and their histopathological correlation is as follows:

- *In early lesions*:
  Dermoscopy: Red-brownish or red-coppery background is brighter or more clearer with a few red dots, and globules (Fig. 5).

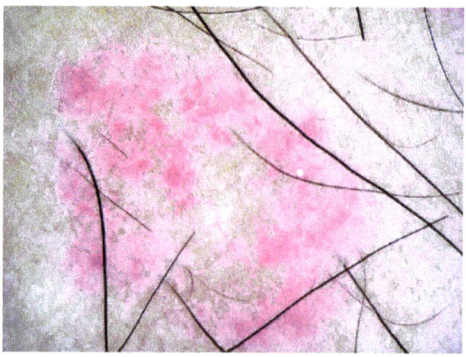

Fig. 5: Dermoscopy of an early lesion of pigmented purpuric dermatosis: Several dark red dots and globules on a coppery-red background.

Histopathology: Perivascular infiltrate of lymphocytes and macrophages around superficial small blood vessels.

- *In established lesions*:

  Dermoscopy: Red-brownish or red-coppery background, red dots, globules, and patches (Fig. 6) are seen prominently, which suggest active inflammation. Some gray dots and a network of brownish to gray interconnected lines, which are less prominent.

  Histopathology: Perivascular infiltrate of lymphocytes and macrophages around superficial small blood vessels, which are dilated and swollen. There is also extravasation of red blood cells (RBCs).

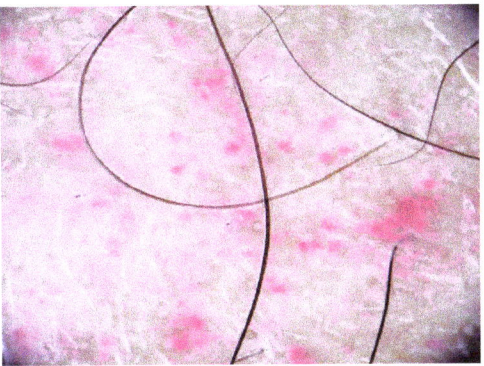

Fig. 6: Dermoscopy of an established lesion of pigmented purpuric dermatosis: Red dots and globules more in number as compared to an early lesion (compare with Figure 5).

- *In resolving lesions*:
  Dermoscopy: The background becomes more brownish and coppery and the reddish tinge reduces. Central red globules with dark-brown pigment deposit indicate hemosiderin deposits at the periphery. Gray dots and a network of brownish to gray interconnected lines are seen (Figs. 7A and B).

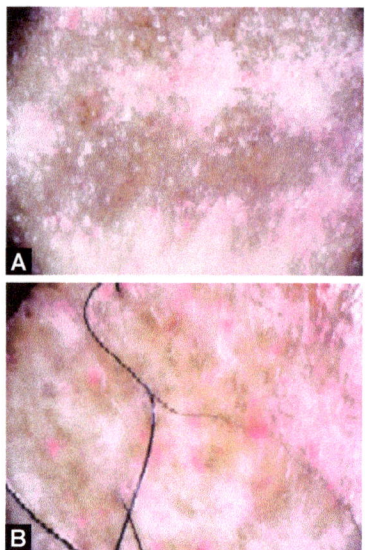

Figs. 7A and B: Dermoscopy of a resolving lesion: More brownish and coppery background as compared to early and established lesions (compare with Figures 5 and 6). Higher magnification shows a few scattered red dots and globules and surrounding brown discoloration. The brown discoloration indicates hemosiderin deposition.

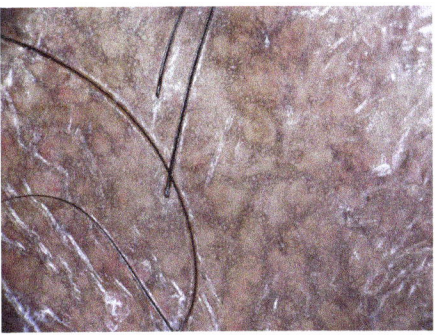

Fig. 8: Dermoscopy of inactive lesion of Schamberg's disease: The pseudo-reticular pattern of pigmentation is more pronounced as also the normal pigment network within the pigmented bands; red dots and globules are absent (Compare with Figures 5 to 7)

Histopathology: Less number of RBCs, less infiltration of lymphocytes and hemosiderin laden macrophages (siderophages).
- *In old or completely resolved lesions*:
Dermoscopy: Pigment deposits appear blackish brown. There are no red globules and dots (Fig. 8).

How is PPD Differentiated from Other Skin Conditions on Dermoscopy?

- *Senile or steroid-induced purpura*: PPD is a type of inflammatory purpura, which can be differentiated from noninflammatory purpura, such as senile or steroid-induced purpura. Senile or steroid-induced purpura show large, irregular-shaped homogeneous purpuric patches

devoid of definite rounded globules and dots since there is no perivascular infiltrate of lymphocytes and macrophages around blood vessels.
- *Stasis dermatitis*: The presence of glomerular vessels and a scaly surface is the characteristic pattern of venous stasis dermatitis. Hemosiderin deposition is deeper in dermis in venous stasis, whereas it is superficial in PPD. Hence, background of lesions appears more grayish-blue in venous stasis compared to PPD.
- *Lichen planus*: Reticular whitish striae with red lines and dots surrounding the striae are seen in lichen planus.
- *Angioma serpiginosum*: Numerous small, relatively well-demarcated, round-to-oval red lacunas without the brownish background are determined with dermoscopy in angioma serpiginosum.

LIMITATIONS

The findings on dermoscopy-like presence of red dots, globules, and patches, with a red-brownish pigmentation in the background may not be solely limited to PPD, as we can find a similar dermoscopic pattern in other inflammatory purpuras like urticarial vasculitis, LCV, and old lesions of lichen planus. Vázquez–López et al.[5] found a pattern composed of purpuric or reddish dots and globules in a patchy, orange-brown background in two cases of urticarial vasculitis[6] and also described a similar pattern composed of reddish or brownish globules in diffuse brownish areas in some cases of pigmented lichen planus. Clinical examination and biopsy help differentiate between urticarial vasculitis and PPD.

CONCLUSION

Dermoscopy is a valuable noninvasive tool in diagnosis, to judge activity of and to monitor response to treatment in PPD. All types of PPD show similar pattern on dermoscopy.[4-6] Awareness regarding use of dermoscopy and more data with respect to PPD need to be created.

REFERENCES

1. Cox NH, Piette WW. Purpura and microvascular occlusion. In: Burns T, Breathnach S, Cox N, Griffiths C (Eds). Rook´s Textbook of Dermatology. Oxford: Blackwell Publishing Ltd; 2004.
2. McKee PH. Superficial and deep perivascular inflammatory dermatoses. In: McKee PH, Calonje E, Granter SR (Eds). Pathology of the Skin with Clinical Correlations. China: Elsevier Mosby; 2005.
3. Sardana K, Sarkar R, Sehgal VN. Pigmented purpuric dermatoses: an overview. Int J Dermatol. 2004;43:482-8.
4. Zaballos P, Puig S, Malvehy J. Dermoscopy of pigmented purpuric dermatoses (lichen aureus): a useful tool for clinical diagnosis. Arch Dermatol. 2004;140(10):1290-1.
5. Vázquez-López F, Fueyo A, Sánchez-Martín J, et al. Dermoscopy for the screening of common urticaria and urticaria vasculitis. Arch Dermatol. 2008;144:568.
6. Vázquez-López F, Maldonado-Seral C, López-Escobar M, et al. Dermoscopy of pigmented lichen planus lesions. Clin Exp Dermatol. 2003;28:554-64.

CHAPTER 12

Becker's Nevus versus Café au lait Macules: A Dermoscopic Analysis

Mary Thomas, Uday S Khopkar

INTRODUCTION

Becker's nevus (BN) was first described by S. William Becker in 1949. It is an androgen-dependent epidermal nevus typically appearing in the second decade of life over the upper half of trunk and/or on the proximal upper extremities.[1,2] The patch usually starts as a subtle hyperpigmentation and expands during the first several years. New irregular pigmented macules and patches develop at the periphery of the lesion and coalesce with the larger patch resulting in a geographic configuration. Hypertrichosis appears months to years after the onset of the lesion in most cases (Fig. 1). Lesions at atypical sites and with atypical presentations, e.g. early onset, absence of hair may misguide the clinician.[3]

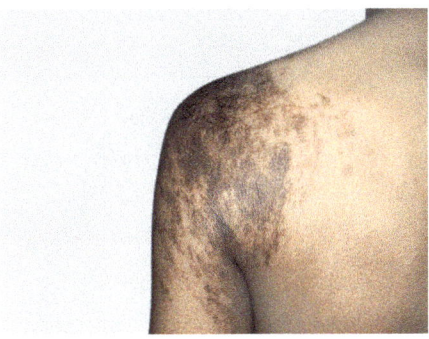

Fig. 1: Becker's nevus in a young man: Hyperpigmented lesion on the upper trunk with hypertrichosis.

Histopathology has been routinely resorted to for differentiating it from its common mimics, e.g. congenital melanocytic nevus (CMN), café au lait macules (CALMs), etc. Typically, the histological findings of BN include acanthosis, papillomatosis and clubbing of the rete ridges with flat tips. There is increase in basal layer pigmentation with large terminal follicles with thick arrector muscle bundles. However, these findings may not be present in all cases.[4]

A close differential diagnosis of BN is the CALM. These lesions may be present at birth or appear in early childhood. They present as light brown to dark brown macules with smooth or irregular borders. There is also a large variation in the size, depth of color, and location of these lesions (Fig. 2). Histologically, increased pigmentation of the basal layer and the occasional presence of giant melanosomes characterize

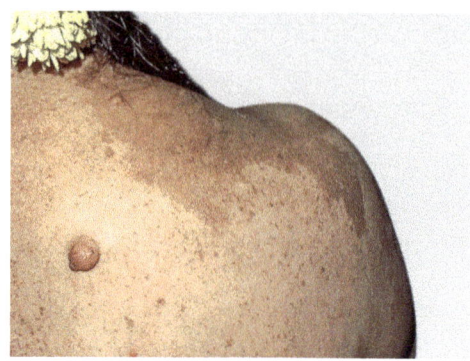

Fig. 2: Café au lait macule on the shoulder of a woman with neurofibromatosis: Hyperpigmentated macule with an irregular border.

> **Box 1:** Syndromes associated with café au lait macules.
>
> - McCune–Albright syndrome
> - Tuberous sclerosis
> - Fanconi anemia
> - Bloom syndrome
> - Ataxia telangiectasia
> - Russell–Silver syndrome
> - Multiple lentigines (LEOPARD) syndrome
> - Multiple endocrine neoplasia type 2b
> - Bannayan–Riley–Ruvalcaba syndrome

CALMs. Though classically associated with neurofibromatosis, CALMs are found in 19% of normal individuals as well and can mimic BN.[5] In such cases, the only method of differentiating the two was believed to be a histological analysis. However, dermoscopy can offer a noninvasive alternative method to differentiate between these two conditions (Box 1).

DERMOSCOPIC FINDINGS OF BECKER'S NEVUS

Center of the Lesions

There is uniform thickening of the normal pigment network throughout the lesion. Blotchy areas of hyperpigmentation (ill-defined pigmented clods) with irregular margins, not restricted to the pigment network, are characteristically seen in the center of the lesions. Intermediate and terminal hair may be seen dermoscopically and can easily be differentiated from the nonpigmented vellus hair (Fig. 3).

In early lesions, it must be noted that the terminal hair may be absent and the blotchy pigmentation, though present, may not be prominent. These features tend to develop as the lesion progresses.

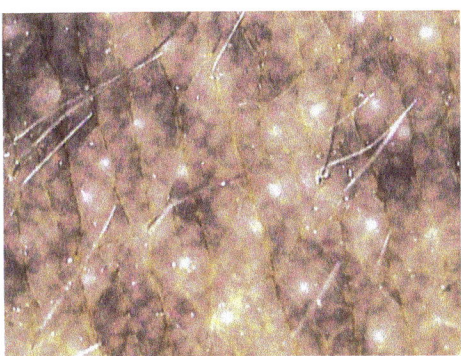

Fig. 3: Becker's nevus: Dermoscopic examination of the center of the lesion reveals blotchy areas of pigmentation with irregular margins not restricted to the pigment network.

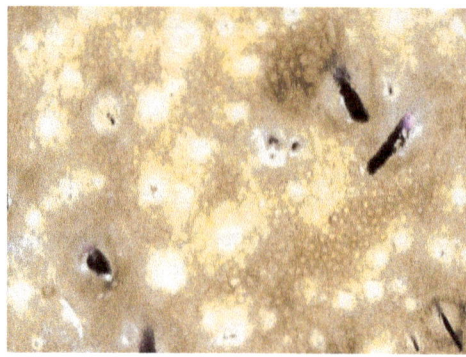

Fig. 4: Becker's nevus: Dermoscopic examination of the periphery of the lesion shows prominent perifollicular hypopigmentation and parafollicular hyperpigmentation.

Periphery of the Lesions

Similar to the center of the lesions a focal prominence of the pigment network can be observed in the periphery of BN. Focal areas of perifollicular hypopigmentation with parafollicular hyperpigmentation are distinctive findings at the periphery. The blotchy hyperpigmentation is less commonly observed peripherally. Terminal hair may or may not be visualized (Figs. 4 and 5) (Table 1).

DERMOSCOPY OF CAFÉ AU LAIT MACULES

The CALMs can be differentiated from classical lesion of BN by the presence of a focal areas of irregular thickening of the normal pigmentary network lines as compared to the uniform

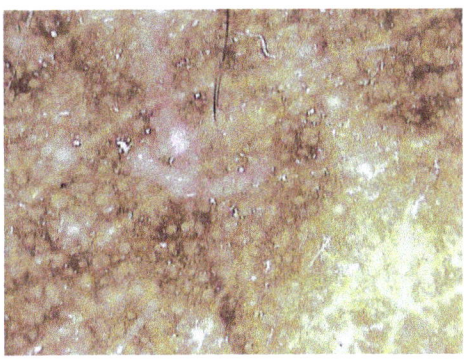

Fig. 5: Becker's nevus: Dermoscopic examination of the periphery of the lesion shows a focal prominence of the pigment network without blotchy hyperpigmentation.

Table 1: Dermoscopic differences between Becker's nevus and café au lait macules.

	Becker's nevus		CALMs
	Center	*Periphery*	*Center and periphery*
Pigmentary network	Prominent	Normal	Focal thickening
Hyperpigmentation	Blotchy	Nil	Nil
Hair follicles	Terminal hair present	Terminal hair present	No terminal hair
Parafollicular hyperpigmentation	Present	Present	Absent

(CALMs: café au lait macules)

thickening seen in BN. In light-colored CALMs, these focal thickenings are seen as tiny arcuate lines (Fig. 6), which in darker

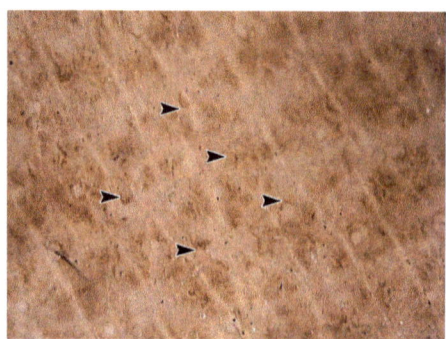

Fig. 6: Café au lait macules: Dermoscopy of light brown lesions reveals focal arcuate areas of irregular thickening of the normal pigment network.

Fig. 7: Café au lait macules: Dermoscopy of darker lesions reveals a snail-track appearance.

lesions join to form snail-track pattern (Fig. 7). In very dark CALMs, there is uniform thickening of the pigment network

CHAPTER 12: Becker's Nevus versus Café au lait Macules... 163

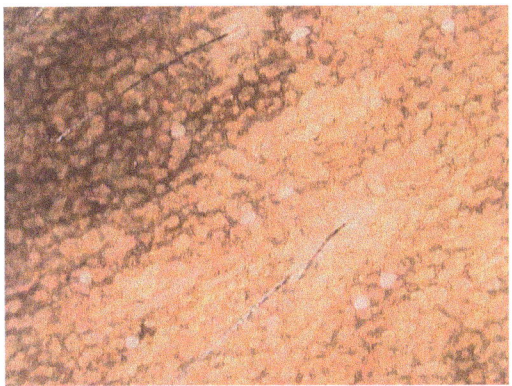

Fig. 8: Café au lait macules: Dermoscopy of deeply pigmented lesions reveals a uniform thickening of the pigment network throughout the lesion.

(Fig. 8). However, confluence of the pigmentation leading to irregular blotches seen in the center of BN does not occur. CALMS are not associated with the presence of terminal hair. There are no areas of focal or parafollicular hyperpigmentation within CALMs (Table 1).

OTHER CONDITIONS WITH MACULAR HYPERPIGMENTATION

Congenital melanocytic nevi (CMN): Two dermoscopic patterns are described in CMN:
- *A globular pattern*: Globules arranged in regular blotches. This is common in small lesions (Fig. 9).

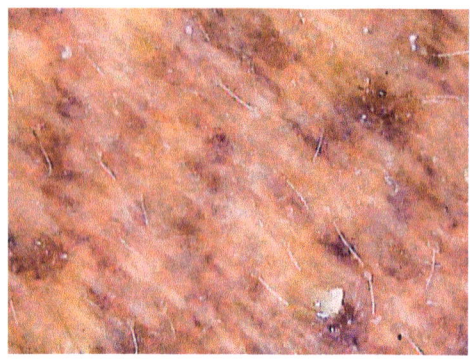

Fig. 9: Congenital melanocytic nevus: Dermoscopy reveals large regular pigmented blotches.

- *A reticular pattern*: Thin pigmentary network interrupted by homogeneous round achromic areas. This pattern is seen in larger lesions.

Postinflammatory pigmentation (PIH): The pattern of pigmentation seen in PIH varies widely from multiple dots with different sizes and colors to a diffuse network of pigment. Blotchy homogeneous pigmentation and varied vascular features may also be observed. Dermoscopic findings for PIH are not diagnostic.

Nevus spilus (NS): Dermoscopy of NS shows dark brown areas with a reticuloglobular pattern on a background of light brown, reticular pigmentation.

Lentiginosis: Delicate pigment network in a regular mesh distributed evenly throughout the lesion.

SUMMARY

Dermoscopy is a quick, noninvasive, easy to use, and effective tool to differentiate Becker's nevus from CALMs particularly in cases where clinical presentation is puzzling. It can substitute a skin biopsy in such cases especially in cosmetically important areas.

REFERENCES

1. Becker SW. Concurrent melanosis and hypertrichosis in distribution of nevus unius lateris. Arch Dermatol 1949;60:155-60.
2. Happle R, Koopman RJ. Becker's nevus syndrome. Am J Med Genet. 1997;68:357-61.
3. Tymen R, Forestier JF, Boutet B, et al. Late Becker's nevus: one hundred cases. Ann Dermatol Venereol. 1981;108:41-6.
4. Elder D, Elenitsas R. Benign pigmented lesions and malignant melanoma. In: Elder D, Elenitsas R, Jaworsky C, (Eds). Lever's Histopathology of the Skin, 8th edition. Philadelphia: Lippincott-Raven; 1997. p. 631.
5. Whitehouse D. Diagnostic value of café au lait spot in children. Arch Dis Child. 1996;41:316-9.

Section 3: Disorders of Hypopigmentation

CHAPTER 13

Dermoscopy in Vitiligo: Utility for Early Diagnosis, Assessing Stability and Monitoring Therapy

Laxmisha Chandreshekhar

The diagnosis of vitiligo is although primarily clinical, the challenge arises when the lesion has to be differentiated from its clinical mimics like contact leukoderma, pityriasis alba, guttate lichen sclerosus, nevus depigmentosus, progressive macular hypomelanosis, and idiopathic guttate hypomelanosis, etc. The role of dermoscope in vitiligo has evolved with time, as it is not only helpful in early diagnosis of vitiligo but also assessing its stability and response to therapy. In addition, it aids in diagnosis of blue and nail trichrome vitiligo.[1-10]

One of the earliest features described in vitiligo was the perifollicular retention of pigment. However, it has become apparent now that this finding has been reported in many other conditions.

CHAPTER 13: Dermoscopy in Vitiligo: Utility for Early Diagnosis... 167

In early vitiligo, the following features have been described: reduced/absent (Fig. 1) or reversed pigment network, perifollicular retention of pigmentation (Fig. 2) and a diffuse white glow (Fig. 3) under ultraviolet (UV) light.[1] The perifollicular retention of pigment can be explained by the early loss of melanocytes in the interfollicular compartment followed by loss of melanocytes in the perifollicular compartment in the active phase of the disease.

Sonthalia et al.[2] described features like perifollicular depigmentation (Fig. 4) and evolving leukotrichia as the marker of impending vitiligo.

The various dermoscopic features described for progressive vitiligo are trichrome vitiligo (three zones brown, tan, and white; Fig. 2), polka dot or confetti-like lesion [depigmented dots distributed in a polka dot pattern (Fig. 5)], comet tail (micro-Koebner's phenomenon; Fig. 6), starburst pattern

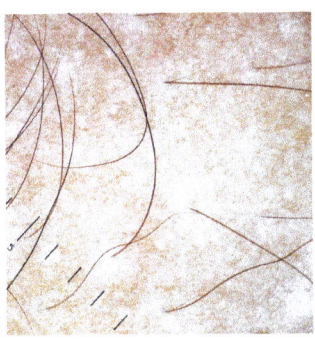

Fig. 1: Loss/reduction of pigment network.

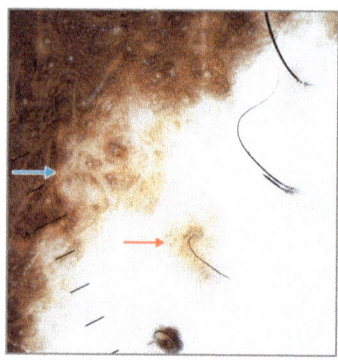

Fig. 2: Perifollicular retention of pigmentation (red arrow) and trichrome sign (blue arrow).

Fig. 3: Diffuse white glow.

CHAPTER 13: Dermoscopy in Vitiligo: Utility for Early Diagnosis... 169

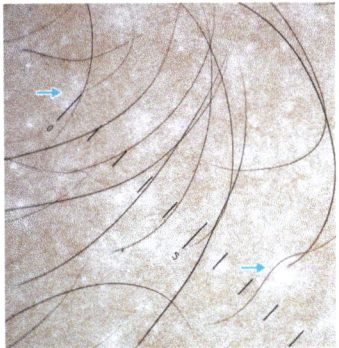

Fig. 4: Perifollicular depigmentation (arrows).

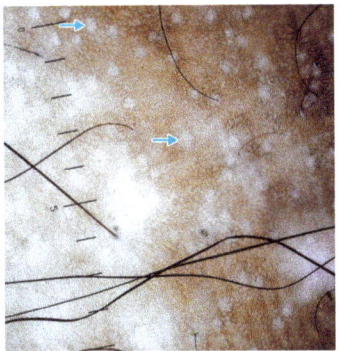

Fig. 5: Polka dots (confetti macules) in active lesions of vitiligo (arrows).

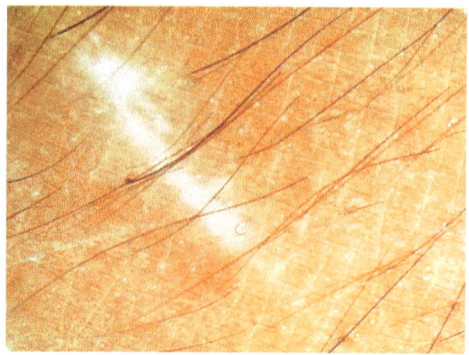

Fig. 6: Comet tail-like projection.

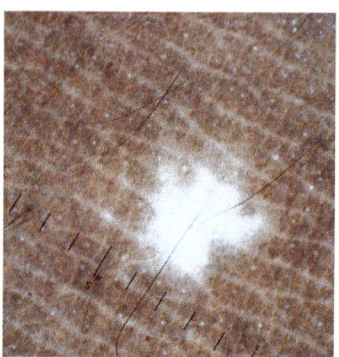

Fig. 7: Starburst appearance with absent pigmentary network in progressive vitiligo.

(Fig. 7), "tapioca sago" appearance, amoeboid (well-defined pattern with hyperpigmented margin and amoeba-like

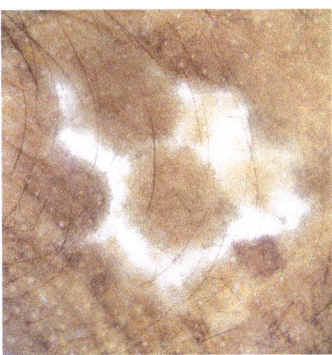

Fig. 8: Marginal reticular hyperpigmentation in a stable vitiligo.

pseudopods), and nebulous pattern (white pattern with indistinct margins merging into the surroundings) and salt and pepper pattern.[3-5] The presence of residual perifollicular pigmentation is commonly found in progressive vitiligo than stable vitiligo.[4,6] Dermoscopic features like lesional reticular pigmentation (well-defined pigment network within the depigmented macule) and marginal reticular pigmentation (Fig. 8), perifollicular hyperpigmentation (Fig. 9), erythema, and telangiectasia (Fig. 10) are suggestive of stable and repigmenting vitiligo.[3,4,7] The presence of telangiectasia, early reservoirs of pigmentation, and perilesional hyperpigmentation are related to the stage of vitiligo and treatment history of patients.[6]

Demonstration of clinically inapparent leukotrichia by a dermoscope in a segmental vitiligo can be an indicator of poor response to medical therapy and the patient can be counseled for surgical modality.[8]

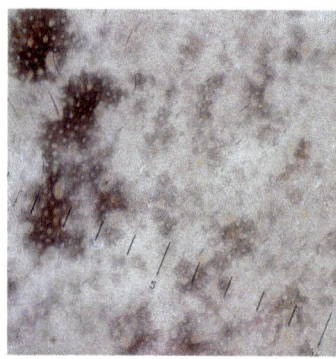

Fig. 9: Perifollicular hyperpigmentation in a case of stable repigmenting vitiligo.

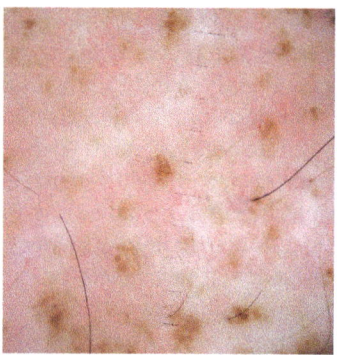

Fig. 10: Erythema and telangiectasia.

The dermoscopic features described for blue vitiligo are a central linear depigmented macule with multiple blue dots and reticular telangiectasia within the white patches. The blue color may be due to the melanin of dermal melanocytes.[9,10]

Dermoscope helps in better recognition of trichrome vitiligo of the nail unit, i.e. brown, light brown, and achromic areas; indicator of disease progression.[11]

Four dermoscopic patterns namely nebulous, feathery (feathery margins and irregular pigmentation associated with perifollicular pigmentation), amoeboid, petaloid (pigmentation well-defined pattern with irregular polycyclic margin) have been described in both guttate vitiligo and idiopathic guttate hypomelanoses, but presence of cloudy or cloudy sky-like pattern supports the diagnosis of the latter as reported by Errichetti and Stinco.[12,13]

REFERENCES

1. Thatte SS, Khopkar US. The utility of dermoscopy in the diagnosis of evolving lesions of vitiligo. Indian J Dermatol Venereol Leprol. 2014;80:505-8.
2. Sonthalia S, Sarkar R, Arora R. Novel dermoscopic findings of perifollicular depigmentation and evolving leukotrichia in areas of clinically unaltered pigmentation: An early predictive sign of impending vitiligo. Pigment Int. 2014;1:28-30.
3. Chandrashekhar L. Dermoscopy: A tool to assess stability in vitiligo. In: Khopkar U (Ed). Dermoscopy and trichoscopy in diseases of the brown skin: Atlas and Short Text. New Delhi, India: Jaypee Brothers Medical Publishers (Pvt) Ltd; 2012. pp. 112-3.
4. Jha AK, Sonthalia S, Lallas A. Dermoscopy as an evolving tool to assess vitiligo activity. J Am Acad Dermatol. 2018;78:1017-9.

5. Jha AK, Sonthalia S, Lallas A, et al. Dermoscopy in vitiligo: diagnosis and beyond. Int J Dermatol. 2018;57(1):50-4.
6. Meng RS, Guang Z, RuiKang C, et al. Application of polarized light dermoscopy in the early diagnosis of vitiligo and its differential diagnosis from other depigmented diseases. Chinese J Dermatol. 2009;42(12):810-3.
7. Chuh AA, Zawar V. Demonstration of residual perifollicular pigmentation in localized vitiligo—a reverse and novel application of digital epiluminescence dermoscopy. Comput Med Imaging Graph. 2004;28(4):213-7.
8. Lee DY, Kim CR, Park JH, et al. The incidence of leukotrichia in segmental vitiligo: implication of poor response to medical treatment. Int J Dermatol. 2011;50:925-7.
9. Chandrashekar L. Dermatoscopy of blue vitiligo. Clin Exp Dermatol. 2009;34:e125-6.
10. Zhang JA, Yu JB, Lv Y, et al. Blue vitiligo following intralesional injection of psoralen combined with ultraviolet B radiation therapy. Clin Exp Dermatol. 2015;40(3):301-4.
11. Di Chiacchio NG, Ferreira FR, de Alvarenga ML, et al. Nail trichrome vitiligo: case report and literature review. Br J Dermatol. 2013;168(3):668-9.
12. Bambroo M, Pande S, Khopkar US. Dermoscopy in the differentiation of idiopathic guttate hypomelanosis (IGH). In: Khopkar U (Ed). Dermoscopy and trichoscopy in diseases of the brown skin: Atlas and Short Text. New Delhi, India: Jaypee Brothers Medical Publishers (Pvt) Ltd; 2012. pp. 97-103.
13. Errichetti E, Stinco G. Dermoscopy of idiopathic guttate hypomelanosis. J Dermatol 2015;42(11):1118-9.

CHAPTER 14

Differential Diagnosis of Hypopigmented Lesions

Ankit H Bharti, Uday S Khopkar

INTRODUCTION

Appreciation of pigmentary changes plays an important role in the diagnosis of skin diseases in brown skin. Dermoscopy magnifies the subtle clinical surface features and unveils some helpful subsurface features to aid in diagnosis. The three-way options of polarized light, ultraviolet light, and white light multiply the utility of dermoscopy in hypopigmentary disorders.[1]

The disorders of hypopigmentation develop either due to damage to epidermal melanocytes, follicular melanocytes, reduction or absence of melanin synthesis or due to failure of melanin transfer to adjacent keratinocytes.[2] The disorders associated with hypopigmentation, with well-documented dermoscopic features such as vitiligo, idiopathic guttate hypomelanosis (IGH), postinflammatory hypopigmentation, chemical and pharmacologic hypomelanosis, hypopigmented mycosis fungoides, pityriasis lichenoides chronica, hypomelanosis from physical agents or bacterial infections (like leprosy) and parasitic infection (like leishmaniasis).

DISORDERS OF HYPOPIGMENTATION

Vitiligo

Dermoscopy can serve as an invaluable tool in assessing the status of vitiligo, its stability, and repigmentation, which can be difficult to discern only on clinical examination.[3] Some of the commonly observed signs associated with dermoscopy of vitiligo are given in Table 1.[4,5]

Hypopigmented macules of vitiligo can be distinguished from other hypopigmented macules as they get accentuated on UV exposure. The loss of epidermal melanin in vitiligo lesions produces a window through which UV light-induced autofluorescence of dermal collagen can be seen resulting in the bright blue–white glow.

Certain patterns, which are common to both vitiligo and IGH such as perifollicular pigmentation, presence of pigment network with central, peripheral, or global, and homogeneity of patterns.[5,6] The evolving vitiligo macule (Figs. 1A and B) displays multiple depigmented areas with loss of pigment network (Fig. 2). Confluence of such areas forms islands of depigmentation including perifollicular depigmentation along with unmasking of subtle leukotrichia, that is otherwise unrecognizable to the naked eye. Vitiligo macules lack microscaling

CHAPTER 14: Differential Diagnosis of Hypopigmented Lesions

Table 1: Dermoscopic patterns observed in vitiligo.

Dermoscopic signs in vitiligo	Explanation
"Polka-dot" or "salt and pepper" appearance	Perifollicular repigmentation
Comet-tail appearance	Sign of Koebner's phenomenon
Trichrome pattern	Darker perilesional and perifollicular repigmentation or hypopigmentation
Reduced pigmentary network	At the edge of evolving lesions of vitiligo due to gradual reduction in amount of pigment in the reticular network
Absent pigmentary network	Loss of the normal reticular pigment network
Reversed pigmentary network	Loss of pigmentary network leading to development of whitish areas
Nebulous (Starburst) pattern	White macule with rounded margins gradually merging with the periphery
Feathery pattern	Partially well-demarcated macules with irregular feathery margin
Petaloid pattern	Fairly well-defined macule with irregular polycyclic pigmented margin
Ameboid pattern	Well-defined pattern with hyperpigmented margin and ameba like pseudopod formation

which is usually observed in some cases of leprosy and post-inflammatory hypopigmentation.[7,8] Reversed pigmentary network is documented in dermoscopy of melanoma and melanocytic nevus, though it is also observed in vitiligo.[9-11] In

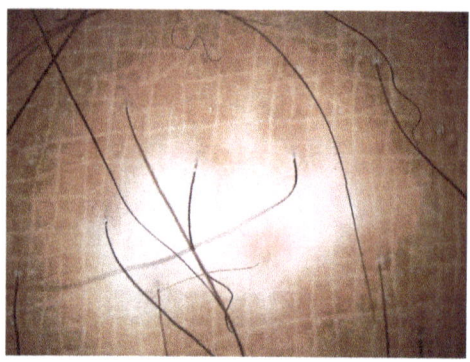

Fig. 1A: Evolving lesion of vitiligo displays loss of pigment network in an ill defined area showing "galaxy sign" with retention of pigment around the hair follicle.

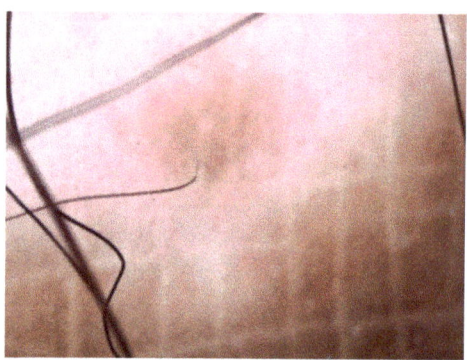

Fig. 1B: Higher magnification of the same lesion shows reversed pigmentary network within the lesion.

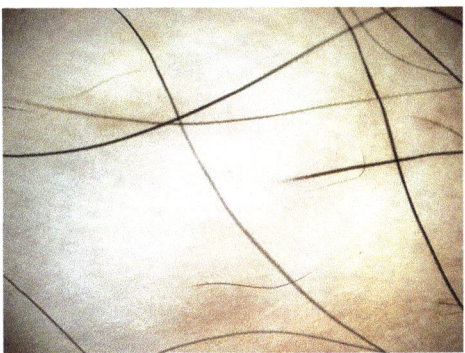

Fig. 2: Dermoscopy of an established lesion of vitiligo with loss of pigment network and patchy retention of pigment.

conclusion, dermoscopy scores over routine histopathology in the diagnosis of evolving lesions of vitiligo and can obviate the need for a skin biopsy in many doubtful cases.

Idiopathic Guttate Hypomelanosis

Four dermoscopic patterns seen in guttate vitiligo or evolving lesions of vitiligo have also been described by Bambroo et al. in IGH namely nebuloid, petaloid (Figs. 3A and B), feathery (Fig. 4), and ameboid.[5] The nebuloid pattern of IGH is observed usually in early lesions as well as among older patients. The feathery, ameboid, and petaloid patterns are more commonly seen in older lesions of IGH. Ankad et al. have described the histopathology features of IGH in a study and observed the whitish areas (yellow diamond) in the center of feathery

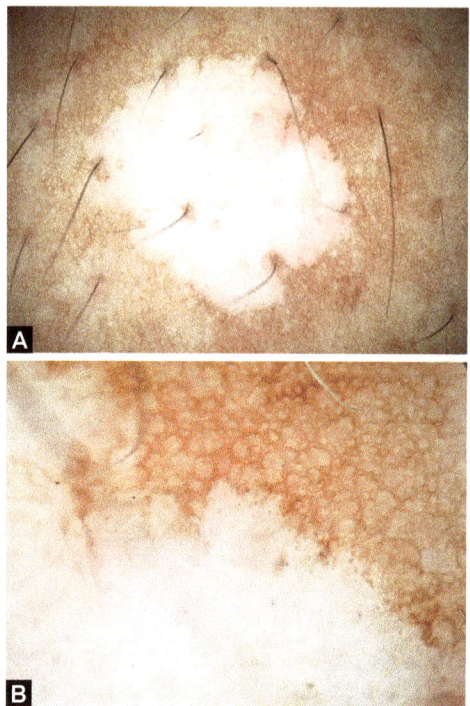

Figs. 3A and B: Petaloid pattern of idiopathic guttate hypomelanosis (IGH) with well-defined loss of pigment network and preserved perifollicular pigment which on high magnification (200×) reveals abrupt loss of pigment network with brown granules of pigment in the depigmented areas.

patterned lesions to correlate with epidermal hyperkeratosis which may denote long-standing disease.[12]

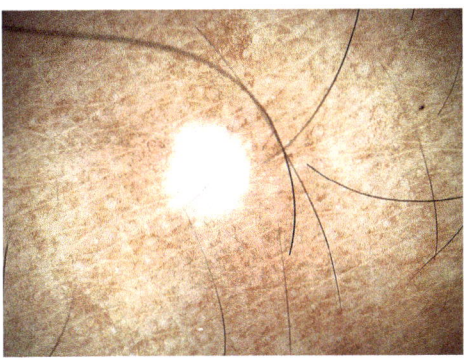

Fig. 4: Dermoscopy of idiopathic guttate hypomelanosis (IGH) shows a "starburst" pattern with circumscribed loss of pigment network with radiating pattern along the margins.

Lichen Sclerosus et Atrophicus (Fig. 5)

The major findings described by Garrido-Rios et al in extragenital lichen sclerosus atrophicus (LS) include white structureless areas (WSA) and comedo-like openings (CLO) are statistically significant in LS, whereas fibrotic bands are more common in morphea. Nevertheless, comma-shaped vessels, hairpin-like vessels, and dotted vessels were exclusively seen in LS. They correlated dermoscopic patterns with histopathology: WSA representing epidermal atrophy and CLO representing follicular plugging in histopathology.

Early lesions of LSA reveal predominant CLO and WSA, conversely these are less prominent in late lesions. This is probably due to reduced hyperkeratosis and destruction of

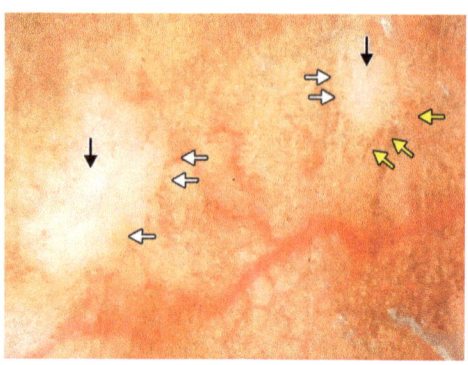

Fig. 5: Dermoscopy of a lesion of lichen sclerosus et atrophicus reveals areas with loss of pigment network, radiating white streaks (white arrows), microscaling and white structureless areas (black arrows) along with prominent linear and arborizing vessels. Brown globules indicating acrosyringeal plugging (yellow arrows).

follicles in the late stages. Another important finding of LS is white chrysalis-like areas (WCLA), which are described as shiny, bright white, parallel or orthogonal or disordered linear streaks, seen on polarized light dermoscopy. Telangiectasias of different lengths and calibers and WCLA have been reported in a histopathologically proven case of LS coexisting with lichen planus and morphea in addition to above mentioned dermoscopic patterns.[13,14]

Dermoscopy of a lesion of cutaneous lichen sclerosus et atrophicus reveals areas with loss of pigment network, radiating white streaks, microscaling and structureless areas

CHAPTER 14: Differential Diagnosis of Hypopigmented Lesions

along with prominent linear and arborizing vessels. Brown globules indicate acrosyringeal plugging.[15,16]

Hypopigmented Mycosis Fungoides

Mycosis fungoides (MF) is the most common primary cutaneous T-cell lymphoma. Dermoscopic evaluation of hypopigmented patch (Figs. 6 and 7) of MF displays—(1) dotted vessels; (2) fine short linear vessels; (3) spermatozoa-like structures; (4) orange–yellowish patchy areas; (5) white scales; and (6) yellow scales.[17]

The variable dermoscopic pattern of vessels observed includes variably sized dotted and linear vessels. A characteristic vascular pattern observed viz. dotted and short, curved linear

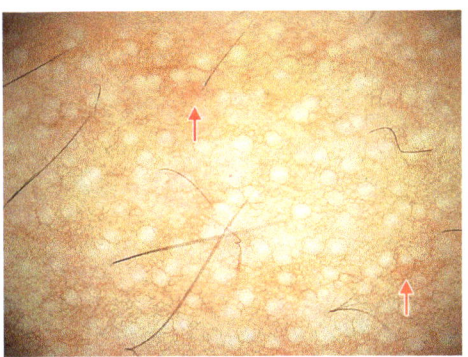

Fig. 6: Dermoscopy of evolving lesion hypopigmented mycosis fungoides reveals well-preserved pigment network with patchy areas of lighter colored pigment network with prominent white dots (acrosyringia) and reddish ill-defined blotches indicating deeper telangiectasia (red arrows).

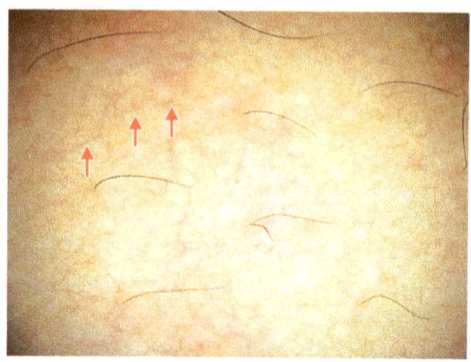

Fig. 7A: A fully evolved lesion of hypopigmented mycosis fungoides reveals areas of loss of pigment network with prominent telangiectasia (red arrows) and focally preserved pigment network.

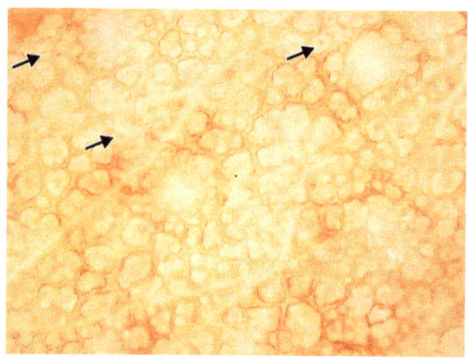

Fig. 7B: Higher magnification shows irregular loss of pigment network and dotted vessels (black arrows).

vessel is also a feature of MF. Another feature "orange-yellowish patchy areas" was described by Xu et al.[18]

Pityriasis Lichenoides

Pityriasis lichenoides is a lesser studied and described entity in dermoscopy. In a study, the findings described were white structureless areas arranged in a haphazard pattern with vague glomerular and dotted vessels in the periphery (Fig. 3), central white crust, and structureless rim with scaling, focal bluish-gray areas or centrifugal strands irregularly distributed along the periphery, and yellow structures and red dots and hemorrhage within the centrally crusted plug.[19] Dermoscopy (Figs. 8 and 9) of an active lesion, one can observe irregularly distributed patchy areas with loss of pigment network and microscaling with a prominent diffuse orangish erythema in background. On higher magnification, it reveals linear, curvilinear, and dotted vessels with diffuse erythema in the background and prominent microscaling with small islands of preserved pigment network.

Pityriasis Versicolor

Pityriasis versicolor white light image (Fig. 10) of pityriasis versicolor shows a sharply delineated lesion with microscaling. The same lesion on polarized light imaging (Figs. 11A and B) displays gradient of reduction of the pigment network toward the center of the lesion and perifollicular accentuation of the pigment loss. On dermoscopy of a hypopigmented macule following pityriasis versicolor displays gradual loss of pigment

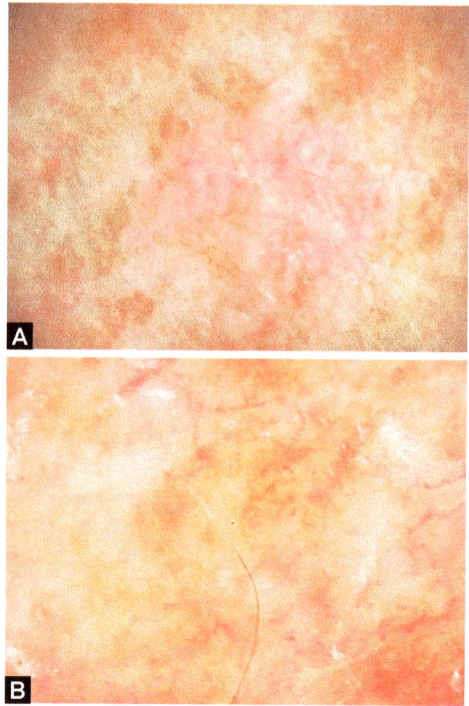

Figs. 8A and B: Dermoscopy of an active lesion of pityriasis lichenoides chronica (A) reveals patchy areas with loss of pigment network and microscaling and orangish red diffuse erythema in background; (B) On higher magnification, it reveals linear, curvilinear, and dotted vessels with diffuse erythema in the background and prominent microscaling with small islands of preserved pigment network.

CHAPTER 14: Differential Diagnosis of Hypopigmented Lesions

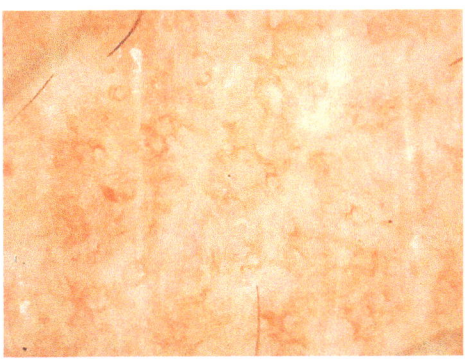

Fig. 9: Postinflammatory hypopigmentation following pityriasis lichenoides chronica (PLC) shows patchy loss and accentuation of pigment network including periappendageal pigment loss with microscaling and occasional dotted vessels and mild erythema in background indicating a healed lesion.

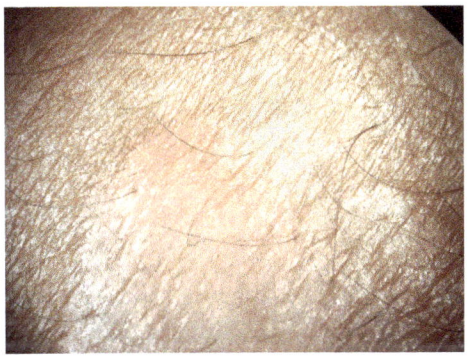

Fig. 10: White light image of pityriasis versicolor showing microscaling and sharp delineation of the lesion.

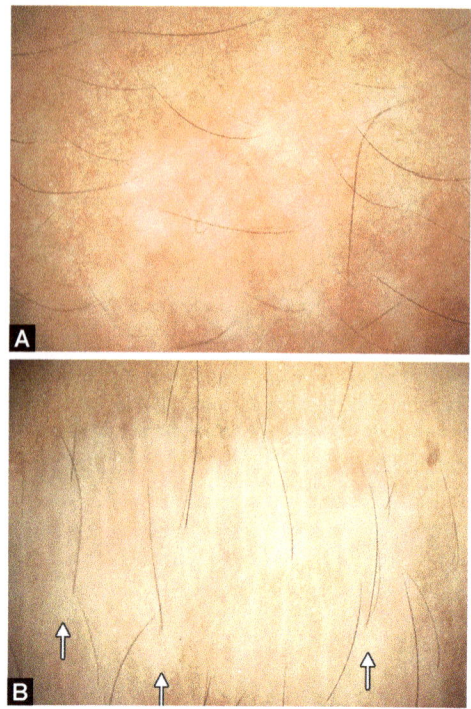

Figs. 11A and B: Polarized light image of the same lesion of pityriasis versicolor (A), post-inflammatory hypopigmentation following pityriasis versicolor (B) displays gradual reduction of the pigment network toward the center of the lesion and perifollicular accentuation of the pigment loss (white arrows).

network, which shows confluence in the central region with particular accentuation in perifollicular region (white arrow).[20,21]

Hansen's Disease: Hypopigmented Patches

Evolving lesions of vitiligo and leprosy usually present with hypopigmented macules and patches. Dermoscopy in such cases can aid clinical diagnosis. Polarized light dermoscopy of a hypopigmented patch of Hansen's disease shows partially obliterated pigment network without any white or depigmented islands nor is there any perifollicular hypo or hyperpigmentation. Additionally, reduced number of white dots that represent appendages and occasional linear telangiectasia are seen in a hypopigmented patch of leprosy (Fig. 12). For dermoscopic signs of vitiligo refer to the chapter 12.

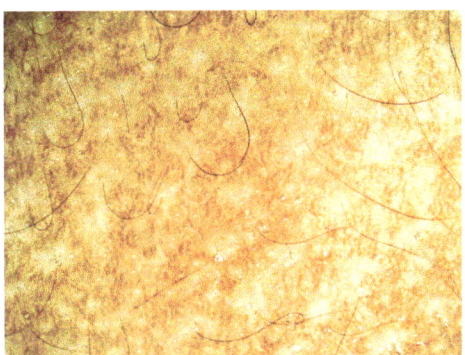

Fig. 12: Dermoscopy of a hypopigmented patch of leprosy displaying partially obliterated pigment network without any island of hypopigmentation or loss of pigment network.

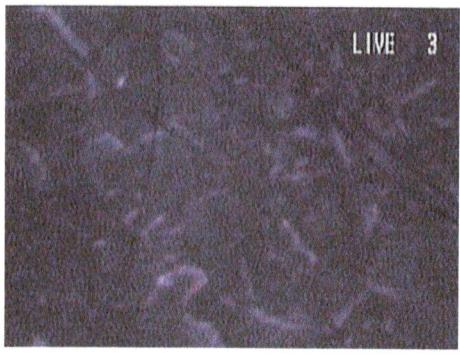

Fig. 13: UV light dermoscopy of a hypopigmented patch of Hansen's disease displaying absence of accentuation of hypopigmentation but easy visualization of scaling.

On UV light dermoscopy, the hypopigmented patches of leprosy do not show accentuation but microscaling due to anhidrosis becomes more apparent (Fig. 13). Hypopigmented patches of vitiligo show accentuation of patches with diffuse whitish glow and nebula-like appearance. Thus perifollicular pigmentation, UV accentuation, scaling, and leukotrichia can serve as important indicators to distinguish leprosy from vitiligo.

Leishmaniasis (Described in Chapter 24)

Cutaneous leishmaniasis (CL) is a parasitic infestation caused by various species of the genus *Leishmania*, which are transmitted by the arthropod vector sandfly. Some of the common dermoscopic features of hypopigmented patches of post kala azar dermal leishmaniasis include "yellow tears-like" structures and "white starburst-like" patterns.[22,23]

CHAPTER 14: Differential Diagnosis of Hypopigmented Lesions

Post-kala-azar dermal leishmaniasis (PKDL) is a complication of visceral leishmaniasis (VL); mainly found in Sudan, Bangladesh, and India.[24] Differentiating early lesions of PKDL from lepromatous leprosy is difficult and so dermoscopy can be instrumental in diagnosing PKDL.

The early/evolving lesions of cutaneous leishmaniasis show erosion, thrombotic vessel, yellow tears, white starburst-like pattern, hyperkeratosis, both erosion and hyperkeratosis together. In advanced lesions, the vascular structures were: linear irregular vessels, hairpin vessels, comma-shaped vessels, dotted vessels, arborizing telangiectasia, glomerular-like vessels but no corkscrew vessels.[25]

Postinflammatory Hypopigmentation (Fig. 14)

Postinflammatory hypopigmentations often present some dermoscopic findings, which are typical of the pre-existing

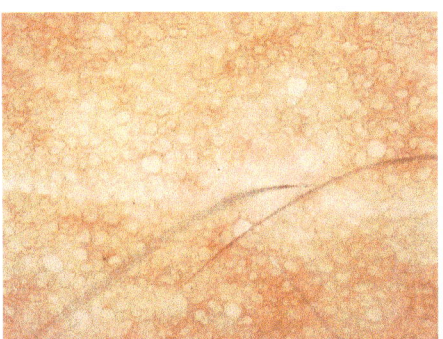

Fig. 14: Postinflammatory hypopigmentation on dermoscopy shows patchy loss of pigment network with patchy accentuation of pigment network as in top right corner with reduction in number of appendages.

original lesions, e.g. nondotted vessels or orangish structureless areas in pityriasis lichenoides,[26,27] dotted vessels in guttate psoriasis and star-like depigmentation in prurigo nodularis, thereby assisting the "retrospective" diagnosis.[28] Postinflammatory hypopigmentation on dermoscopy typically shows patchy loss of pigment network along with patchy accentuation of pigment network with variable reduction in number of appendages.

Nevus Depigmentosus

The hypopigmented macules of nevus depigmentosus on dermoscopy (Figs. 15A and B) display a pattern of sulcus cutis and crista cutis, which are usually continuous in a normally pigmented to a hypopigmented area. The main difference is

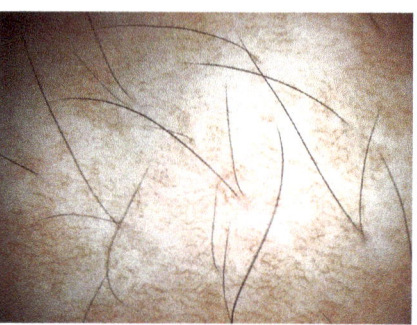

Fig. 15A: Dermoscopy of nevus depigmentosus displays patchy loss of pigment network leading to a pattern of parallel running sulci and cristae instead of the normal reticulate pigmentary network. This pattern merges with the surrounding reticulate network of the normal skin.

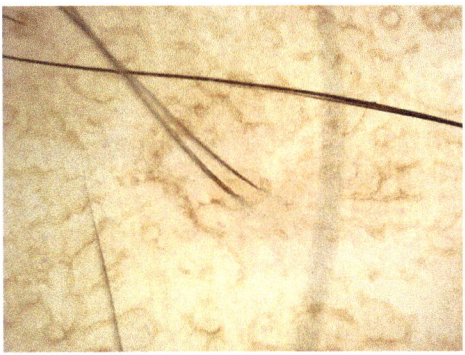

Fig. 15B: Nevus depigmentosus at higher magnification shows the sulci and cristae pattern of pigment network.

the intensity of the pigmentation along with a serrated and irregular border. Dermoscopy illustrated that the reticulate pigmented spots along with the border of the normal skin were in accordance with the serrated and irregular border of nevus depigmentosus.[29,30]

Dermoscopy is useful for evaluating the precise structure and distribution of pigmentation in pigment anomalies. Its frequent use in hypopigmented lesions can yield excellent results sometimes obviating the need for a biopsy.

REFERENCES

1. Nischal KC, Khopkar U. Focus dermoscope. Indian J Dermatol Venereol Leprol. 2005;71(4):300-4.
2. Bolognia JL, Jorizzo JL, Schaffer JV. Dermatology, 3rd edition. China: Elsevier Inc.; 2012.

3. Burns DA, Breathnach S, Cox N, et al. Rook's Textbook of Dermatology, 8th edition, Volume 1. London: Wiley-Blackwell; 2010.
4. Laxmisha C. Dermoscopy: A Tool to Assess Stability in Vitiligo. Dermoscopy and Trichoscopy in Diseases of the Brown Skin: Atlas and Short Text, Volume 27. New Delhi: Jaypee Brothers Medical Publishers (P) Ltd.; 2012. pp. 91-6.
5. Monica B, Pande S, Khopkar US. Dermoscopy in the Differentiation of Idiopathic Guttate Hypomelanosis (IGH) and Guttate Vitiligo. In: Khopkar US (Ed). Dermoscopy and Trichoscopy in Diseases of the Brown Skin: Atlas and Short Text, Volume 30. New Delhi: Jaypee Brothers Medical Publishers (P) Ltd.; 2012. pp. 97-103.
6. Marghoob AA, Malvehy, Braun RP. Atlas of Dermoscopy, 2nd edition. London, UK: Informa Healthcare; 2012.
7. Rameshwar G, Khopkar US. Dermoscopy: Differentiating Evolving Vitiligo from a Hypopigmented Patch of Leprosy. In: Khopkar US (Ed). Dermoscopy and Trichoscopy in Diseases of the Brown Skin: Atlas and Short Text, Volume 2. New Delhi: Jaypee Brothers Medical Publishers (P) Ltd.; 2012. pp. 104-13.
8. Thatte SS, Khopkar US. The utility of dermoscopy in the diagnosis of evolving lesions of vitiligo. Indian J Dermatol Venereol Leprol. 2014;80(6):505.
9. Atul D, Khopkar US. Genodermatoses. In: Khopkar US (Ed). Dermoscopy and Trichoscopy in Diseases of the Brown Skin: Atlas and Short Text, Volume 453. New Delhi: Jaypee Brothers Medical Publishers (P) Ltd.; 2012. pp. 257-63.
10. Balakrishnan N, Dongre AM, Khopkar US. Dermatoscopic features of hyper and hypopigmented Lesions of dowling-degos disease. Indian J Dematol. 2016;61(1):125.

11. Thatte SS, Dongre AM, Khopkar US. Reversed pigmentary network pattern in evolving lesions of vitiligo. Indian Dermatol Online J. 2015;6(3):222.
12. Ankad BS, Beergouder SL. Dermoscopic evaluation of idiopathic guttate hypomelanosis: A Preliminary Observation. Indian Dermatol Online J. 2015;6(3):164-7.
13. Garrido-Ríos AA, Álvarez-Garrido H, Sanz-Muñoz C, Aragoneses-Fraile H, Manchado-López P, Miranda-Romero A. Dermoscopy of extragenital lichen sclerosus. Arch Dermatol. 2009;145(12):1468.
14. Larre Borges A, Tiodorovic-Zivkovic D, Lallas A, Moscarella E, Gurgitano S, Capurro M, Apalla Z, Bruno J, Popovic D, Nicoletti S, Pérez J. Clinical, dermoscopic and histopathologic features of genital and extragenital lichen sclerosus. J Eur Acad Dermatol and Venereol. 2013;27(11):1433-9.
15. Lacarrubba F, Pellacani G, Verzì A, Pippione M, Micali G. Extragenital lichen sclerosus: clinical, dermoscopic, confocal microscopy and histologic correlations. J Am Acad Dermatol. 2015;72(1).
16. Shim WH, Jwa SW, Song M, Kim HS, Ko HC, Kim MB, Kim BS. Diagnostic usefulness of dermatoscopy in differentiating lichen sclerous et atrophicus from morphea. J Am Acad Dermatol. 2012;66(4):690-1.19.
17. Lallas A, Apalla Z, Lefaki I, et al. Dermoscopy of early stage mycosis fungoides. J Eur Acad Dermatol Venereol. 2013;27(5):617-21.
18. Xu P, Tan C. Dermoscopy of poikilodermatous mycosis fungoides (MF). J Am Acad Dermatol. 2016;74(3):e45-7.
19. Ankad BS, Beergouder SL. Pityriasis lichenoides et varioliformis acuta in skin of color: new observations by dermoscopy. Dermatol Pract Concept. 2017;7(1):27.
20. Zhou H, Tang X, De Han J, Chen MK. Dermoscopy as an ancillary tool for the diagnosis of pityriasis versicolor. J Am Acad Dermatol. 2015;73(6).

21. Bonifaz A, Gómez-Daza F, Paredes V, Ponce RM. Tinea versicolor, tinea nigra, white piedra, and black piedra. Clinics in dermatology. 2010;28(2):140-5.
22. Salman A, Yucelten AD, Seckin D, et al. Cutaneous leishmaniasis mimicking verrucous carcinoma: a case with an unusual clinical course. Indian J Dermatol Venereol Leprol. 2015;81(4):392.
23. Caltagirone F, Pistone G, Arico M, et al. Vascular patterns in cutaneous leishmaniasis: a videodermatoscopic study. Indian J Dermatol Venereol Leprol. 2015;81(4):394-8.
24. Zijlstra EE, Musa AM, Khali EA, et al. Post-kala-azar dermal leishmaniasis. Lancet Infect Dis. 2003;3(2):87-98.
25. Taheri AR, Pishgooei N, Maleki M, et al. Dermoscopic features of cutaneous leishmaniasis. Int J Dermatol. 2013;52(11):1361-6.
26. Errichetti E, Stinco G. The practical usefulness of dermoscopy in general dermatology. G Ital Dermatol Venereol. 2015;150(5):533-46.
27. Errichetti E, Lacarrubba F, Micali G, et al. Differentiation of pityriasis lichenoides chronica from guttate psoriasis by dermoscopy. Clin Exp Dermatol. 2015;40(7):804-6.
28. Meng R, Zhao G, Cai RK, et al. Application of polarized light dermoscopy in the early diagnosis of vitiligo and its differential diagnosis from other depigmented diseases. Chin J Dermatol. 2009;42:810-3.
29. Naoki OI, Kawada A. The diagnostic usefulness of dermoscopy for nevus depigmentosus. European Journal of Dermatology. 2011;21(4):639-40.
30. R, Zhao G, Cai RK, et al. Application of polarized light dermoscopy in the early diagnosis of vitiligo and its differential diagnosis from other depigmented diseases. Chin J Dermatol. 2009;42:810-3.

CHAPTER 15

Dermoscopy in the Differentiation of Idiopathic Guttate Hypomelanosis and Guttate Vitiligo

Monica Bambroo, Sushil Pande, Uday S Khopkar

INTRODUCTION

Use of dermoscopy for evaluation of inflammatory diseases of the skin has not been sufficiently explored. F Vazquez-Lopez et al. did pioneering work in assessing dermoscopic patterns in inflammatory conditions.[1-2] Not much work has been done previously for application of digital dermoscopy in hypopigmented lesions, which are of great relevance in Indian set-up. Chuh and Zawar reported "reverse" application of dermatoscopy in localized vitiligo.[3]

NEED FOR DERMOSCOPY

Disorders of pigmentation, both hypopigmentation and hyperpigmentation constitute a significant number of dermatology outpatients. Many of them look alike by clinical examination. Wood's lamp although used frequently has many limitations especially for evaluation of diseases of hypo- and hyperpigmentation in Indian skin. Diagnosing and differentiating common hypopigmented conditions like idiopathic guttate hypomelanosis (IGH) and guttate vitiligo in a routine dermatological practice could pose a diagnostic dilemma to the clinician. Although similar morphologically, their clinical course and response to treatment varies significantly. In India, this has immense psychosocial implications as vitiligo is associated with considerable social stigma. Differences in the histopathology of vitiligo and idiopathic guttate hypomelanosis are subtle and no single clinicopathological criterion separates the two. Hence, any additional criteria for differentiation that dermoscopy could offer would be helpful.

DERMOSCOPIC PATTERNS

On analyzing multiple dermoscopic images, each patient with lesions of guttate vitiligo and IGH, following four patterns were consistently identified. Classification of patterns was done based on the margin, pigment distribution, and digital appearance of the lesions.

1. Pattern I oval or round cloudy dense white pattern with indistinct margins merging into the surrounding skin. It was named as "nebular pattern" (also called galaxy sign) (Fig. 1).
2. Pattern II appeared slightly more defined with feathery margins and irregular pigmentation and was named as *"feathery pattern"* (Fig. 2).

CHAPTER 15: Dermoscopy in the Differentiation of Idiopathic Guttate...

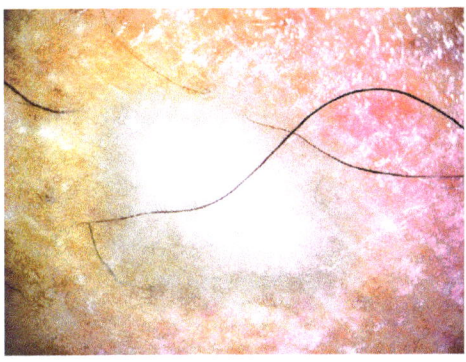

Fig. 1: Nebulous pattern: A dense white pattern within distinct margins merging into the surroundings. "Nebulous pattern", usually seen with unstable vitiligo (also called galaxy sign).

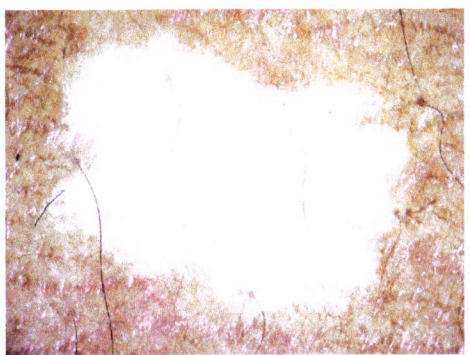

Fig. 2: Feathery pattern with perifollicular pigmentation: Slightly more defined with feathery margins and irregular pigmentation. Perifollicular pigmentation on dermoscopy is also seen (guttate vitiligo).

3. Pattern III was fairly well defined with irregular pigmented margin and was called as *"petaloid pattern"* (Fig. 3).
4. Pattern IV was a very well-defined pattern with hyperpigmented margin and pseudopod-like extensions that enclosed some of the unaffected or hyperpigmented margin and hence was called *"amoeboid pattern"* (Fig. 4).

Other expected dermoscopic features of vitiligo-like perifollicular pigmentation, Koebner's phenomenon, presence of pigment network, distribution of pigment network whether central, peripheral, or global and homogeneity of pattern were also noted.

In our experience, all the four dermatoscopic patterns are found in both IGH and vitiligo. Multiple patterns are seen in a single individual irrespective of diagnosis (Fig. 5). Nebular

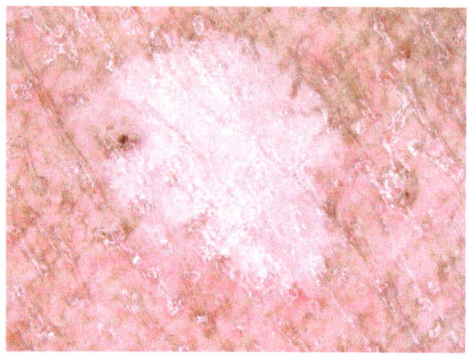

Fig. 3: Petaloid pattern: Fairly well defined with irregular polycyclic pigmented margin and was called as "petaloid pattern".

CHAPTER 15: Dermoscopy in the Differentiation of Idiopathic Guttate...

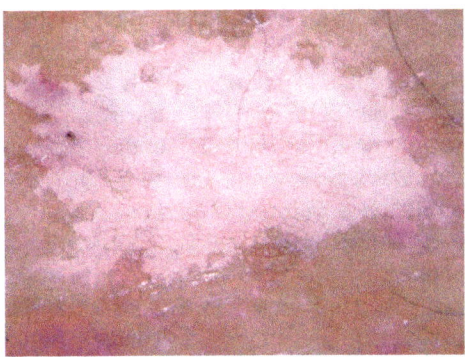

Fig. 4: Ameboid pattern: Well-defined pattern with hyperpigmented margin containing the lesion and amoeba-like pseudopod "amoeboid pattern".

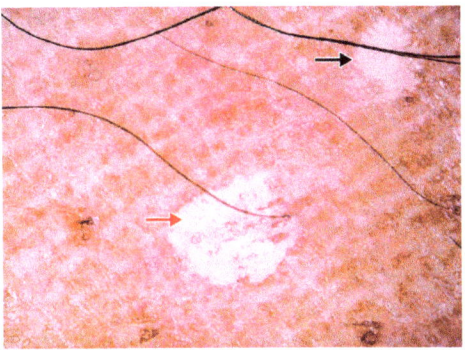

Fig. 5: Multiple patterns in a single individual "amoeboid" (black arrrow) and "petaloid" pattern (red arrow).

pattern was found usually in cases of guttate vitiligo and rarely in IGH while the reverse was true for amoeboid lesions.

Perifollicular pigmentation, which is considered a hallmark of the lesions of vitiligo[3] was surprisingly also noted in the dermatoscopic images of IGH although the intensity of pigmentation was less as compared with vitiligo (Figs. 2 and 6). The only difference being that perifollicular pigmentation in guttate vitiligo was better defined and deeply pigmented. While repigmentation is not demonstrated to occur in IGH, perifollicular pigmentation as a finding on dermoscopy needs to be validated in further studies and explained in pathogenesis of IGH.

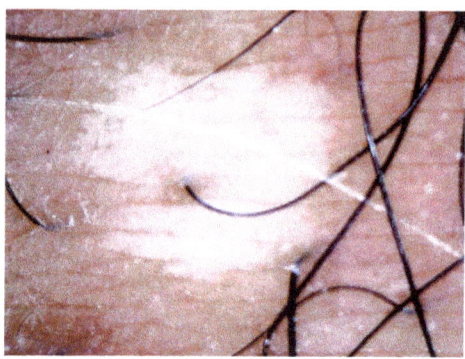

Fig. 6: Perifollicular pigmentation: Perifollicular pigmentation a hallmark of vitiligo can also be seen in idiopathic guttate hypomelanosis (IGH).

SYNTHESIS AND UNANSWERED QUESTIONS

Vitiligo and IGH seem to have overlapping dermoscopic patterns as well as clinical and light microscopy features probably indicating that they both represent similar endpoints of different pathogenetic processes. Dermoscopic patterns provide additional diagnostic criteria for differentiation of the two conditions in clinical practice. Detailed pathogenesis of IGH is yet to be elucidated and may hold clues for therapeutic intervention in vitiligo.

REFERENCES

1. Vázquez-López F, Manjón-Haces JA, Maldonado-Seral C, et al. Dermoscopic features of plaque psoriasis and lichen planus: new observations. Dermatology. 2003;207:151-6.
2. Vázquez-López F, Marghoob AA. Dermoscopy vs capillaroscopy of nontumoral dermatoses. Arch Dermatol. 2004;140:617.
3. Chuh AA, Zawar V. Demonstration of residual perifollicular pigmentation in localized vitiligo—a reverse and novel application of digital epiluminescence dermoscopy. Comput Med Imaging Graph. 2004;28:213-7.

Section 4: Papulosquamous Disorders

CHAPTER

16

Dermoscopy in Lichen Planus and Differential Diagnosis

Sunanda Mahajan

INTRODUCTION

Lichen planus (LP) shows specific and pathognomonic dermatoscopic features and is the first inflammatory skin disease for which dermoscopy was found to be of some value.[1] The surface of LP lesions shows clinically pathognomonic white lines or dots in a variable configuration called Wickham striae (WS), which can be easily recognized by the use of dermoscope. WS are highly sensitive and specific criteria for the diagnosis of LP.[2,3]

PURPOSE OF DERMOSCOPY IN LICHEN PLANUS

- Exploration with a handheld dermoscope allows easy and rapid recognition of WS and facilitates the diagnosis of LP.

WS can be used to monitor activity as they disappear after treatment.[4]
- Dermoscopy helps in monitoring the evolution of LP, its treatment outcome, and in determining the prognosis.[1,5]
- The characteristic WS helps in differentiating LP from other conditions and may avoid unnecessary biopsies.

Typically various evolutions of the lesions of LP can be seen in the same patient at various sites and the dermoscopic findings vary depending on the duration, size, and morphology of the lesions as well as type of LP, site of the lesion, any physical factors like rubbing/scratching, local applications of steroids, etc. The lesions of LP appear over a period of time and as the lesions age the dermoscopy features change.[4] Complete evolution and regression of LP could be followed with dermoscope on a noninvasive basis.[5]

The three main components—(1) WS, (2) vascular structures, and (3) pigmentation visualized in variations according to evolution of lesions.

Three main features seen in dermoscopy of LP lesions:
1. *Wickham striae:* WS can appear as pearly-whitish and rarely as yellow or blue–white opaque structures on the surface of the lesions in several patterns or configurations on dermoscopy namely (Figs. 1A to I):[1,4-7]
    - Arboriform or reticular WS
    - Linear WS
    - Round WS
    - Radial streaming—starburst pattern or spokes of a wheel pattern

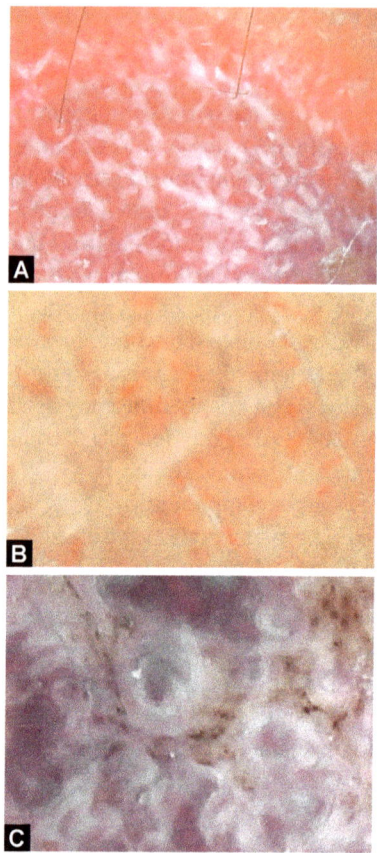

Figs. 1A to C: Patterns of Wickham striae (WS). (A) Arboriform or reticular WS; (B) Linear WS; (C) Round or circular WS.

CHAPTER 16: Dermoscopy in Lichen Planus and Differential Diagnosis

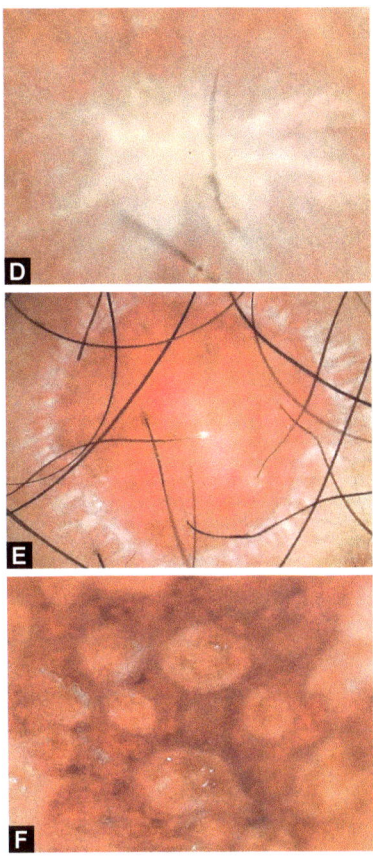

Figs. 1D to F: Patterns of Wickham striae (WS). (D) Radially arranged, starburst or spokes of wheal pattern; (E) Annular WS; (F) Globular WS.

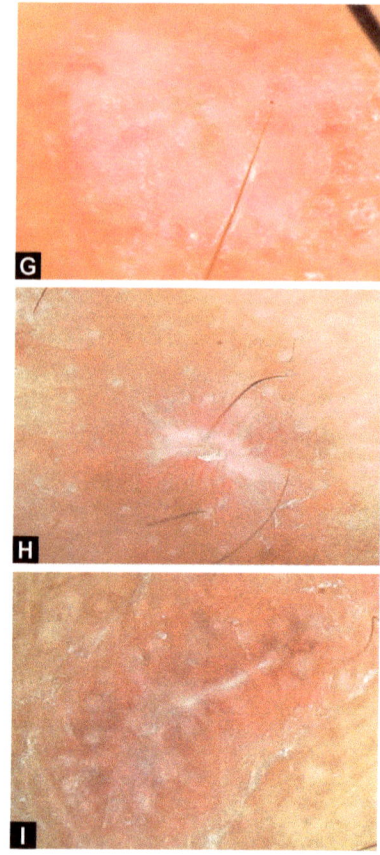

Figs. 1G to I: Patterns of Wickham striae (WS). (G) Veil like structureless WS; (H) Leaf venation with starry sky pattern; (I) Fern leaf like pattern.

- Annular WS
- Globular
- Veil-like structureless
- Leaf venation pattern
- Fern leaf pattern
- Starry sky pattern term used to describe: clustered, follicular white dots of WS.[6]

2. *Vascular structures* are relatively more prominent in early and mature lesions of LP and become inconspicuous in late lesions—appear as red lines and red globules.[5]
3. *Pigmentation* tends to increase gradually as the lesions mature and is maximum in the resolved lesions—brownish, and bluish, violaceous or blackish dots, globules or blotches.

DERMOSCOPIC EVALUATION OF LICHEN PLANUS[1,4,5]

Early papules: Pinhead sized skin coloured or violaceous papules on dermoscopy display whitish or violaceous veil-like structureless[4] or diffuse ill-defined WS, or show dense whitish opaque structures that are sometimes radially arranged, in starburst pattern or spokes of a wheel pattern with reddish linear structures intermingled within the whitish striae. Many of the lesions also demonstrate yellowish brown globules or blotches in the center of the lesions[5] (Figs. 2A to D) and ill-defined violaceous blotchy pigmentation in the background.

Some of the early papules on dermoscopy display elongated structures (Micro-Koebner's) with central linear white WS

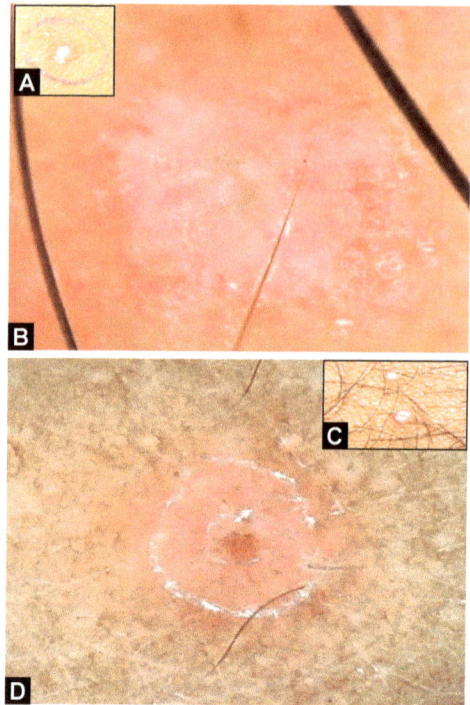

Figs. 2A to D: Early lesion of LP. (A) Pinhead size papule; (B) Whitish structure less WS with blotchy pigmentation in center and linear vessels at periphery; (C) Violaceous pinhead sized papule; (D) Central brownish pigmentation with radiating WS and a peripheral collarette of scale.

(Figs. 3 and 4) from which comb-like white structures project also described as leaf venation pattern or fern leaf pattern.[9]

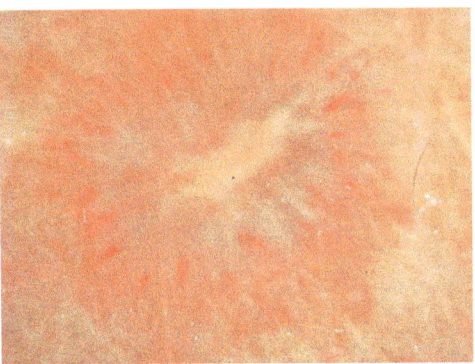

Fig. 3: Micro-Koebner's showing radially arranged, comb-like Wickham striae (WS) with linear vessels.

Mature Violaceous Papules and Plaques

Typical violaceous polygonal flat topped papules on dermoscopy display pearly whitish or yellowish WS in various patterns. WS border shows comb-like projections to broad arboriform ramifications (Figs. 5 to 7) departing from periphery to form a network (reticular or annular WS). Prominent vascular structures seen as linear vessels surrounding the WS border projections (radial capillaries) in radial horizontal oriented lines or red globules/dots.

Koebner's phenomenon which is clinically as coalescing papules in linear fashion on dermoscopy shows comb-like projections from center with linear vessels in between the WS (Fig. 8).

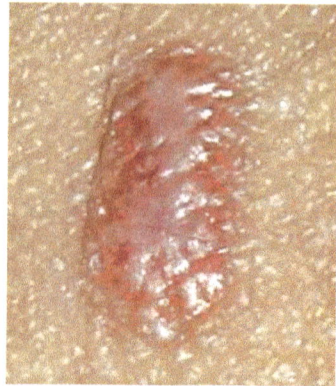

Fig. 4A: White light image of a classic lesion of lichen planus: Violaceous elongated papule.

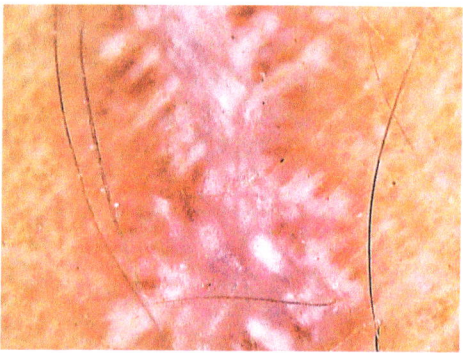

Fig. 4B: Polarized dermoscopy image of the same lesion as in Figure 4A: Linear Wickham's striae with radially arranged streaks.

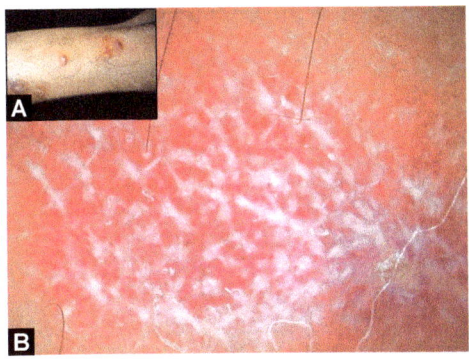

Figs. 5A and B: Mature lesion. (A) Violaceous flat topped papules; (B) Reticulate or arboriform WS with multiple irregularly arranged red globules.

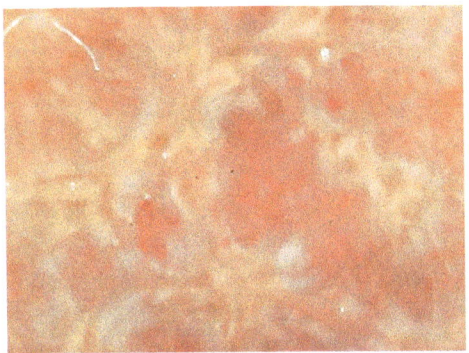

Fig. 6: Yellowish reticulate WS with only a few red globules.

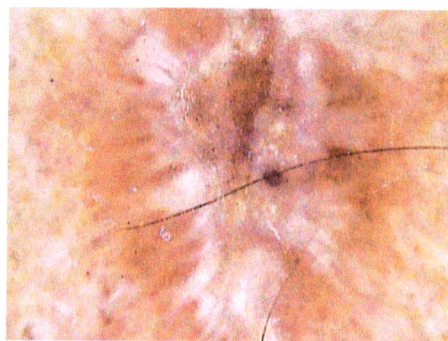

Fig. 7: Dermoscopic image of a classic lesion of lichen planus: Center with yellowish brown globules with surrounding reticulate dense WS showing radiating projections at periphery. Red lines and globules seen along edges. As lesion matures brown globules predominate over red globules.

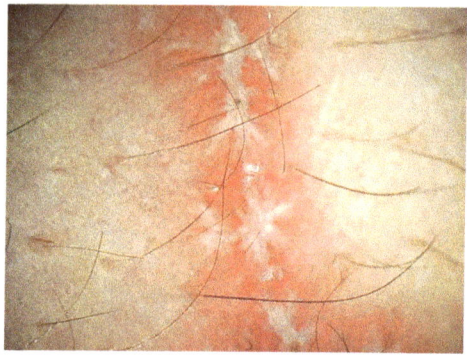

Fig. 8: Classical Koebner's phenomenon with comb-like projections of WS from center showing linear vessels in between the projections.

Longstanding Lesions

Chronic lesions of LP show WS that are more reticular or network like less dense and thin, fade in the center and appear more conspicuous at the periphery of the lesions with or without prominent peripheral vessels (Figs. 9A and B). Pigmentary

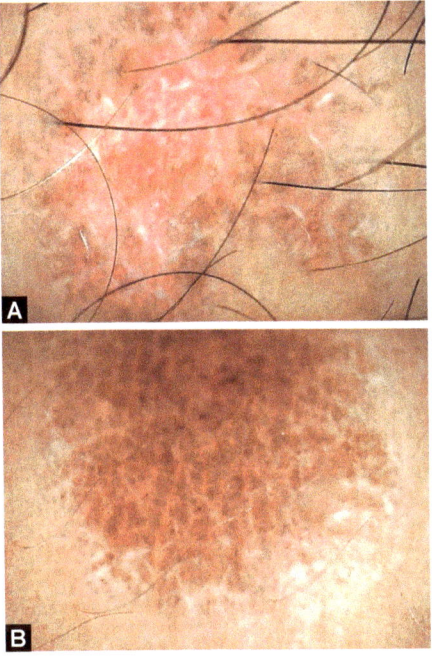

Figs. 9A and B: Long-standing lesion (A, B) Less prominent and less dense WS mainly at periphery with pigmentation.

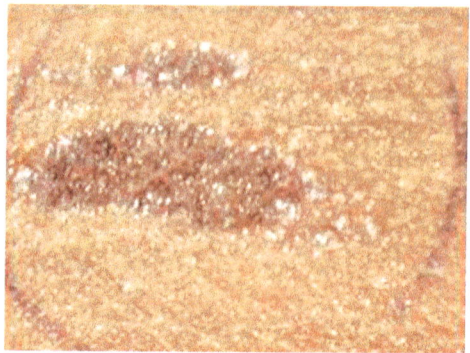

Fig. 10: Lichen planus lesion nearing resolution.

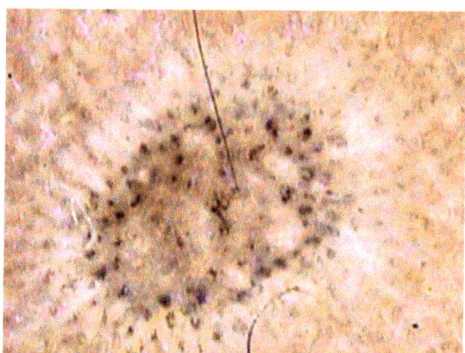

Fig. 11: Dermoscopic image of the lesion seen in Figure 10: Multiple brown and greyish blue globules and radially arranged WS at periphery.

CHAPTER 16: Dermoscopy in Lichen Planus and Differential Diagnosis 217

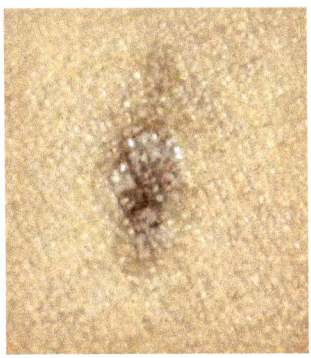

Fig. 12: Lichen planus lesion nearing resolution.

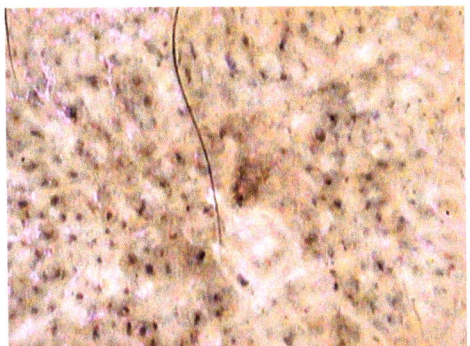

Fig. 13: Dermoscopic image of the lesion seen in Figure 12: Center with multiple brown and grayish blue globules, faint annular WS and radially arrange WS at periphery.

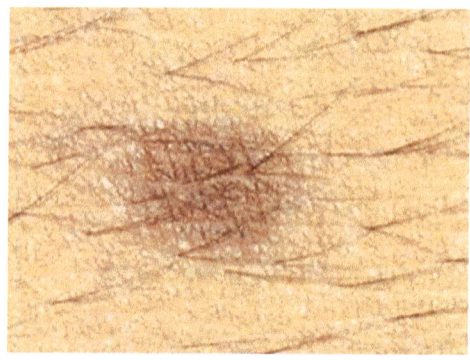

Fig. 14: Subsided lesion of lichen planus with postinflammatory hyperpigmentation.

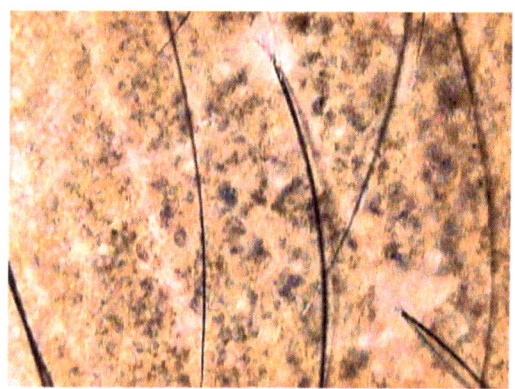

Fig. 15: Dermoscopic image of the lesion seen in Figure 14 shows dark brown dots and globules of pigment distributed irregularly within the lesion.

changes increase in the form of brownish or bluish gray granules, globules, and blotches mainly in the center of the lesions and around the WS. Also, few comedones or plugged follicles may be seen in the center of the lesion.

Resolving lesions (pigmented lesions of LP): Dermoscopy of resolving lesions of LP displays brownish or bluish–gray globules (Figs. 10 to 15) or blotches in the center of the lesion. The pattern of this pigment may be any of the following:
- *Diffuse*: Diffuse structureless brownish areas
- *Dotted*: Fine or coarse gray-blue or brown dots or globules arranged in various configurations
- *Mixed*: Diffuse brownish areas and dotted structures.

These findings help in determining the prognosis because those lesions with largest number of grey-blue-brown granules seem to be more persistent in comparison to lesions with brownish structureless areas.[10]

In addition, white dots (follicular openings surrounded by dermal melanophages) and yellow dots (correspond to hyperkeratosis and acanthosis histopathologically) have been described to occur in some chronic LP, regressing LP and lichen planopilaris.[4]

Annular Lichen Planus[4,5]

Central homogeneous pigmentation with peripheral WS (Figs. 16 and 17) and vascular structures can be visualized in the early lesions and later the vascular structures disappear.

Edge of the lesion shows ring-shaped WS with radially arranged projections from the ring and linear, tortuous red

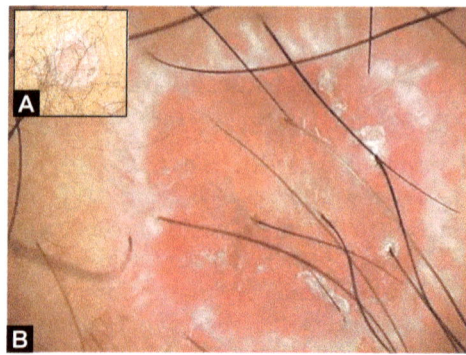

Figs. 16A and B: Annular LP. (A) Annular lesion of LP; (B) Ring shaped WS at periphery with comb-like projections, centre shows erythema and follicular plugs.

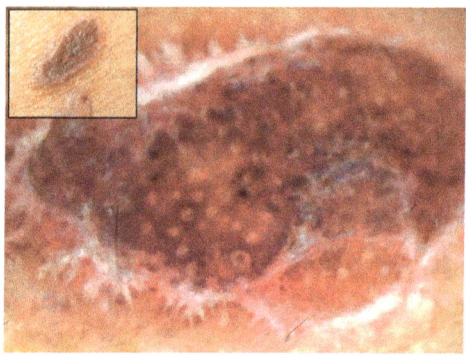

Fig. 17: Annular lesion. Ring shaped WS at periphery with bluish black and brownish globules and blotches in the center.

vessels in-between/parallel to the projections, whereas center shows erythema, perifollicular scale, brownish pigment, and ill-defined grayish black pigmented blotches.

Hypertrophic Lichen Planus

Keratin-filled craters or comedo-like structures filled with yellow plugs or round corneal structures (corn pearls) dot (Figs. 18 to 20) the surface of the lesions, which may also display, albeit to a smaller extent, Wickham striae (WS), vascular findings, and interspersed areas of brownish or bluish pigmentation.[1,5]

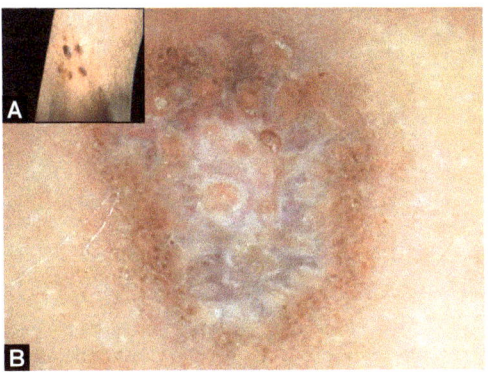

Figs. 18A and B: Hypertrophic LP. Keratin filled craters and comedo like structures with scanty WS and bluish and brownish pigmentation.

SECTION 4: Papulosquamous Disorders

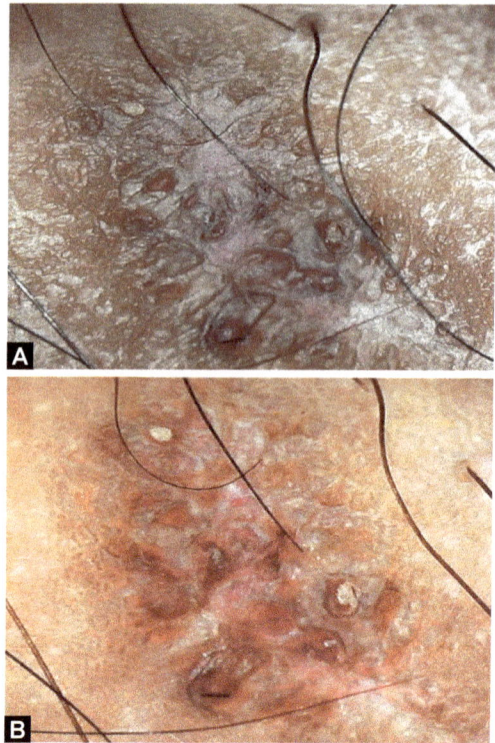

Figs. 19A and B: Hypertrophic LP. (A) Nonpolarized dermoscopy—shows craters and comedo-like openings very well; (B) Polarized dermoscopy shows the scanty WS and pigmentation.

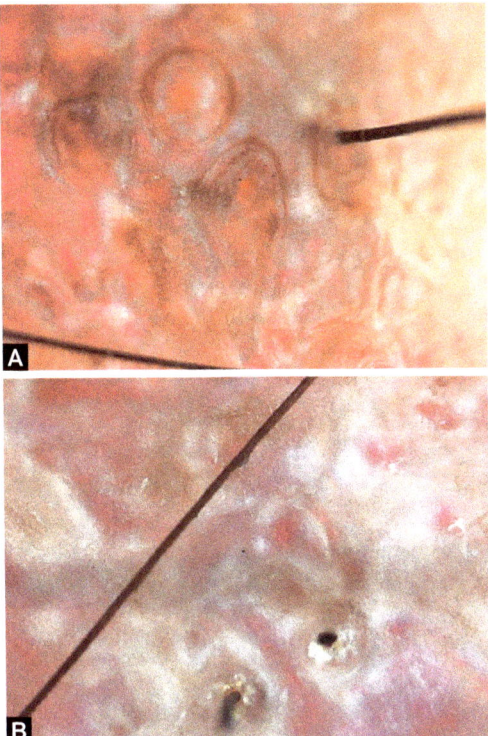

Figs. 20A and B: Hypertrophic LP. (A) Close up of the crateriform areas with blotchy pigmentation; (B) Corn pearls with few red globules and WS.

Follicular Lichen Planus/Lichen Planopilaris[4,9]

Early lesion shows whitish ill-defined grayish white veil-like structureless WS or whitish globular WS against erythematous background[4] and perifollicular yellowish areas and scaling (Figs. 21A to C).

Older lesions (Figs. 22A and B) show irregular whitish dots with fine coarse gray–blue or brown dots and globules in different shapes, with ill-defined grayish blue blotches mainly distributed around the hair follicle openings, absent follicles may appear as structureless white areas.

Palmoplantar Lesions

These are clinically seen as keratotic plaques and punctate keratoses (Fig. 23A).

Dermoscopy of keratotic papules shows (Figs. 23B, C, E) ill-defined or roundish, yellowish, or brownish areas some with peripheral projections[11] that may create a star-like appearance sometimes with a purplish background. Some lesions show irregular craters with scales in polycyclic pattern or a lacy reticular pattern (Fig. 23D).[12]

Mucosal Lichen Planus—Lips

Clinically LP lesions on lip are commonly seen as whitish or hyperpigmented papules, plaques or annular lesions with lacy pattern on surface. On dermoscopy the WS show linear parallel arrangement with linear or tortuous vessels (Figs. 24A to C) in-between the WS or reticulate WS with pigment globules and reddish globules in-between the network of WS.

CHAPTER 16: Dermoscopy in Lichen Planus and Differential Diagnosis

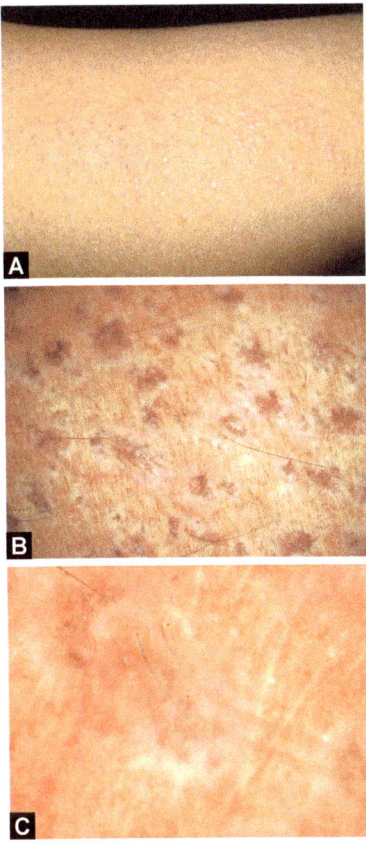

Figs. 21A to C: Follicular LP. (A) Grouped follicular papules over forearm; (B and C) Dermoscopy-structureless veil like WS with perifollicular grayish pigmentation.

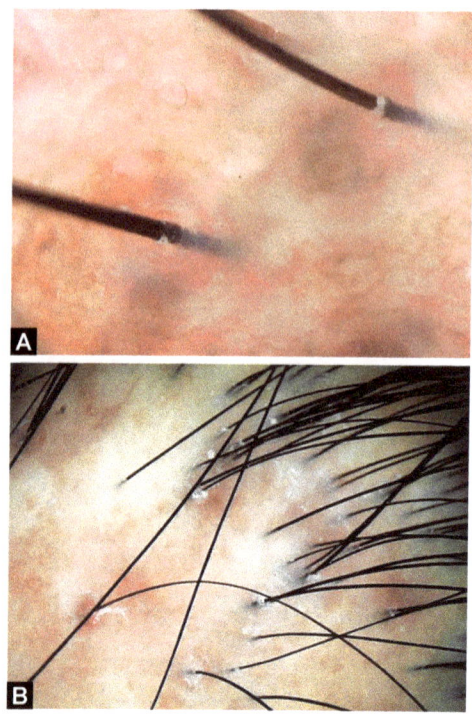

Figs. 22A and B: Lichen planopilaris scalp. (A) Perifollicular scale with bluish gray pigmented globules around the follicle and erythema; (B) Absent follicles seen as structureless white areas, perifollicular scale and pigmentation.

Dermoscopy of early lesions shows WS and vascular component predominantly, mature lesions (Fig. 24D) in

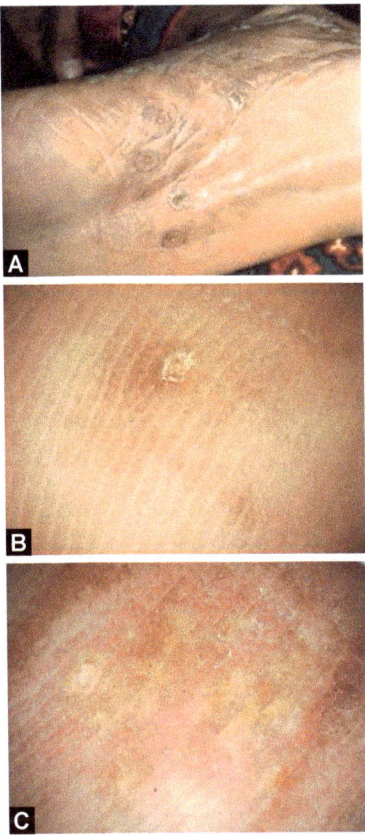

Figs. 23A to C: (A) Plantar lesions; (B) Puncted keratoses with surrounding brownish pigmentation; (C) Ill-defined yellowish white blotches with brownish pigmentation.

228 SECTION 4: Papulosquamous Disorders

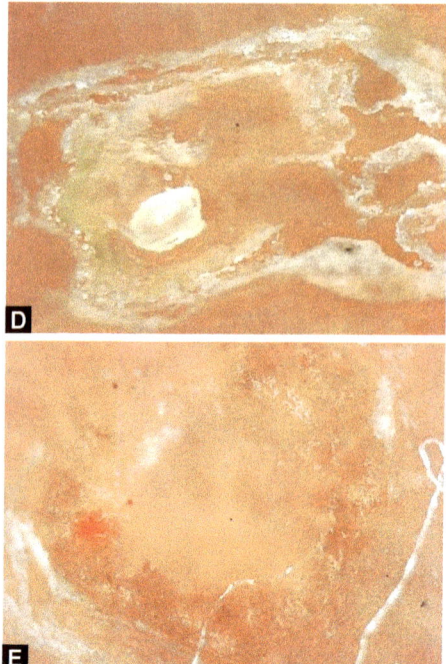

Figs. 23D and E: (D) Crater filled with keratin in concentric layers; (E) Higher magnification of keratotic lesion showing yellowish white areas surrounded by scaling and pigmentation.

addition display pigmentation in the form of brown or bluish black globules and dots preominantly along the margins of the WS, and bluish blotches in the background of the WS.

CHAPTER 16: Dermoscopy in Lichen Planus and Differential Diagnosis

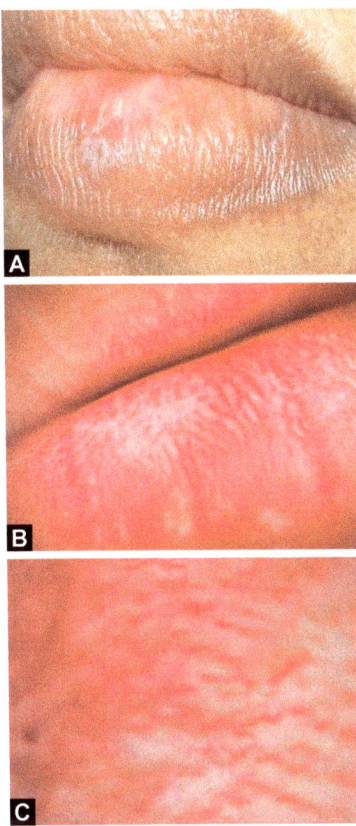

Figs. 24A to C: (A) LP affecting lip mucosa; (B) Dermoscoy showing reticulate and linear parallel WS with red lines and globules; (C) Higher power shows parallel linear WS with linear vessels in between the WS.

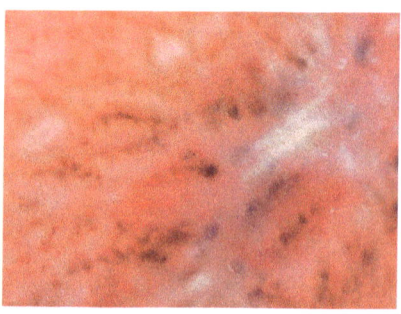

Fig. 24D: Late lesion shows few reticulate WS with multiple bluish black globules.

HISTOPATHOLOGICAL CORRELATION (TABLE 1)

Vascular Structures[5]

- Red globules (RG—rounded, dilated, red structures) are the tortuous capillaries within the thin, elongated dermal papillae and are related with epidermal hyperplasia and elongated papillae.
- *Red dots*: Rounded punctate, red structures represent normal papillary vessels.
- *Red lines*: Linear red structures represent the deeper ectatic horizontal subpapillary capillaries.
- Linear vessels in LP have also been termed as radial capillaries.

Nonvascular Structures[5]

- *Wickham striae*—appear as pearly-whitish structures in polymorphic configurations correspond histologically

CHAPTER 16: Dermoscopy in Lichen Planus and Differential Diagnosis

Table 1: Dermoscopy features with histopathological correlation.

Dermoscopy feature	Histopathological correlation
Wickham striae: Pearly-whitish structures in polymorphic configurations	Compact orthokeratosis above the zones of wedge-shaped hypergranulosis
Central yellow-brown areas	Vacuolar alterations of basal keratinocytes and spongiosis in the spinous zone
The comedo-like openings	Hyperplastic, dilated, hypergranulotic infundibula with orthokeratosis
Corn pearls	Transepidermal elimination
Red globules: Rounded, dilated, red structures	Tortuous capillaries within the thin, elongated dermal papillae (epidermal hyperplasia)
Red dots—rounded punctate, red structures	Normal papillary vessels
Red lines—linear red structures	Deeper ectatic horizontal subpapillary capillaries
A brownish diffuse pigmentation pattern	Pigmentation within the epidermis
The gray-blue dots	Pigment in dermal melanophages
Blue-white veils	A reflection of deep-seated melanophages or veins in the dermis[6]

  to compact orthokeratosis above the zones of wedge-shaped hypergranulosis, centered around acrosyringia and acrotrichia.
- Central yellow–brown areas seem to be related to vacuolar alterations of basal keratinocytes and to spongiosis in the spinous zone.

- The gray–blue dots or brown punctate areas represent melanophages in dermis, and
- The comedo-like openings may be related with the hyperplastic, dilated, hypergranulotic infundibula with orthokeratosis.
- Corn pearls seen as rounded, solid, corned structures over some comedo-like openings of hypertrophic LP suggested transepidermal elimination.

DIFFERENTIAL DIAGNOSIS

Chronic Plaque Psoriasis[5,8]

Early erythematous scaly papule shows homogeneously distributed reddish globules on a red background and absence of WS (Figs. 25A and B). The globules on higher magnification show tortuous, coiled capillaries. Long-standing hyperpigmented plaques display diffuse hyperpigmentation with brown globules, whitish globules and scaling (Figs. 26 and 27).

Lupus Erythematosus

Erythematous papules and plaques display irregular whitish streaks with multiple red globules. Some lesions showed brown granular pigmentation with red spots and globules in the center (Figs. 28 to 31). Chronic lesions show pigmentation in the form of brownish granules or globules.

Lichenoid Drug Eruption

Displays purplish white streaks and globules with multiple brown and red dots mainly in the center of the lesion (Figs. 32A and B). The characteristic WS patterns are absent.

CHAPTER 16: Dermoscopy in Lichen Planus and Differential Diagnosis

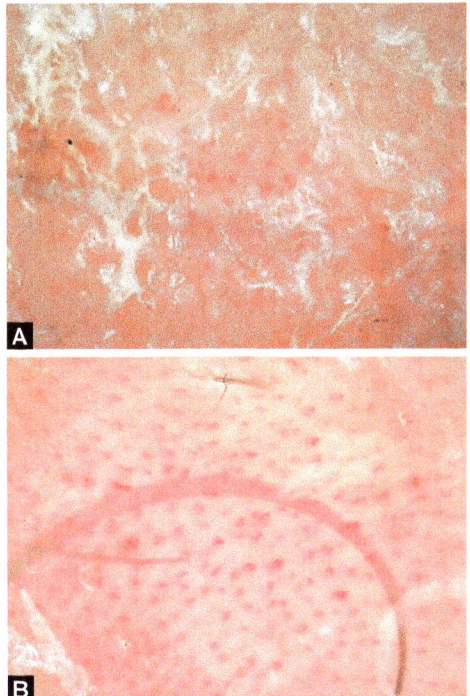

Figs. 25A and B: Psoriasis: (A) Regularly distributed red globules with white scales; (B) Close up showing the red globules.

Pityriasis Rosea[2,8]

Active lesion shows characteristic peripheral collarette of scale (hanging curtain sign) and reddish globules or puncta, which

234 **SECTION 4:** Papulosquamous Disorders

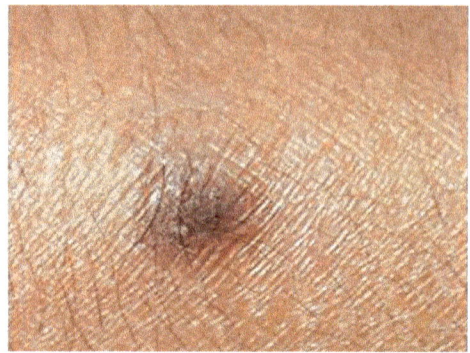

Fig. 26: Clinical image of a chronic plaque of psoriasis.

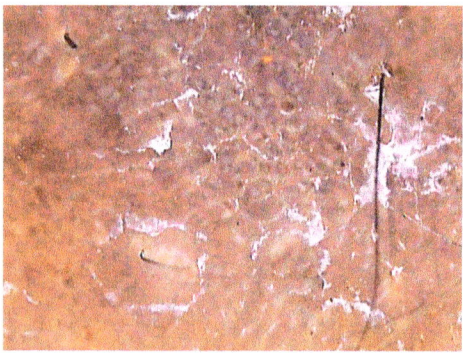

Fig. 27: Dermoscopic image of the lesion in Figure 26: Reticulate brownish and bluish pigmentation with white globules and scaling.

CHAPTER 16: Dermoscopy in Lichen Planus and Differential Diagnosis

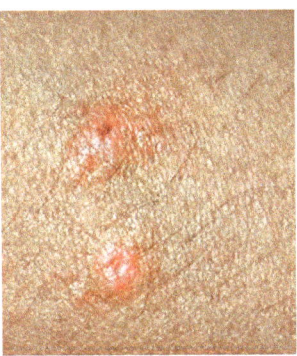

Fig. 28: Early lesion of lupus erythematosus.

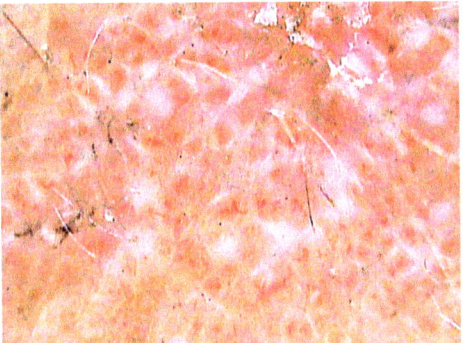

Fig. 29: Dermoscopic image of the lesion in Figure 28: Multiple red globules in center with reticulate whitish network resembling Wickham's striae.

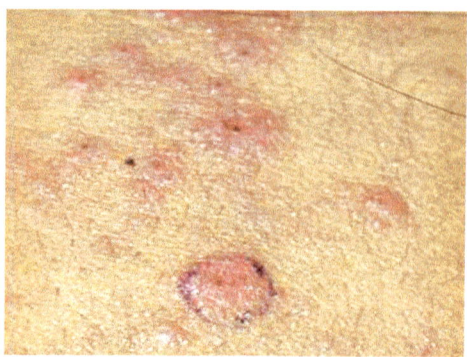

Fig. 30: Lupus erytheamatosus: Clinically presenting with erythematous papule.

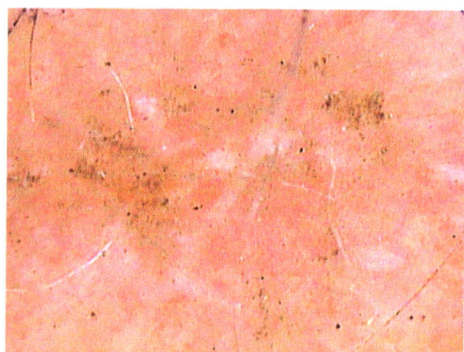

Fig. 31: Dermoscopy of Lesion in Figure 30: Multiple brown dots and globules interspersed with irregular whitish streaks on background of erythema.

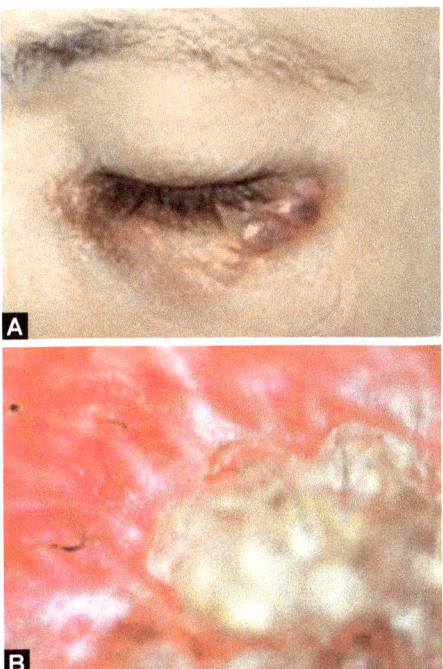

Figs. 32A and B: (A) Lichenoid drug eruption: clinical picture of papules; (B) Thick adherent scale, irregular purplish white streaks and red globules, lines and blotches.

are irregularly or focally distributed (Figs. 33A and B). Whereas, older lesions show granular or globular yellowish brown pigmentation in the center (Figs. 34A and B). The classical WS are absent.

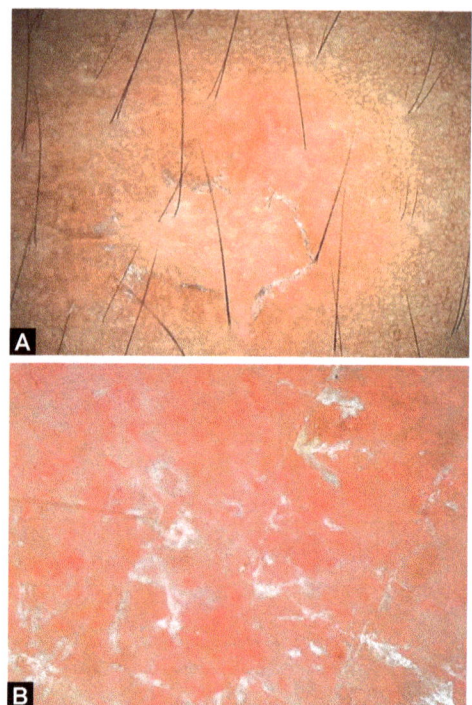

Figs. 33A and B: Pityriasis rosea: (A) Collarette scale with erythema and brownish pigmentation; (B) Higher magnification showing irregularly distributed red dotted vessels.

Lichen simplex chronicus or chronic eczema displays (Figs. 35A to C) patchily distributed dotted vessels within the lesion with brown crusts and brown globules.[2,13]

CHAPTER 16: Dermoscopy in Lichen Planus and Differential Diagnosis

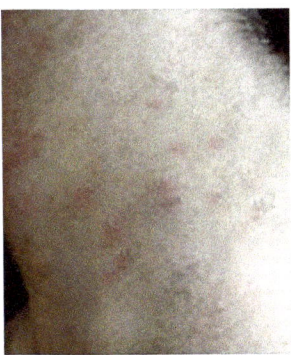

Fig. 34A: Clinical photograph of pityriasis rosea.

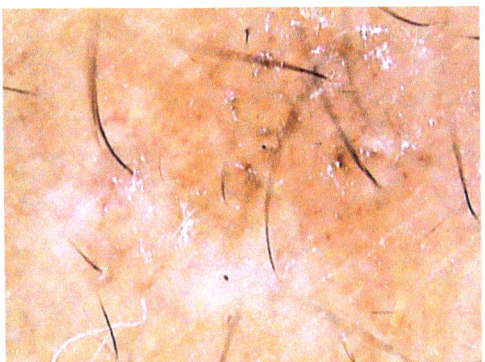

Fig. 34B: Dermoscopic image of the lesion shown in Figure 34A: Central brown dots and globules with background erythema and peripheral microscales.

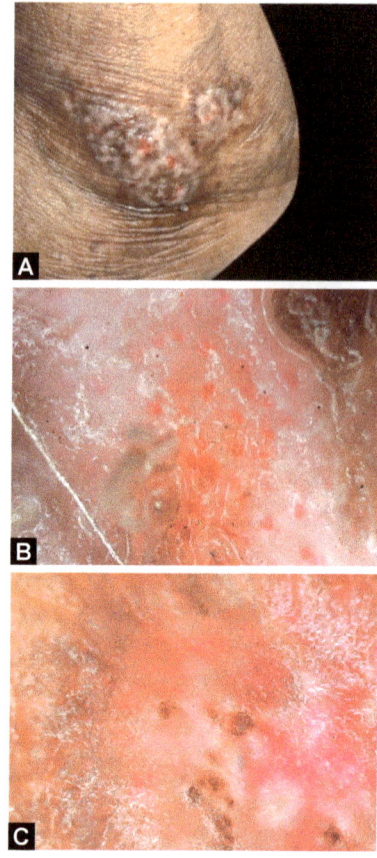

Figs. 35A to C: Lichen simplex chronicus. (A) Clinical photo; (B) Irregularly distributed red globules; (C) Irregularly distributed red and white blotches with scattered red globules and brown crusts.

Prurigo Nodularis

Clinically seen as pruritic hyperpigmented nodules on dermoscopy show central yellowish brown (Figs. 36A and B) or reddish brown crust, erosion, and/or scales with radially

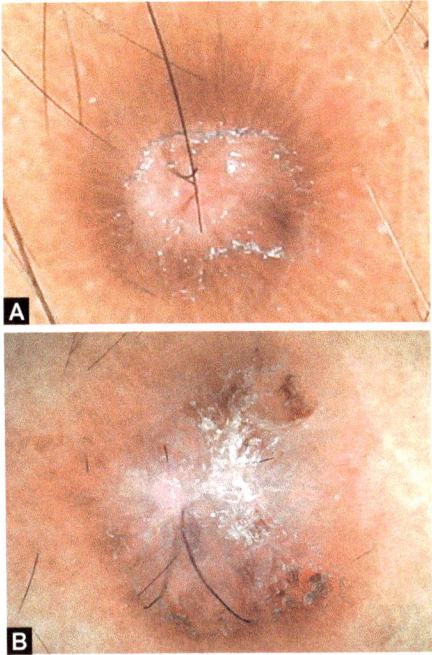

Figs. 36A and B: Prurigo nodularis: (A) Radially arranged white lines giving white starburst pattern on a brownish background; (B) Reddish brown crusts with radially arranged white lines and surrounding brownish pigmentation.

arranged whitish lines forming "white starburst pattern" on a brownish and/or reddish background.[11]

Plane Warts

Plane warts clinically appear as flat skin colored papules with Koebner's phenomenon (Fig. 37A). Dermoscopy of the papules

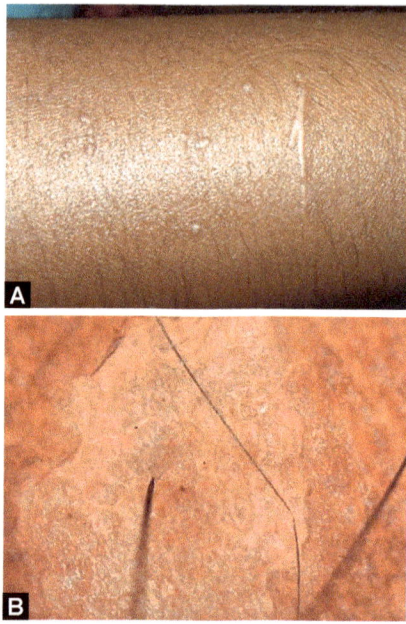

Figs. 37A and B: Verruca plana. (A) Clinical photo showing skin colored papules and Koebner's phenomenon; (B) Dermoscopy of papule showing regularly distributed red dots surrounded by whitish reticular pseudonetwork.

CHAPTER 16: Dermoscopy in Lichen Planus and Differential Diagnosis 243

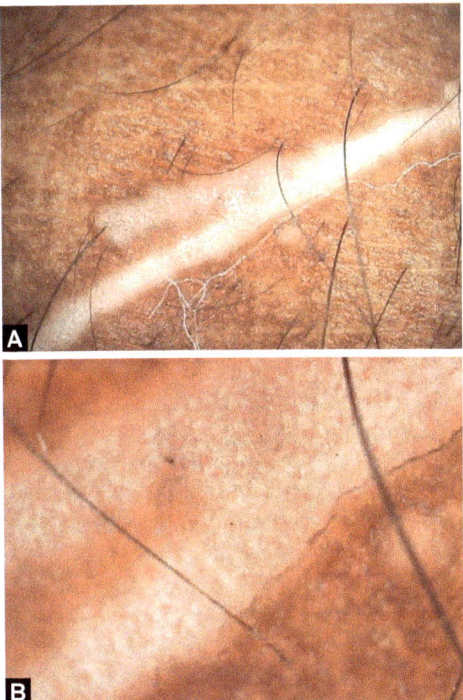

Figs. 38A and B: Dermoscopy of Koebner's phenomenon in verruca plana-multiple regularly distributed red dots, absent WS.

show multiple small, regularly distributed red dots on a whitish background, which correspond to small vessels in the papillary dermis and orthohyperkeratosis (Figs. 37B and 38).[14,15]

CONCLUSION

Dermoscopy is a simple, economical, noninvasive tool to diagnose LP enhancing the demonstration of WS. Further, the evolution of the disease can be monitored and different patterns of postinflammatory pigmentation can be noted with their prognostic implications. Dermoscopy has a potential diagnostic value especially in dark-skinned individuals to differentiate it from other lichenoid dermatoses. However, more experience with the technique is needed before it can be used reliably for this purpose. Hence, it must be combined with history, naked eye examination, and in appropriate cases histology, rather than being used in isolation.

REFERENCES

1. Vázquez-López F, Pineda FV. Lichen planus. In: Micali G, Lacarrubba F (Eds). Dermatoscopy in Clinical Practice: Beyond Pigmented Lesions, 2nd edition. Boca Raton, FL: CRC Press; 2016.
2. Lallas A, Kyrgidis A, Tzellos TG, et al. Accuracy of dermoscopic criteria for the diagnosis of psoriasis, dermatitis, lichen planus and pityriasis rosea. Br J Dermatol. 2012;166(6):1198-205.
3. Zalaudek I, Argenziano G. Dermoscopy subpatterns of inflammatory skin disorders. Arch Dermatol. 2006;142(6):808.
4. Güngör Ş, Topal IO, Göncü EK. Dermoscopic patterns in active and regressive lichen planus and lichen planus variants: a morphological study. Dermatol Pract Concept. 2015;5(2):45-53.
5. Vázquez-López F, Manjón-Haces JA, Maldonado-Seral C, et al. Dermoscopic Features of Plaque Psoriasis and Lichen Planus: New Observations. Dermatology. 2003;207(2):151-6.

6. Tan C, Min ZS, Xue Y, et al. Spectrum of dermoscopic patterns in lichen planus: A case series from China. J Cutan Med Surg. 2014;18(1):28-32.
7. Lallas A, Kyrgidis A, Tzellos TZ, et al. Accuracy of dermoscopic criteria for the diagnosis of psoriasis, dermatitis, lichen planus and pityriasis rosea. Br Assoc Dermatol. 2012;166:1198-205.
8. Papakonstantinou E, Raap U. Alternative uses of dermoscopy in general dermatology. J Surg Dermatol. 2017;2(2):67-74.
9. Friedman P, Cohen Sabban E, Marcucci C, et al. Dermoscopic findings in different clinical variants of lichen planus. Is dermoscopy useful? Dermatol Pract Concept. 2015;5(4):13.
10. Vázquez-López F, Maldonado-Seral C, López-Escobar M, et al. Dermoscopy of pigmented lichen planus lesions. Clin Exp Dermatol. 2003;28(5):554-5.
11. Errichetti E, Stinco G. The practical usefulness of dermoscopy in general dermatology. G Ital Dermatol Venereol. 2015;150(5):533-46.
12. Madke B, Gutte R, Doshi B, et al. Hyperkeratotic palmoplantar lichen planus in a child. Indian J Dermatol. 2013;58:405.
13. Navarini AA, Feldmeyer L, Tőndury B, et al. The yellow clod sign. Arch Dermatol. 2011;147(11):1350.
14. Vázquez-López F, Kreusch J, Marghoob AA. Dermoscopic semiology: Further insights into vascular features by screening a large spectrum of nontumoral skin lesions. Br J Dermatol. 2004;150(2):226-31.
15. Teoli M, Di Stefani A, Botti E, et al. Dermoscopy for treatment monitoring of viral warts. Dermatology. 2006;212:318.

CHAPTER 17

Lichen Planus Pigmentosus versus Ashy Dermatosis: Through a Dermoscope

Shekhar S Haldar, Uday S Khopkar

INTRODUCTION

Acquired dermal hypermelanoses due to fixed drug eruption, erythema dyschromicum perstans (EDP), lichen planus pigmentosus (LPP) and other postinflammatory hyperpigmentations are a common diagnostic and management problem in the brown-skinned Indians. Of these, EDP or ashy dermatosis and LPP are of great concern to patients due to its obscure etiology and the cosmetic and psychological implications of a long-drawn skin malady. According to current literature, these conditions have slightly different clinical presentations, without any specific differentiating histological features.[1] These have, therefore, been a topic of debate over the past several years. Several experts believe that

CHAPTER 17: Lichen Planus Pigmentosus versus Ashy Dermatosis...

they should be considered variants of a single entity while others believe that they are different from one another, each occurring in a different set of individuals having a particular ethnic background and environmental exposure. However, it is important to distinguish between these two, as they vary in their prognosis. EDP usually is asymptomatic with slow evolution and slower but surely evolving course while LPP is often symptomatic with pruritus and accompanied by frequent relapses and remissions.[2]

Current modality of diagnosis is a clinicohistopathological correlation (Table 1). Dermatoscopic examination of these

Table 1: Clinicohistopathological features of ashy dermatosis and lichen planus pigmentosus in our patients.

Clinical findings	Ashy dermatosis (n = 10)	Lichen planus pigmentosus (n = 20)
Color of macules Blue–gray	10/10 (100%)	7/20 (35%)
Dark brown	3/10 (30%)	20/20 (100%)
Color distribution within patch	Uniform	Heterogeneous
Symmetrical distribution	9/10 (90%)	11/20 (55%)
Active red border	1/10 (10%)	0
Residual hypopigmented halo	1/10 (10%) (Fig. 1)	0
Border of macules	Ill-defined and rounded	Well-defined irregular (Fig. 2)
Lichenoid papules	0	2/20 (10%)
Perifollicular hyperpigmentation (Fig. 3)	0	4/20 (20%)
Pruritus	0	9/20 (45%)

Contd...

Contd...

Clinical findings	Ashy dermatosis (n = 10)	Lichen planus pigmentosus (n = 20)
Hyperkeratosis	0	2/20 (10%)
Hypergranulosis	0	2/20 (10%)
Focal epidermal hyperplasia	5/10 (50%) (Fig. 4)	14/20 (70%)
Focal epidermal atrophy	0	20/20 (100%) (Fig. 6)
Rete ridge pattern of hyperplasia	Intermittent "finger-like" projection with rounded tip (Fig. 5)	Intermittent "arrow head" like projections with pointed tip (Fig. 7)
Basal cell degeneration	8/10 (80%)	18/20 (90%)
Colloid bodies	6/10 (60%)	15/20 (75%)
Perivascular infiltrate	9/10 (90%)	18/20 (90%)
Pigment incontinence	10/10 (100%) (Fig. 4)	20/20 (100%) (Fig. 6)
Perifollicular lymphocytic infiltrate	0/10 (Fig. 8)	4/20 (20%)

conditions reveals a particular pattern, which can be correlated with the clinical and histopathological findings. This kind of a three-way correlation can serve as a platform for formulating diagnostic criteria to distinguish these similar and long-debated conditions (Figs. 1 to 8).

CHAPTER 17: Lichen Planus Pigmentosus versus Ashy Dermatosis...

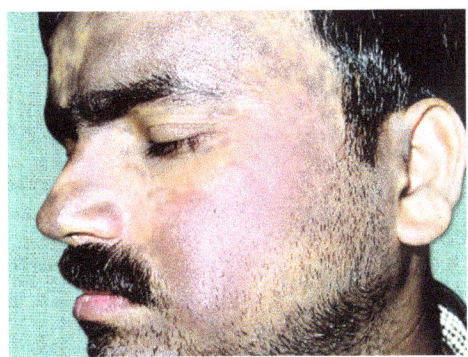

Fig. 1: Distribution of pigmentation: Involvement of face and neck, the most common distribution in both ashy dermatosis and lichen planus pigmentosus.

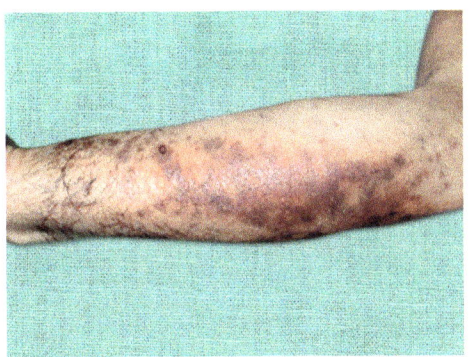

Fig. 2: Morphology of lesions of lichen planus pigmentosus: Macules and patches with well-demarcated, irregular borders.

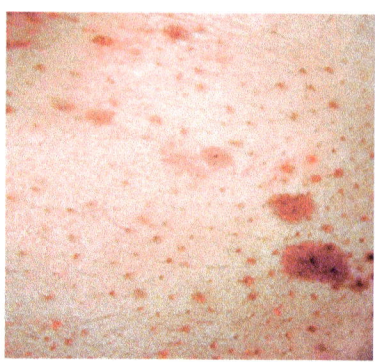

Fig. 3: Perifollicular involvement in lichen planus pigmentosus (LPP): Perifollicular hyperpigmentation along with patches of LPP, which are dark-brown in color. Note the absence of any erythematous border.

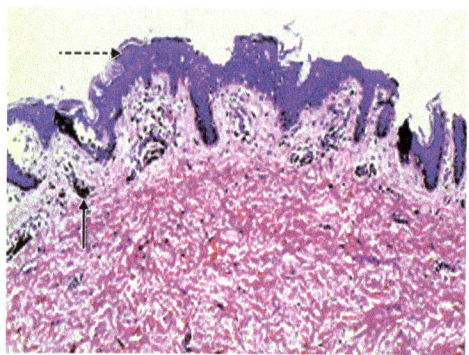

Fig. 4: Histopathology in ashy dermatosis: Mild-epidermal hyperplasia (dotted arrow) with superficial perivascular infiltrate of heavily pigmented melanophages and lymphocytes (solid arrow).

CHAPTER 17: Lichen Planus Pigmentosus versus Ashy Dermatosis...

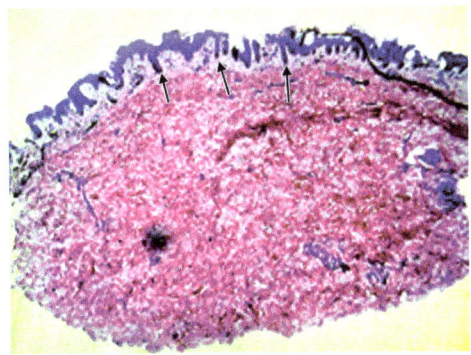

Fig. 5: Rete ridge pattern in ashy dermatosis: Rete ridges appear as finger-like projections with rounded tips having uniform width from the base to the tip.

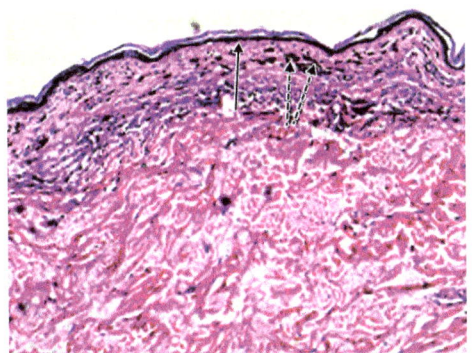

Fig. 6: Histopathology in lichen planus pigmentosus: Epidermal atrophy (solid arrow) with perivascular infiltrate of heavily pigmented melanophages (dotted arrows).

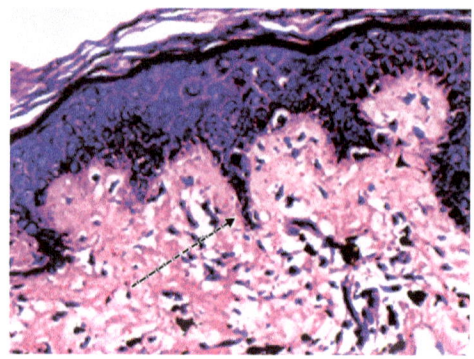

Fig. 7: Rete ridge pattern in lichen planus pigmentosus: Areas of focal hyperplasia showing a characteristic rete ridge pattern where they appear like "arrowheads" with a broad base and a pointed tip.

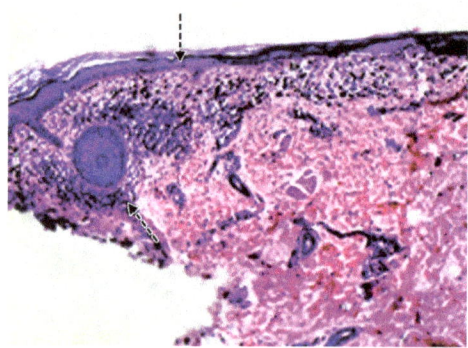

Fig. 8: Perifollicular involvement in lichen planus pigmentosus (LPP): Perifollicular cellular infiltrate by lymphocytes with pigment incontinence within the infiltrate (dotted arrows).

DERMOSCOPY

Ashy Dermatosis

Face

- The uniform reticular pattern of pigment network is accentuated. The pigmented lines, which form the reticular pattern, are more thickened than usual and the lines are granular rather than linear (Fig. 9). Sometimes, the granules appear to be superimposed on lines. The granules probably correlate with clusters of melanophages commonly found in the papillary dermis in this condition.
- The reticular pattern is complete at places, whereas at other places they disintegrate into more discrete speckled, granular, linear, angulated bluish-gray deposits (Fig. 10).

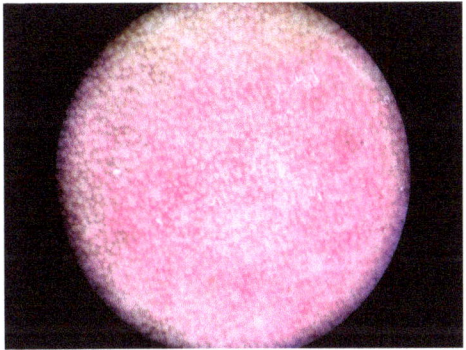

Fig. 9: Dermoscopy of ashy dermatosis: The uniform reticular pattern is accentuated. The pigmented lines, which form the reticular pattern, are more thickened than usual and the lines are granular rather than linear.

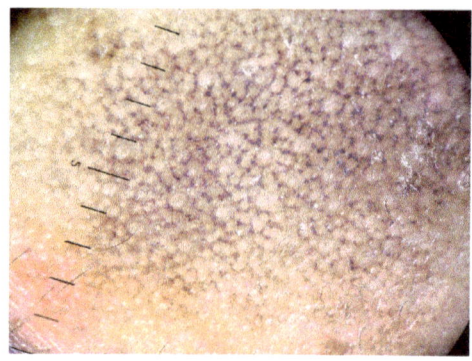

Fig. 10: Dermoscopy of ashy dermatosis: The reticular pattern is complete at places, whereas at other places they disintegrate into more discrete speckled, granular, linear, angulated bluish–gray deposits.

Extremities

- Normal reticular pattern of pigment and the pigment surrounding the acrosyringeal openings are blunted (Fig. 11).
- Rounded, linear, granular discrete bluish-gray pigment deposits evenly spaced and at places tending to form a curvilinear pattern.
- The pigment clusters are limited by skin surface markings and do not cross them.
- Pigment deposits do not encircle the follicular openings.

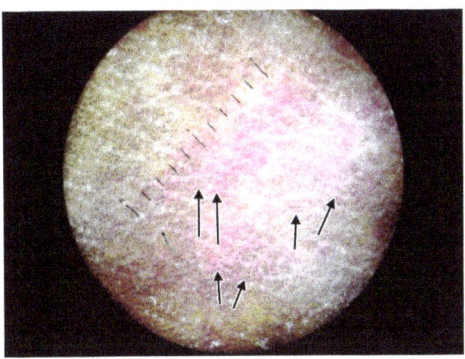

Fig. 11: Dermoscopy of ashy dermatosis:
- Normal reticular pattern of pigment and the pigment surrounding the acrosyringeal openings is blunted.
- Rounded, linear, granular discrete bluish–gray pigment deposits evenly spaced and at places tending to form a curvilinear pattern (arrows)
- The pigment clusters are limited by skin surface markings and do not cross them.

Lichen Planus Pigmentosus

Face

The reticular pattern is not uniformly accentuated, at places the quantity of pigment appears to be more at certain places than the other (Fig. 12).

Extremities

1. A "hem-like" regular distribution of clusters of pigment is seen (Fig. 13).

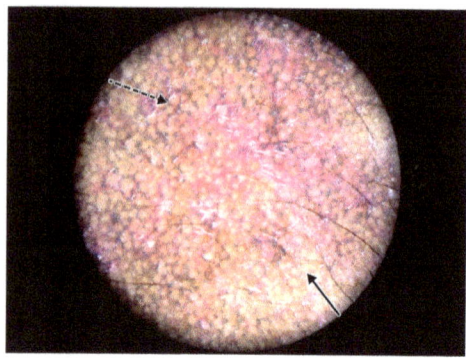

Fig. 12: Dermoscopy of lichen planus pigmentosus: The reticular pattern is not uniformly accentuated; at places, the quantity of pigment appears to be more (dotted arrow). Other places it appears to be less (solid arrow).

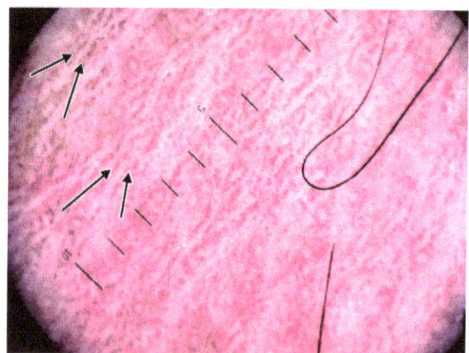

Fig. 13: Dermoscopy of lichen planus pigmentosus: A "hem-like" regular distribution of clusters of pigment is seen.

2. There is a tendency for the pigment to be deposited around the acrosyringeal openings (Fig. 14) and around follicular openings (Fig. 15).

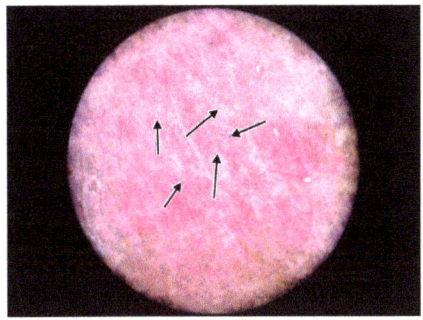

Fig. 14: Perieccrine involvement in lichen planus pigmentosus: There is a tendency for the pigment to be deposited around the acrosyringeal openings (arrows).

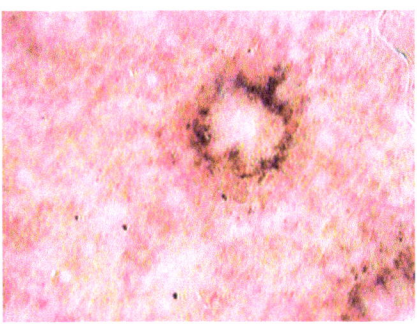

Fig. 15: Perifollicular involvement in lichen planus pigmentosus: Pigment deposition around the follicular opening.

Table 2: Comparative study of dermoscopic features.

Findings	Ashy dermatosis	Lichen planus pigmentosus
Face	Uniform accentuation of the reticular pattern	Reticular pattern not uniformly accentuated
Extremities	Normal deposition of pigment around acrosyringium is blunted Pigment granules deposited in a curvilinear pattern	Deposition of pigment around acrosyringium is accentuated Pigment granules deposited in a "hem-like" pattern

Ashy dermatosis and LPP can be reliably differentiated from one another based on their clinical, histopathological, and dermoscopic features (Table 2). Small sample size and short duration were limitations of our study. In order to make the differentiating criteria more robust and reliable, similar studies with larger sample size are needed to validate these findings. This could in the future obviate the need for a biopsy.

REFERENCES

1. Vega ME, Waxtein L, Arenas R, et al. Ashy dermatosis and lichen planus pigmentosus: a clinicopathologic study of 31 cases. Int J Dermatol. 1992;31(2):90-4.
2. Torrelo A, Zaballos P, Colmenero I, et al. Erythema dyschromicum perstans in children: a report of 14 cases. J Eur Acad Dermatol Venereol. 2005;19(4):422-6.

CHAPTER 18

Dermoscopy: Eczema versus Psoriasis

Manas Chatterjee, Ruchi Hemdani

INTRODUCTION

Psoriasis is a chronic relapsing papulosquamous dermatosis presenting as well-circumscribed erythematous, pruritic, plaques with silvery-white scaling.

Eczema is a pattern of inflammation with widely diverse etiology, characterized by pruritus and with oozing at some point in its history.

Accurate clinical distinction between psoriasis and eczema might be difficult requiring histological analysis, which also, at times, may be inconclusive. Dermoscopy is a noninvasive tool of aid in such scenario as many dermoscopic features exist to distinguish psoriasis from eczema.

DERMOSCOPY IN PSORIASIS

Plaque Psoriasis

Homogeneous vascular pattern, red dots and light red background are some of the significant dermoscopic features. Accurate diagnostic probability is 99% if all three are present simultaneously.[1] Commonly seen features are diffuse white scales, red globules (vessels) regularly distributed in honeycomb or sieve-like pattern (Fig. 1). It is advised to remove scales with liquid paraffin prior to dermoscopy.

Nail Psoriasis

Irregular depressions, purple striae, white areas with smooth red rim corresponding to reddish-orange stain surrounding

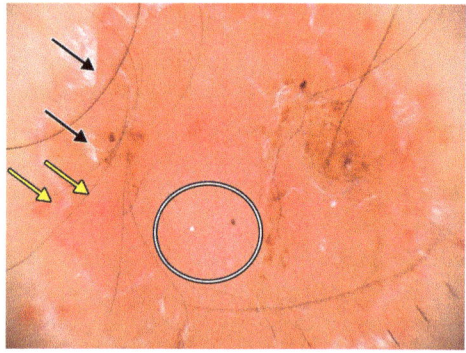

Fig. 1: Plaque psoriasis—red globules (vessels) regularly distributed in honeycomb (circle), light red background (yellow arrows), diffuse white scales (black arrows).

the area of onycholysis are seen (Figs. 2A and B). This finding is specific to onycholysis in nail psoriasis.[2]

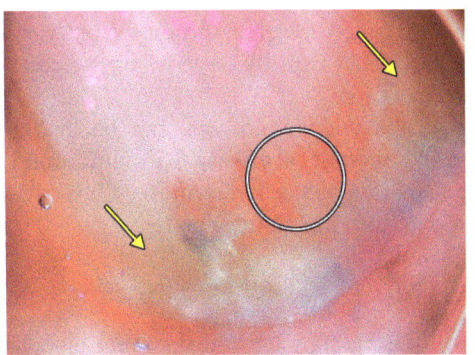

Fig. 2A: Nail psoriasis: Smooth reddish-orange stain surrounding the white area of onycholysis (yellow arrows), regular nail bed capillaries (circle).

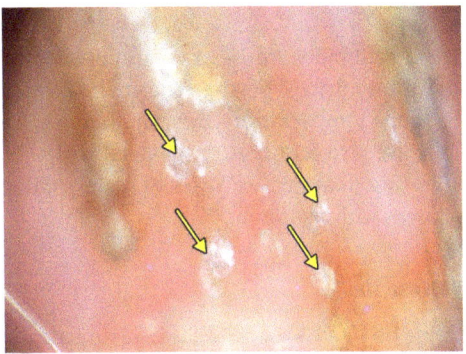

Fig. 2B: Nail psoriasis: Irregular depressions—pits (yellow arrows).

Dermoscopy of the hyponychium is essential to confirm the diagnosis of psoriasis in cases with mild hyperkeratosis of the nail bed or only onycholysis.[3] Findings include dilated, irregularly distributed, long and tortuous capillaries. Capillary density is associated with the severity of the condition and response to treatment.[4]

Proximal nail fold dermoscopy can be instrumental in evaluation of the severity of disease. The number and diameter of the capillaries are reduced in psoriasis.[5-7] It is advised to use linkage fluid to study nail features better.

Scalp Psoriasis

Findings on dermoscopy are red dots and globules (RDG), atypical red vessels (ARV), structureless red areas (SRA), hidden hair (HH), twisted red loops (TRL), glomerular vessels (GV), signet ring vessels (SRV) and perifollicular pigmentation (PP)[8] (Fig. 3).

Red dots and globules are the most common feature in scalp psoriasis and absent in seborrheic dermatitis. Interfollicular twisted red loops represent tortuous capillaries in the dermal papilla. They are also found in uninvolved scalp.[9] It is useful in the monitoring treatment in cases of scalp psoriasis, as the number reduces with treatment.[10]

Guttate Psoriasis

Monomorphic picture (Fig. 4) similar to plaque psoriasis.[11]

CHAPTER 18: Dermoscopy: Eczema versus Psoriasis

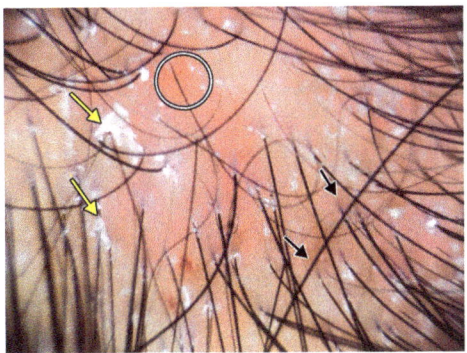

Fig. 3: Scalp psoriasis—regularly arranged vessels (circle), white scales (yellow arrows), perifollicular pigmentation (black arrows).

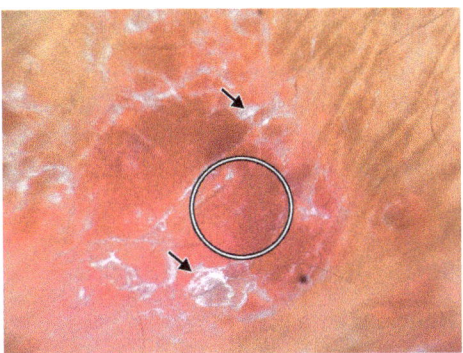

Fig. 4: Guttate psoriasis—regularly arranged vessels (circle), diffuse white scales (black arrows)

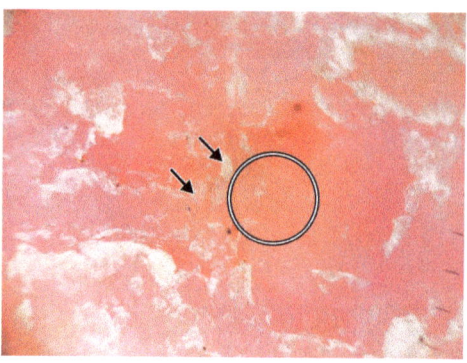

Fig. 5: Palmar psoriasis—white scales on erythematous background (black arrows), regular distributed dotted vessels (circle).

Palmar Psoriasis

White scales on erythematous background in a diffuse or patchy distribution, with regular distributed dotted vessels are seen (Fig. 5). Also, monomorphic, homogeneously distributed, "bushy" capillaries are present, which is a highly specific feature.[12]

DERMOSCOPY IN ECZEMA

Chronic Hand Eczema (CHE)

Focally distributed yellow scales, brownish-orange dots and/or globules on an erythematous background are commonly seen dermoscopic findings. Other features include focally distributed dotted vessels, patchily distributed white scales

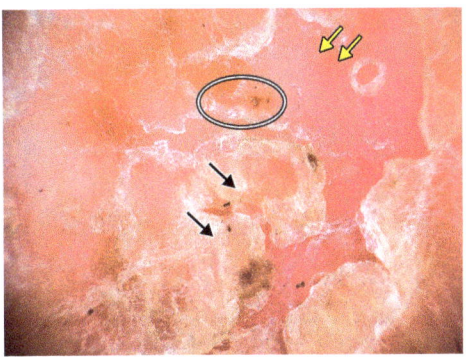

Fig. 6: CHE—focally distributed yellow scales (black arrows), brownish-orange dots and/or globules on an erythematous background (circle), normal capillary pattern (yellow arrows).

and sparse yellow-orangish crusts, normal or dilated capillaries without tortuosity (Fig. 6).

Similar features are displayed on dermoscopy in chronic hand eczema (CHE), eczema on other sites as well as in contact dermatitis.[13]

Pompholyx

The tiny spongiotic vesicles appear as brownish-orange dots/globules (Fig. 7), with increased thickening of the stratum corneum at these sites.[14]

Nummular Eczema

No specific feature. We have to rule out psoriasis which is the closest clinical mimic.

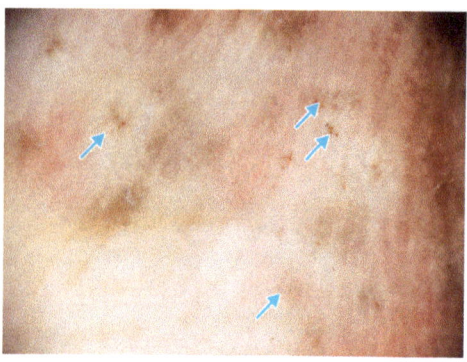

Fig. 7: Pompholyx—brownish-orange dots/globules (blue arrows).

Atopic Dermatitis

Dermoscopy of atopic dermatitis displays scanty white crusts, yellowish scales, patchy groups of red dotted vessels on a pinkish background (Fig. 8).[15]

Stasis Dermatitis

Glomerulus-like tortuous vessels distributed in clusters or throughout the lesion are seen at high magnification (×30 magnification). Red globules are seen at low magnification (×10 magnification) along with a scaly surface (Fig. 9). This dermoscopic pattern is also seen in Bowen disease.[16]

Seborrheic Dermatitis

Dermoscopic features include arborizing red lines, hidden hairs, perifollicular white scale, twisted red loops, atypical

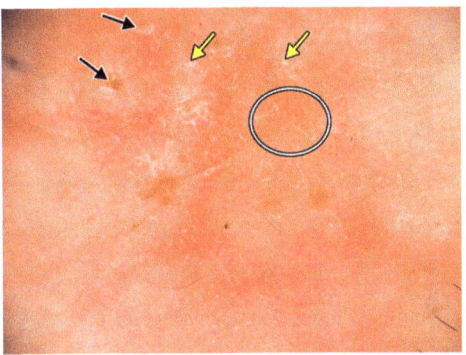

Fig. 8: Atopic dermatitis—yellowish sero-crusts (black arrows), sparse whitish scales (yellow arrows), and patchily distributed dotted vessels on a pinkish background (circle).

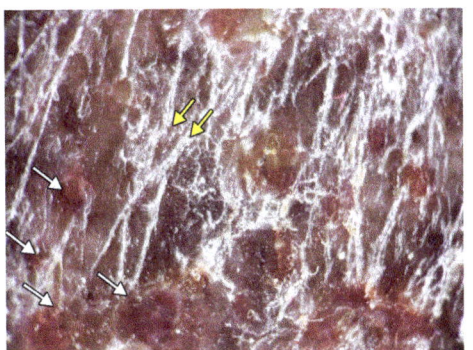

Fig. 9: Stasis dermatitis—red globules and purpurae (white arrows), scaly surface (yellow arrows).

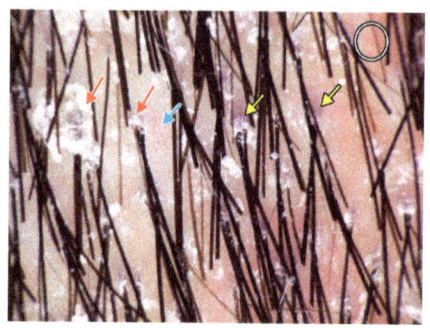

Fig. 10: Seborrheic dermatitis—perifollicular white scale (red arrows), atypical red vessels (blue arrow), structureless red areas (circle), perifollicular pigment (yellow arrows).

red vessels (ARV), structureless red areas, glomerular vessels, yellow dots (YD), perifollicular pigmentation, signet ring vessels, comma vessels (CV), honeycomb pigment pattern and brown dots (BD)[8] (Fig. 10).

In sebopsoriasis-like forms of seborrheic dermatitis, diffuse interfollicular TRL can be seen.

SALIENT DIFFERENTIATING FEATURES (TABLE 1)[1]

Table 1: Dermoscopic features of psoriasis and eczema.

Dermoscopic feature	Psoriasis	Eczema
Background color	Dull red > Light red	Dull red
Type of vessels	Dotted	Dotted + Linear
Pattern of vessels	Regular > Rings	Peripheral > Patchy
Scale color	White	White + Yellow
Scale distribution	Diffuse	Patchy

CONCLUSION

In conclusion, dermoscopy is a noninvasive, rapid and cheap test that serves as a perfect tool in differentiation of psoriasis from eczema in indecisive cases and thus improves the follow-up of patient with respect to his/her response to treatment.
(Note: All images are taken in polarized light (×10 magnification).

REFERENCES

1. Lallas A, Kyrgidis A, Tzellos TG, et al. Accuracy of dermoscopic criteria for the diagnosis of psoriasis, dermatitis, lichen planus and pityriasis rosea. Br J Dermatol. 2012;166:1198-205.
2. Farias DC, Tosti A, Chiacchio ND, et al. Dermoscopy in nail psoriasis. An Bras Dermatol. 2010;85:101-3.
3. Tosti A, Pirraccini BM, Farias DC. Nail dermoscopy. In: Micali G (Ed). Videodermatoscopy in Clinical Pratice. London: Informa Healthcare; 2009.
4. Iorizzo M, Dahdah M, Vicenzi C, et al. Videodermoscopy of the hyponychium in nail bed psoriasis. J Am Acad Dermatol. 2008;58:714-5.
5. Ohtsuka T, Yamakage A, Miyachi Y. Statistical definition of nail fold capillary pattern in patients with psoriasis. Int J Dermatol. 1994;33:779-82.
6. Zaric D, Clemmensen OJ, Worm AM, et al. Capillary microscopy of the nail fold in patients with psoriasis and psoriatic arthritis. Dermatologica. 1982;164:10-4.
7. Bhushan M, Moore T, Herrick AL, et al. Nail fold video capillaroscopy in psoriasis. Br J Dermatol. 2000;142:1171-6.
8. Kibar M, Aktan S, Bilgin M. Dermoscopic findings in scalp psoriasis and seborrheic dermatitis; two new signs; signet ring vessel and hidden hair. Indian J Dermatol. 2015;60:41-5.

9. Tosti A, Torres F. Dermoscopy in the diagnosis of hair and scalp disorders. Actas Dermosifiliogr. 2009;100:10104-9.
10. Ross EK, Vincenzi C, Tosti A. Videodermoscopy in the evaluation of hair and scalp disorders. J Am Acad Dermatol. 2006;55:799-806.
11. Lallas A, Apalla Z, Tzellos T, et al. Photoletter to the editor: dermoscopy in clinically atypical psoriasis. J Dermatol Case Rep. 2012;6:61-2.
12. Lacarrubba F, Musumeci ML, Ferraro S, et al. letter to editor: a three-cohort comparison with videodermatoscopic evidence of the distinct homogeneous bushy capillary microvascular pattern in psoriasis vs atopic dermatitis and contact dermatitis. JEADV. 2015;10:1-2.
13. Errichetti E, Stinco G. Dermoscopy in differential diagnosis of palmar psoriasis and chronic hand eczema. J Dermatol. 2016;43:423-5.
14. Errichetti E, Stinco G. Dermoscopy in General Dermatology: A Practical Overview. Dermatol Ther. 2016;6:471-507.
15. Errichetti E, Stinco G, Piccirillo A. Dermoscopy as an auxiliary tool in the differentiation of the main types of erythroderma due to dermatological disorders. Int J Dermatol. 2016;55:616-8.
16. Zaballos P, Salsench E, Puig S, et al. Dermoscopy of venous stasis dermatitis. Arch Dermatol. 2006;142:1526.

Section 5: Nail Disorders

CHAPTER 19

Overview of Onychoscopy

Archana Singal, Deepak Jakhar

INTRODUCTION

Onychoscopy is derived from "onycho" referring to nails and "scopy" meaning visual examination with an instrument, in this context with a dermatoscope or dermoscope. Onychoscopy is a noninvasive, painless, technically easy, and reproducible in vivo imaging technique that permits the visualization of morphological features that are not visible to the unaided eyes.[1] In a way, onychoscopy provides "submacroscopic" observation of the nail features and bridges the gap between naked eye examination and histopathology. Onychoscopy enhances the diagnostic accuracy in the clinical examination of nail lesions. Initially exploited to study the pigmentation of nail and proximal nailfold capillaries in connective tissue diseases,

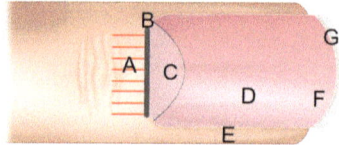

Fig. 1: Different parts of nail unit. A, proximal nailfold with nailfold capillaries; B, cuticle; C, lunula; D, nail plate; E, lateral nailfolds; F, onychodermal band; G, free edge of nail plate beneath; which overlies hyponychium. Two other important components of nail unit are nail matrix and nail bed.

uses of onychoscopy are evolving at a fast pace. These days, it is employed in the diagnosis of inflammatory nail diseases, infections and nail tumors too.[2-4] It is of utmost importance to understand various parts of nail unit before proceeding to perform onychoscopy (Fig. 1).

INSTRUMENTS

Onychoscopy is performed using the handheld dermatoscope/dermoscope that has a transilluminating light source and standard magnifying optics (10–20×). As of now, there is neither a consensus on the superiority of one instrument over the other nor on the type of light source that is best suited for onychoscopy. Both contact and noncontact dermatoscopes can be used. The surface abnormalities are better detailed by nonpolarized light source and a polarized light is best suited to study the pigmentary and vascular lesions of the nail unit. Various interface media have been employed like immersion oil, alcohol solution, distilled water and ultrasound jelly.[5] The ultrasound jelly scores above others by virtue of its increased viscosity and adherence to the nail plate. However, use of a specific interface medium entirely depends on the personal preference and comfort.

INDICATIONS

Flowchart 1 summarizes in brief various indications of onychoscopy.

NAIL PIGMENTATION

Melanonychia

International study group on melanonychia in 2013 published the guidelines for the use of dermatoscope in the study;

Flowchart 1: Indications of onychoscopy.

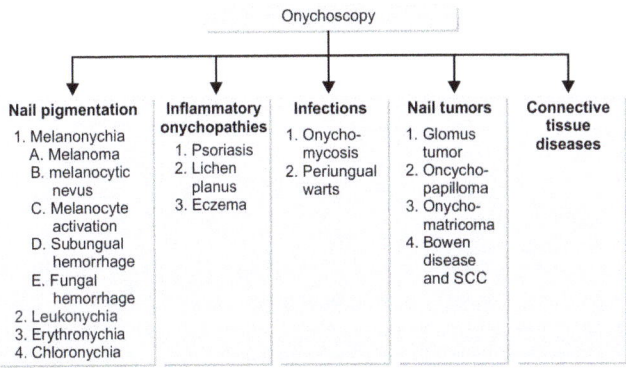

detection and management of nail pigmentation.[6] Flowchart 2 summarizes the step-wise approach for nail pigmentation. The salient onychoscopic features of nail unit melanoma are enlisted in Box 1. Figure 2 shows the characteristic onychoscopic picture of subungual hematoma. The benign longitudinal melanonychia is characterized by the regular, parallel and isochromic pattern (Fig. 3).

Flowchart 2: Step-wise approach to nail unit pigmentation.

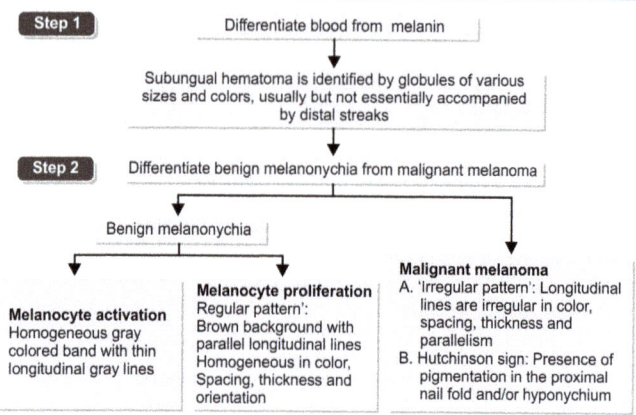

Box 1: Onychoscopic diagnosis of nail unit melanoma.

- Irregular pattern
- Abrupt stoppage of lines
- *Micro-Hutchinson sign*: Pigmentation of cuticle and/or proximal nail fold
- *Triangular pigmentary band*: Proximal end broader than distal
- Hemorrhage
- Erosion and/or microscopic grooving of nail plate

CHAPTER 19: Overview of Onychoscopy

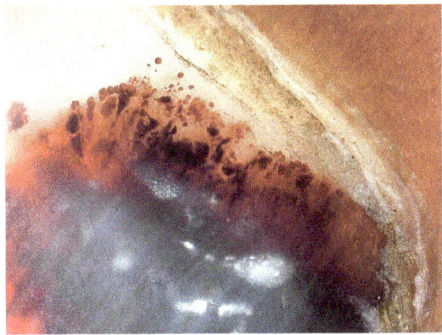

Fig. 2: Subungual hematomas presenting as homogeneous areas of brown black discoloration and showing characteristic round red spots/globules at the periphery representing fresh bleed. There is the peripheral fading of the pigmentation. (DermLite DL3-3Gen;20X)

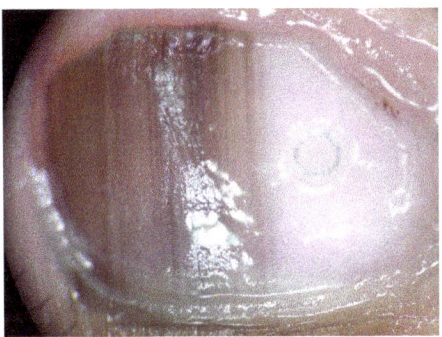

Fig. 3: Benign melanonychia showing the presence of regular pattern characterized by parallel monochromic lines with uniform thickness. (DermLite DL3-3Gen;10X).

Leukonychia

Leukonychia appears as white irregular areas within the nail plate.[7] Longitudinal leukonychia has been described with Darier's disease (Fig. 4), Hailey–Hailey disease, and nail tumors like onychopapilloma and onychomatricoma.

Erythronychia

Longitudinal erythronychia appears as a linear band, pink to red in color. When seen in single digit, the possible differentials include onychopapilloma, glomus tumor, and melanoma in situ whereas when present in multiple digits, the differentials include lichen planus, Darier's disease (Fig. 5), and systemic amyloidosis.[8]

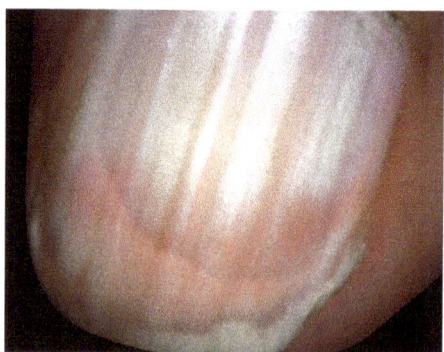

Fig. 4: Longitudinal leukonychia and erythronychia. (DermLite DL3-3Gen;10X)

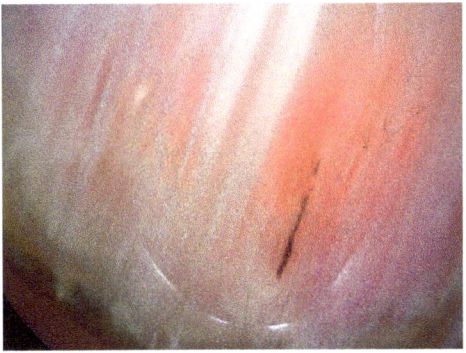

Fig. 5: Longitudinal erythronychia alternating with longitudinal leukonychia in a case of Darier's disease, a splinter hemorrhage is also seen. (DermLite DL3-3Gen;20X)

Chloronychia

The greenish discoloration of nails is seen in *Pseudomonas aeruginosa* or other bacterial infection under the nails usually accompanied by onycholysis and is commonly due to prolonged contact with water, soap, or detergents or other bacterial infection. Occasionally, it may be acquired during overzealous manicure or possibly by use of contaminated instruments (Fig. 6).[1]

INFLAMMATORY DISEASES

Nail Psoriasis

Onychoscopic features observed depend upon the part of the nail unit affected.[9,10]

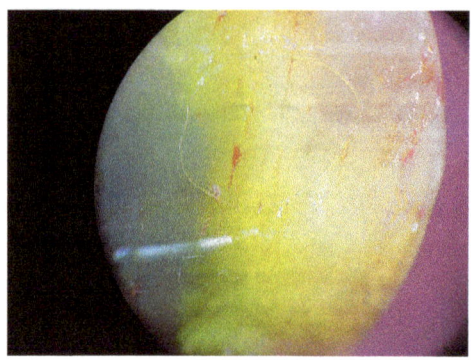

Fig. 6: Chloronychia presenting as greenish discoloration of nail plate. (DermLite DL3-3Gen;20X)

Nail Matrix

- *Pits*: Large, deep and irregular depressions on the nail plate (Fig. 7).
- *Leukonychia*: White irregular areas within the nail plate representing parakeratosis.

Nail Bed

- *Salmon patch*: Red-to-orange–colored patch with irregular shape and size that manifest in the nail plate (Fig. 8).
- *Splinter hemorrhage*: Longitudinal fusiform streaks ranging from bright red to black in color appearing in the distal nail bed (Fig. 8).
- *Onycholysis*: Erythematous border at the proximal end of onycholytic band becomes evident on onychoscopy

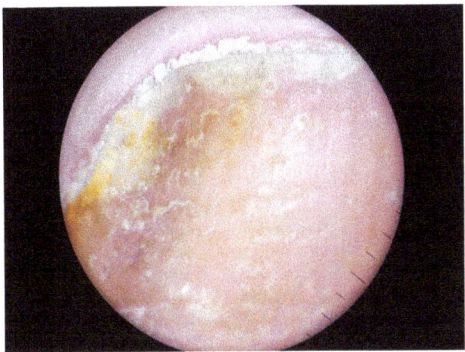

Fig. 7: Nonpolarizing onychoscopy showing the large irregular pits with distal onycholysis and yellowish staining characteristic of psoriasis. (DermLite DL3-3Gen;20X).

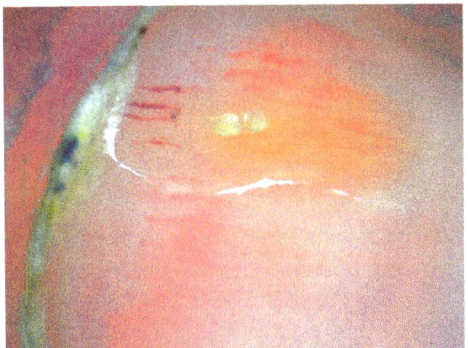

Fig. 8: Salmon patch visible as orange-colored patch with adjacent longitudinal fusiform streaks characteristic of splinter hemorrhage. (DermLite DL3-3Gen;20X)

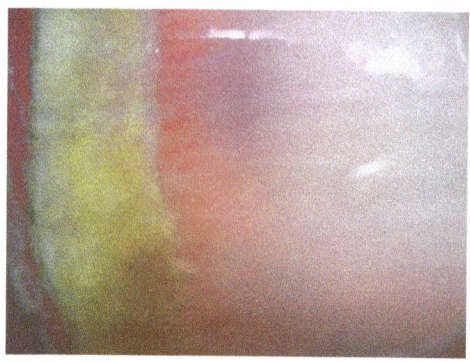

Fig. 9: Onycholysis with characteristic proximal erythematous band. Also note the fusiform dilated nail bed vessels. (DermLite DL3-3Gen;20X)

(Fig. 9). Absence of longitudinal striae helps differentiate psoriasis from onychomycosis.
- *Nail bed vessels*: Fusiform-dilated vessels surrounded by a prominent halo just proximal to the onychodermal band (Fig. 9).

Proximal Nail Fold

Mean capillary is reduced and capillary architecture alterations in the form of dropouts and coiled capillaries are seen.

Hyponychium

Dermoscopy of the hyponychium is very useful to confirm the diagnosis of nail psoriasis in uncertain cases by demonstrating irregularly distributed, dilated, tortuous, twisted capillaries

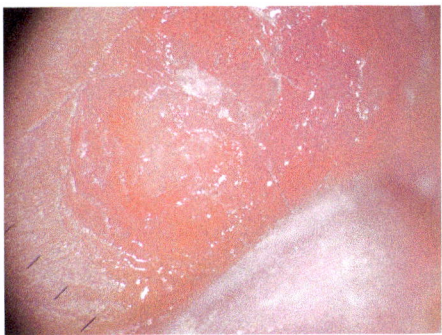

Fig. 10: Dilated vessels in the hyponychium in a case of nail psoriasis. (DermLite DL3-3Gen;40X)

usually on higher magnification. These capillaries correlate with the disease severity (Fig. 10).

Nail pitting, splinter hemorrhages, and onycholysis are the most common findings.

Nail Lichen Planus

Onychoscopic features depend on the site of nail unit affected.[3,11]

Nail Matrix

Manifest on the nail plate as trachyonychia, pitting, pterygium, and red lunula (Fig. 11).

Nail Bed

Chromonychia, splinter hemorrhages, onycholysis, subungual keratosis, longitudinal fissures in a thinned out nail plate (Fig. 12).

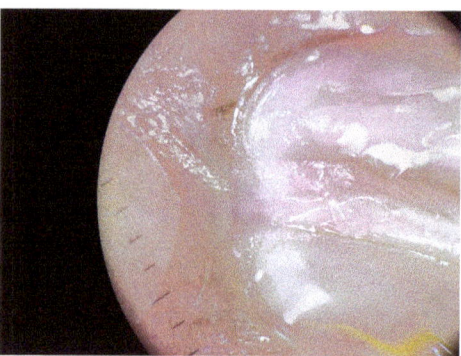

Fig. 11: Nail lichen planus showing thinning and longitudinal fissures in the nail plate. (DermLite DL3-3Gen;10X)

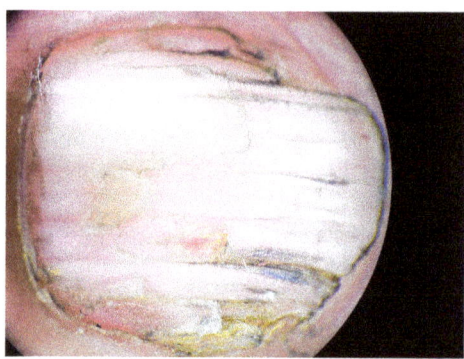

Fig. 12: Nail Lichen Planus: Longitudinal streaks with nail plate splitting, onychoschizia, and distal onycholysis. (DermLite DL3-3Gen;20X)

Proximal Nailfold Capillaries

No changes.

INFECTIONS

Onychomycosis

The typical features of onychomycosis are summarized in Figure 13.[12,13] These features definitely aid in diagnosis of onychomycosis (Figs. 14 and 15) and helps it differentiate from nail psoriasis (Figs. 16 and 17).

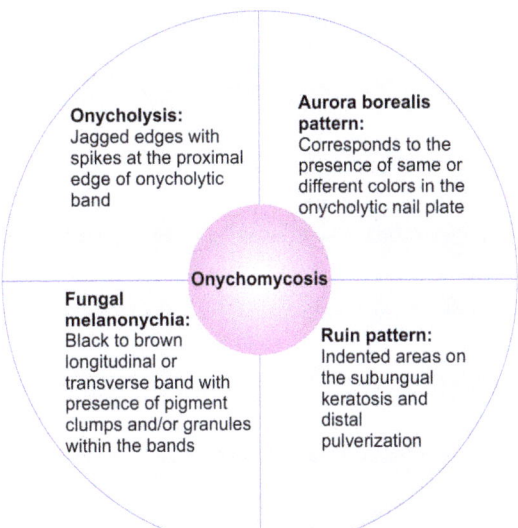

Fig. 13: Onychoscopic patterns observed in onychomycosis.

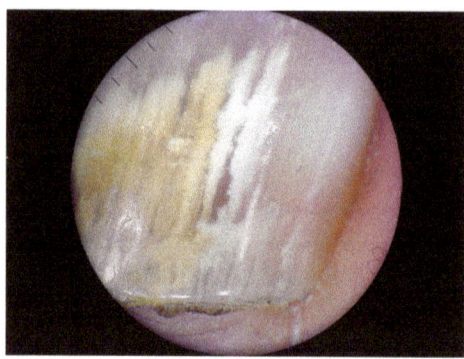

Fig. 14: Onychomycosis: Onycholysis with jagged spikes at the proximal end of onycholytic bands. Also note the different colors of jagged spikes corresponding to the "aurora borealis" pattern. (DermLite DL3-3Gen;20X)

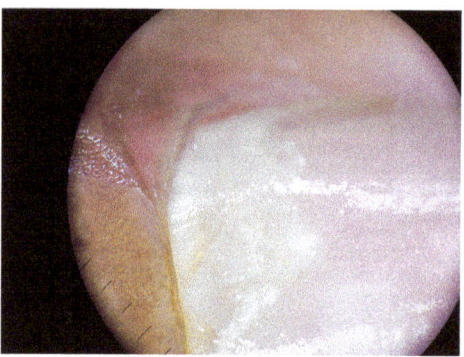

Fig. 15: Proximal subungual onychomycosis displaying irregular proximal onycholysis. (DermLite DL3-3Gen;10X)

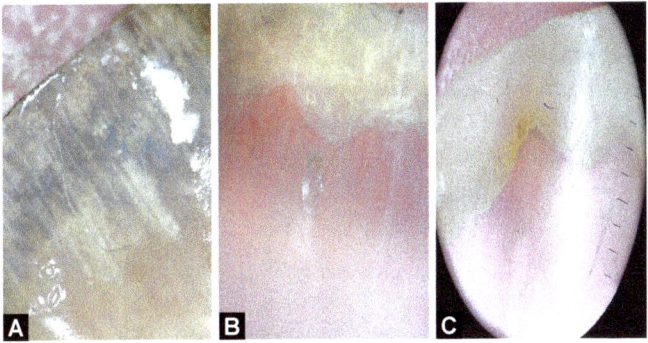

Figs. 16A to C: Different causes of onycholysis: (A) Onychomycosis has a jagged edges/spikes proximal to onycholytic band; (B) Psoriasis has an erythematous band proximal to a regular onycholytic band with dilated nail bed vessels; (C) Traumatic onycholysis is characterized by regular onycholytic band with absence of above described features. (DermLite DL3-3Gen;20X)

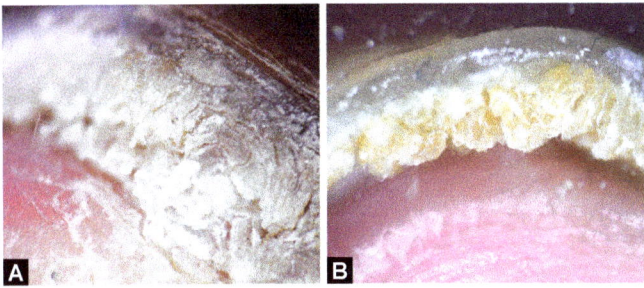

Figs. 17A and B: Distal end onychoscopy showing differences in subungual hyperkeratosis: (A) Onychomycosis has a friable subungual hyperkeratosis, which ultimately leads to the "ruin pattern"; (B) Psoriasis has a compact subungual hyperkeratosis. (DermLite DL3-3Gen;20X)

Periungual Warts

Thrombosed vessels visible as red to black dots within a hyperkeratotic lesion is a typical finding of the warty lesion (Fig. 18).[3] Figure 19 shows the clinical and onychoscopic picture of periungual wart.

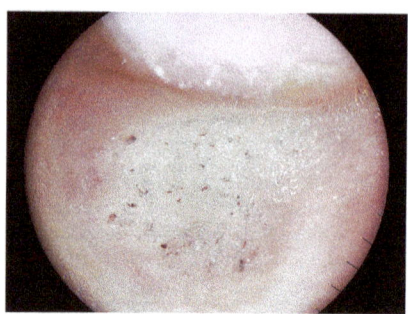

Fig. 18: Periungual wart: Characteristic red to brown dots suggestive of thrombosed vessels. (DermLite DL3-3Gen;10X)

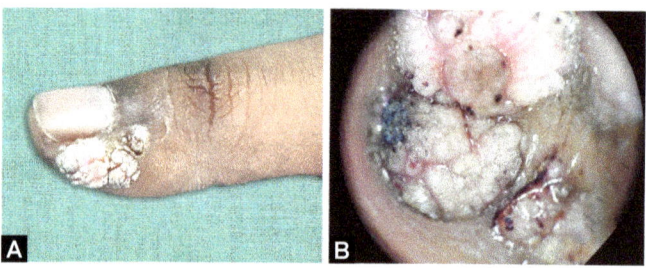

Figs. 19A and B: (A) Multiple coalescing periungual warts; (B) Thrombosed vessels visible as red dots. (DermLite DL3-3Gen;20X)

Nailfold Capillaroscopy

Nailfold capillaroscopy (NFC) is a noninvasive technique of visualizing and assessing the quantitative and qualitative features of proximal nailfold capillaries in connective tissue diseases. It is particularly helpful in differentiating primary Raynaud's phenomenon from secondary causes.[4] In addition, NFC is useful for the assessment of vascular injury and evaluation of therapeutic response.

Systemic Sclerosis

Assessment of microcirculation in systemic sclerosis (SSc) with NFC not only helps in diagnosis, but also in prognosis of the disease. Three different patterns of microvascular involvement are described in SSc (Table 1).[14]

Table 1: Different patterns of microvascular involvement.

Patterns	Features
Early pattern (Fig. 20)	Few dilated and/or giant capillaries, hemorrhages, and preserved capillary distribution without loss of capillaries
Active pattern (Fig. 21)	Large numbers of giant capillaries, hemorrhages, a moderate loss of capillaries, slight derangement, and diffuse pericapillary edema
Late pattern (Fig. 22)	Severe loss of capillaries with extensive avascular areas, bushy and ramified capillaries, or more than one capillary loop in a dermal papilla

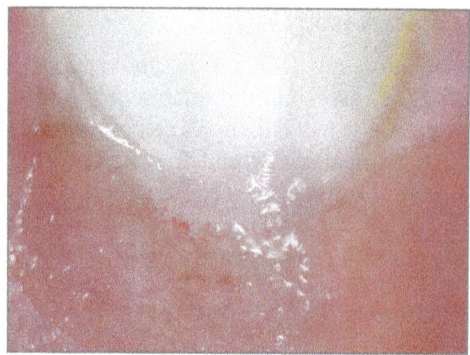

Fig. 20: Scleroderma—early pattern: Nailfold capillaroscopy showing a few dilated and tortuous vessels. (DermLite DL3-3Gen;20X)

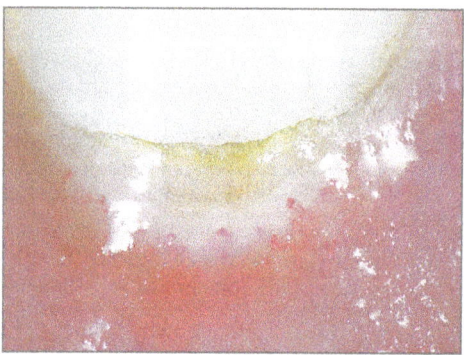

Fig. 21: Scleroderma—active pattern: Large number of dilated vessels with structural alteration. There is moderate loss of capillaries. (DermLite DL3-3Gen;20X)

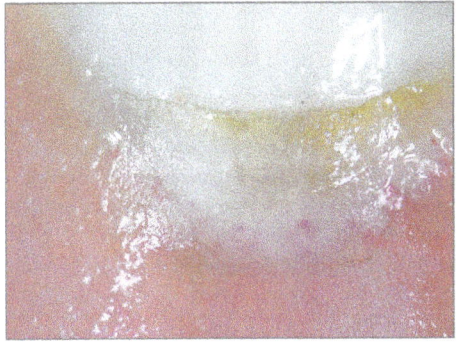

Fig. 22: Scleroderma—late pattern: Severe loss of capillaries with avascular areas and giant capillaries. (DermLite DL3-3Gen;20X)

Dermatomyositis and Polymyositis

Presence of two or more of the following characteristics in two or more nail folds:[15]
- Capillary dilation
- Twisted enlarged capillaries
- Loss of capillaries
- Bushy capillaries
- Disorganization of capillary architecture
- Microhemorrhages.

In contrast to polymyositis (PM), capillary dilation and loss of capillaries are more commonly and severely affected in dermatomyositis (DM).

Onychoscopy is being used increasingly, as it provides important as well as recordable information in the assessment of nail diseases.

REFERENCES

1. Lencastre A, Lamas A, Sá D, et al. Onychoscopy. Clin Dermatol. 2013;31(5):587-93.
2. Ronger S, Touzet S, Ligeron C, et al. Dermoscopic examination of nail pigmentation. Arch Dermatol. 2002;138(10):1327-33.
3. Nakamura RC, Costa MC. Dermatoscopic findings in the most frequent onychopathies: descriptive analysis of 500 cases. Int J Dermatol. 2012;51:483-96.
4. Mannarino E, Pasqualini L, Fedeli F, et al. Nailfold capillaroscopy in the screening and diagnosis of Raynaud's phenomenon. Angiology. 1994;45:37-42.
5. Gewirtzman AJ, Saurat JH, Braun RP. An evaluation of dermoscopy fluids and application techniques. Br J Dermatol. 2003;149(1):59-63.
6. Di Chiacchio ND, Farias DC, Piraccini BM, et al. Consensus on melanonychia nail plate dermoscopy. An Bras Dermatol. 2013;88(2):309-13.
7. Piraccini BM, Bruni F, Starace M. Dermoscopy of non-skin cancer nail disorders. Dermatol Ther. 2012;25(6):594-602.
8. Jellinek NJ. Longitudinal erythronychia: suggestions for evaluation and management. J Am Acad Dermatol. 2011;64(2):167e1-11.
9. Yadav TA, Khopkar US. Dermoscopy to detect signs of subclinical nail involvement in chronic plaque psoriasis: A study of 68 patients. Indian J Dermatol. 2015;60(3):272.
10. Yorulmaz A, Artuz F. A study of dermoscopic features of nail psoriasis. Postepy Dermatol Alergol. 2017;34(1):28-35.
11. Nakamura R, Broce AA, Palencia DP, et al. Dermatoscopy of nail lichen planus. Int J Dermatol. 2013;52(6):684-7.
12. Jesús-Silva MA, Fernández-Martínez R, Roldán-Marín R, et al. Dermoscopic patterns in patients with a clinical diagnosis of onychomycosis—results of a prospective study including data of

potassium hydroxide (KOH) and culture examination. Dermatol Pract Concept. 2015;5(2):5.
13. De Crignis G, Valgas N, Rezende P, et al. Dermatoscopy of onychomycosis. Int J Dermatol. 2014;53(2):e97-9.
14. Cutolo M, Sulli A, Pizzorni C, et al. Nail fold videocapillaroscopy assessment of microvascular damage in systemic sclerosis. J Rheumatol. 2000;27:155-60.
15. Klyscz T, Bogenschutz O, Junger M, et al. Microangiopathic changes and functional disorders of nail fold capillaries in dermatomyositis. Hautarzt. 1996;47:289-93.

CHAPTER 20

Neoplastic Nail Unit Disorders

Ishmeet Kaur, Archana Singal

INTRODUCTION

Nail apparatus is the functional unit of the digital tip. Since, it has a complex structure with attachment to the surrounding tissues like distal interphalangeal joint, tendon, bone, fascia and cartilage, a variety of tumors are known to occur in the nail unit that pose a great diagnostic challenge. In such cases, various noninvasive modalities like dermoscopy, ultrasound and MRI scan can be employed before arriving at a final diagnosis on histopathology. Early diagnosis and treatment is essential in order to prevent permanent nail disfigurement.

CLASSIFICATION OF NAIL UNIT TUMORS

1. Nail tumors can also be classified on the basis of their benign and malignant nature as shown in Table 1.

2. *Site of origin*: A wide variety of tumors arise from different anatomical structures constituting the nail unit as shown in Table 2 and Figure 1.

Table 1: Common benign and malignant tumors of the nail unit.

Benign tumors	Malignant tumors
Verrucae	Bowen's disease
Granuloma pyogenicum	Squamous cell carcinoma
Glomus tumor	Keratoacanthoma
Onychomatricoma	Malignant melanoma
Onychopapilloma	Basal cell carcinoma
Digital fibrokeratoma	Metastatic tumors
Koenen's tumor	
Subungual exostosis	
Digital mucous cyst	
Melanocytic nevus	

Table 2: Site of origin: A wide variety of tumors arise from different anatomical structures constituting the nail unit.

Site of origin	Nail tumor
Nail matrix	• Onychomatricoma • Onychopapilloma • Onychocytic matricoma • Subungual filamentous tumor • SADA (Subungual acantholytic dyskeratotic acanthoma) • Matrix cyst

Contd...

Contd...

Site of origin	Nail tumor
Nail bed	• Onycholemmal horn • Onycholemmal cyst • Onycholemmal carcinoma • Proliferating onycholemmal cyst • Malignant onycholemmal cyst
Periungual tissue	• Granuloma pyogenicum • Wart
Vascular bed	• Granuloma pyogenicum • Glomus tumor
Nail melanin unit	• Malignant melanoma • Melanocytic nevus
Fibrous tissue tumors	• Digital fibrokeratoma • Koenen's tumor
Bone and joint	• Myxoid cyst • Subungual exostosis • Osteochondroma
Metastatic origin	• Lung, genitourinary tract, breast

- Onychocytic matricoma
- Onychomatricoma
- Onychopapilloma
- Subungual filamentous tumor
- SADA (Subungual acantholytic dyskeratotic acanthoma)
- Matrix cyst

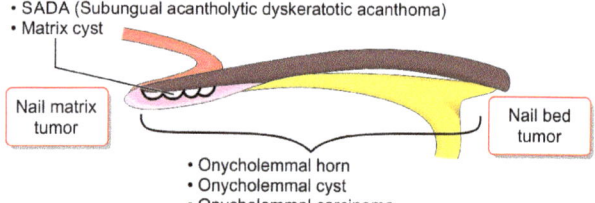

Fig. 1: Nail-specific tumors.

BENIGN NAIL UNIT TUMORS

VIRAL WART

Wart is the most common benign tumor of the nail caused by human papilloma virus (HPV). It is a fibroepithelial tumor that can affect the periungual as well as the subungual region with fingernail involvement more common than toenail.[1]

The wart begins in the periungual region as a rough hyperkeratotic lesion which usually arises from the lateral aspect of the proximal nail fold (PNF), which can further spread and involve the entire nail fold. On the other hand, subungual warts originate from the hyponychium and spread to involve the nail bed resulting in onycholysis.[2] Matricial involvement, although uncommon, can present with longitudinal ridges and grooves due to pressure effect exerted by the wart.[3] In longstanding cases, warts can lead to bony erosions as well as malignant transformation to Bowen's disease and squamous cell carcinoma (SCC).[2]

Diagnosis is usually clinical. On dermoscopy, thrombosed vessels seen as red black dots over a keratotic surface can help differentiate warts from other growths (Figs. 2 and 3).[4]

Treatment options can be either topical (20–60% salicylic acid, TCA and glutaraldehyde), intralesional (Bleomycin 2–3 units/mL, cryosurgery), surgical excision and LASER ablation [CO_2 laser, neodymium-doped yttrium aluminum garnet (Nd:YAG) and erbium-doped yttrium aluminium garnet laser (Er:YAG laser)]. Immunotherapy including topical imiquimod and vaccines like MMR and *Candida* has also been used in recalcitrant cases.[5]

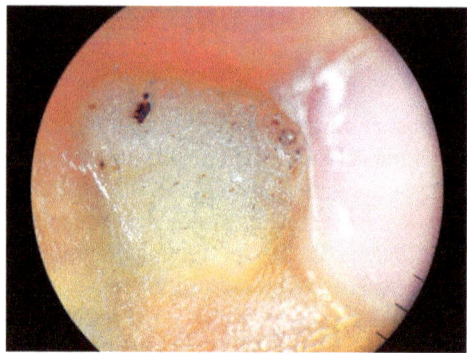

Fig. 2: Periungual warts at proximal nail fold; note characteristic red black dots of thrombosed vessels. (10×)

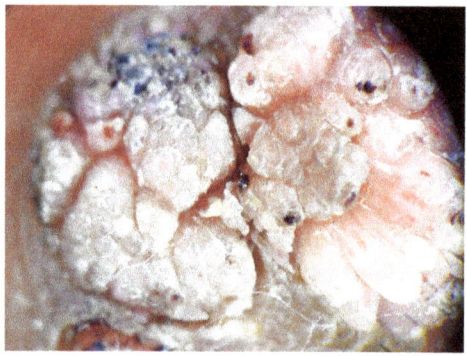

Fig. 3: Fingerlike projections of periungual and subungual warts. (20×)

GRANULOMA PYOGENICUM

Granuloma pyogenicum (lobular capillary hemangioma) is a common benign vascular tumor of the nail involving the periungual tissue and the nail bed.[6] Nail is the site of predilection due to high vascularity and exposure to recurrent trauma.[2] It can present as a rapidly growing red papule, sessile, or pedunculated, seen most frequently in the proximal nail fold followed by hyponychium (Fig. 4) and nail bed with a characteristic collarette scale. Tenderness and bleeding tendency are common presenting complaints.[1] Pyogenic granuloma can occur secondary to various factors such as acute or chronic local trauma, retronychia (in-growing toenail), drugs such as retinoids, cyclosporine, antiretrovirals, antineoplastic

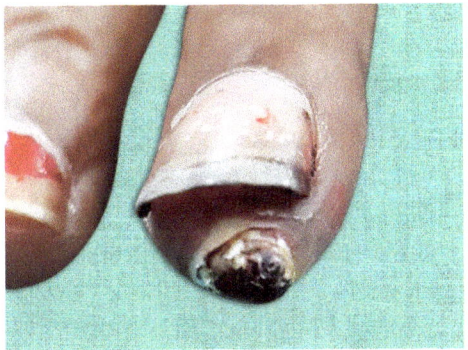

Fig. 4: Granuloma pyogenicum in the hyponychium following repeated needle trauma in a woman.

like epidermal growth factor receptor (EGFR) inhibitors, peripheral nerve injury and pregnancy. Differential diagnoses include granulation tissue, pseudopyogenic granuloma, SCC and amelanotic melanoma.[1]

Dermoscopy shows red discoloration with a milky-red veil with a darker discoloration at the center of the lesion and white collarette. Necrotic areas, brown in color (Fig. 5), can also be seen.[4,7] However, it is not considered specific or diagnostic for pyogenic granuloma. Histopathology, on the other hand, can help in differentiating from other tumors as well as granulation tissue. It shows proliferation of newly formed vessels in lobular fashion separated by fibrous septae with presence of variable amounts of edema, mixed inflammatory infiltrates and collarettes of epidermal hyperplasia.[8] Besides the treatment

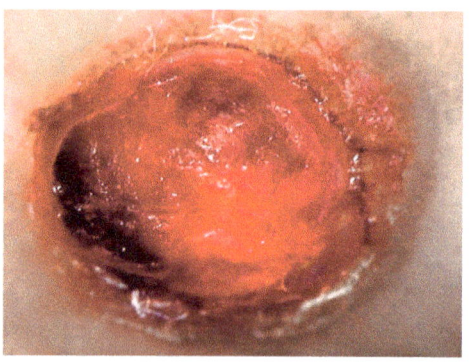

Fig. 5: Highly vascular red central area with necrotic hemorrhagic crust and epidermal collarette (10×; polarizing).

of lesion of pyogenic granuloma, the underlying cause should also be taken care of.

GLOMUS TUMOR

Glomus tumor is a benign vascular tumor arising from the neuromyoarterial plexus called the glomus bodies of the nail bed.[9] About 75% of glomus tumors occur in hands and majority in the subungual region.[1] Glomus tumor usually presents in 3rd to 5th decade with a female preponderance.[1] It presents with a characteristic triad of severe pain, cold temperature sensitivity and localized tenderness seen in 63–100% of the patients along with positive Love's pin test and Hildreth's test. When visible, it can be seen as a reddish blue mass under the nail plate, which can mimic longitudinal erythronychia. Larger lesions can present with distal onycholysis and fissuring.[9]

MRI can reveal the size, location and the extent of the tumor, which can also be detected by ultrasound but only in tumors larger than 3 mm in size. Dermoscopy has significant findings; nail plate shows ramified small and linear blood vessels (Fig. 6). Intraoperative onychoscopy can also help in localizing the tumor and in detecting residual sister lesions. After nail plate removal, the tumor is usually seen as ramified group of vessels over a blue background.[4,10]

Histology of the mass shows proliferating vascular channels lined with endothelial as well as glomus cells with darkly stained nucleus and pale cytoplasm. These glomus cells stain positive for vimentin (a 42-kD muscle actin), smooth muscle actin and myosin, but they stain negative for factor VIII-related

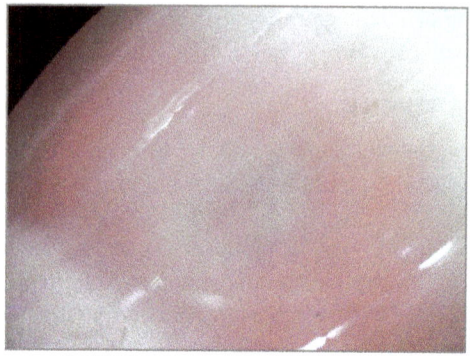

Fig. 6: Ill-defined red-purple patch of glomus tumor (20x magnification).

antigen, desmin, and some other neural markers. Treatment of glomus tumor is complete excision.[1]

ONYCHOMATRICOMA

Onychomatricoma is a rare benign tumor of nail matrix, arising from its epithelium and the connective tissue. It typically occurs in middle-aged women with a predilection for fingernails and presents with a classic tetrad of xanthonychia along with thickening of the nail plate, splinter hemorrhage, and transverse over-curvature of the nail plate.[11]

Diagnosis is usually based on clinical, imaging and histopathological features. Dermoscopy of the distal edge aids in the diagnosis which shows characteristic honeycomb or woodworm holes that correspond to longitudinal tunnels containing the digital processes of the tumor within the nail plate. Other typical dermoscopic findings of onychomatricoma include yellowish discoloration with longitudinal striae and splinter hemorrhages.[4,12] Recently, three signs have been described in onychomatricoma seen on intraoperative dermoscopy. Firstly, Sagrada Familia sign, which corresponds to the crypts in the proximal part of the ventral aspect of the nail plate. Second refers to the digitations seen above the lunula. The symmetrical arrangement of the above two components is known as the mirror sign.[13] Differential diagnoses for onychomatricoma include onychomycosis, fibrokeratoma, glomus tumor, SCC, Bowen's disease and viral warts. Complete excision of the tumor is the treatment of choice.[1,12]

ONYCHOPAPILLOMA

Onychopapilloma is a rare benign tumor arising from the distal nail matrix and the nail bed. Longitudinal erythronychia is the most common presentation with longitudinal deformation of the nail plate in the form of V-shaped nick distally. Larger lesions may appear as a localized subungual growth with onycholysis.[14] Dermoscopy can aid in diagnosis, localization as well as differentiating from other tumors like onychomatricoma. It typically shows thin red band extending from the lunula till the distal margin, often with presence of splinter hemorrhages.[4] The distal edge may show a subungual filiform growth with a linear fissure.[15] Differential diagnoses include glomus tumor, viral warts, Darier's disease, lichen planus and Bowen's disease. Symptomatic lesions, when associated with nail deformity, may be excised.[2]

DIGITAL FIBROKERATOMA

Acquired digital fibrokeratoma (DF) occurs in middle-aged men and involves finger and toes near the interphalangeal joint. Acquired periungual DF presents as a solitary nodule originating from the proximal nail fold or the nail bed.[1] The lesions may sometimes be multiple or grow on the nail plate causing longitudinal grooves. The differential diagnoses include Koenen tumors, supernumerary digits, neurofibroma, verruca vulgaris, and cutaneous horn.[16] Dermoscopy reveals a central pale yellow homogeneous zone with a surrounding collarette (Fig. 7).[17] Some cases show clumps of homogeneous red lacunae divided by a white meshwork-like septal wall with surrounding telangiectasias. Diagnosis can be further confirmed with the help of histopathology. Treatment choices include complete excision or ablation of the lesion.[1,16]

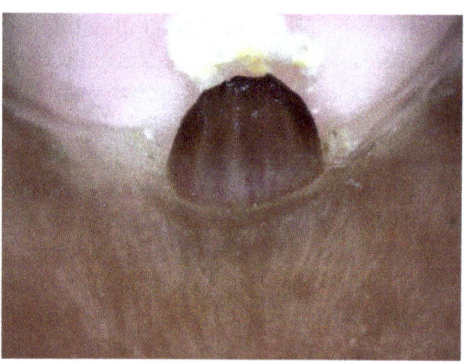

Fig. 7: Acquired digital fibrokeratoma toenail (20×).

KOENEN'S TUMOR

Koenen's tumor also known as periungual or subungual fibroma is a benign pathognomonic manifestation of tuberous sclerosis complex. It is one of the major diagnostic criteria and usually appears after puberty in up to 50% of patients.[18] A typical lesion presents as an asymptomatic smooth fleshy garlic clove-like growth arising from the proximal nail fold (Fig. 8) which may sometimes cause a longitudinal depression in the nail plate or show a hyperkeratotic tip mimicking a fibrokeratoma. It tends to increase in size and number with age. Treatment of choice is simple excision.[1]

SUBUNGUAL EXOSTOSIS

It is the most common bone tumor associated with the nail unit. It typically presents as a subungual bony outgrowth on

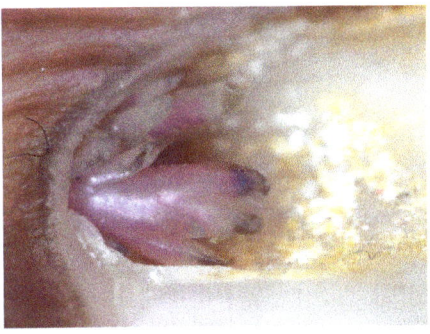

Fig. 8: Garlic clove-like Koenen's tumor on toenail leading to linear band of nail plate depression (20×).

the dorsomedial aspect of the great toe which may cause nail disfigurement and onycholysis. The tumor itself is not painful, but pain can occur due to pressure effect while walking. Trauma is a common trigger factor.[2] Dermoscopy of the tumor may show onycholysis with vascular ectasia associated with hyperkeratosis and ulceration.[19] Radiography must be done in such cases which show a trabeculated osseous outgrowth from the dorsal part of the distal phalanx which may be covered with fibrocartilage. Treatment is surgical excision. Recurrence can be seen in up to 20% cases.[2]

DIGITAL MUCOUS CYST

Digital mucous cyst typically affects middle-aged women with osteoarthritis of the terminal digit. It is believed to arise as a herniation of the joint capsule of the distal interphalangeal joint, forming a localized swelling (Fig. 9) that drains viscous

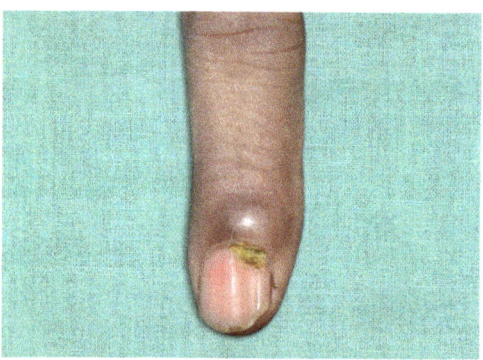

Fig. 9: Clinical picture of a digital mucous cyst in a woman.

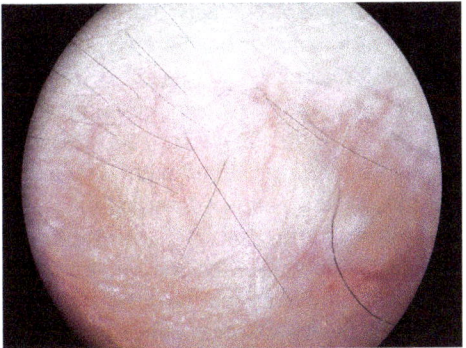

Fig. 10: Serpentine vessels on polarized dermoscopy (20×)

jelly-like synovial fluid. It is usually located under the proximal nail fold and may cause nail plate deformity and groove due to pressure effect on the matrix.[2] Dermoscopy may show presence of linear branched and serpentine vessels when no compression is applied. The vessels may disappear after compression and show white bright areas instead (Fig. 10).[20,21] Treatment of myxoid cyst is difficult with a high recurrence rate and options include incision and drainage, intralesional sclerosant and steroids.[2]

MALIGNANT NAIL UNIT TUMORS

BOWEN'S DISEASE

Bowen's disease, also known as SCC in situ, is the most common malignant tumor of the nail.[2] It is a noninvasive tumor that most frequently affects middle-aged men.[2] It is associated with various predisposing factors such as trauma, immunosuppression and HPV infection, most commonly HPV type 16.[22] The tumor typically presents as a verrucous proliferation arising from the periungual area or nail bed. Subungual involvement presents with onycholysis which usually has an adjacent band of longitudinal melanonychia causing diagnostic confusion with malignant melanoma.[1] Less commonly, subungual erosions with oozing of fluid, erythronychia and fibrokeratoma-like lesions can be seen.[1,2,22] Dermoscopy of Bowen's disease shows melanonychia and warty growth with small hemorrhages. It can help in ruling out acral melanoma by the presence of surface scales and lack of a parallel ridge pattern.[23] Surgical removal with Moh's micrographic surgery is the treatment of choice for Bowen's disease. Other options include excision with a 5-mm margin, photodynamic therapy, topical 5% fluorouracil and 5% imiquimod but have a high risk of recurrence.[2,24]

SQUAMOUS CELL CARCINOMA

The majority of SCCs of the nail unit arise from longstanding lesions of Bowen's disease. Multiple predisposing factors include chronic paronychia, HPV infection, sun exposure and trauma. The tumor affects middle-aged men with a predilection for fingernails.[25] It most commonly presents as a warty growth originating from the lateral nail fold and the nail bed with nail disfigurement. Other associated findings include swelling, bleeding, ulceration and pain. The tumor closely mimics lesions of viral warts, onychomycosis and chronic paronychia leading to a late diagnosis.[25,26] Dermoscopy usually reveals irregular dilated blood vessels and erosions.[2,26] X-ray of the digit is of utmost importance to rule out bony involvement which is seen in 20% of the cases.[27] Moh's micrographic surgery remains the treatment of choice. Other treatment modalities include curettage, electrodessication, cryosurgery, carbon dioxide laser and radiation therapy. Because of low but devastating risk of metastasis tumors with bone invasion, this complication is usually managed with amputation of the distal phalynx.[27,28]

BASAL CELL CARCINOMA

Basal cell carcinoma although being the most common malignancy to occur in skin is the least common malignancy of the nail unit.[29] It usually occurs in the thumb nail and shows a male predilection.[30] Clinical presentation can vary from longitudinal melanonychia with onycholysis and ulceration. Treatment options include topical imiquimod, electrodessication, and Moh's micrographic surgery.[29]

MALIGNANT MELANOMA

Malignant melanoma is a rare condition, seen in around 1.5–2% of the Caucasian population with a higher prevalence in Asian and Afro-Americans.[30] It has two patterns of presentation, namely longitudinal melanonychia and amelanotic melanoma. Longitudinal melanonychia of a single digit is the most common clinical presentation affecting the fingers (Fig. 11) more than toes. An ABCDEF rule has been proposed to help with early diagnosis of subungual melanoma as shown in Table 3.[31]

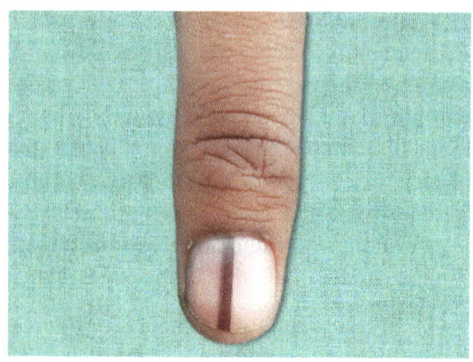

Fig. 11: Clinical picture of longitudinal pigmented band in the fingernail.

Table 3: Diagnostic algorithm for ungual melanoma.[32]

A	Age (5–7 th decade)
B	Border (irregular/blurred) Brown-black pigment Band irregularity Breadth > 3 mm
C	Change—Rapid increase in size/growth of the nail band
D	Dystrophy of nail Digit, i.e. Thumb > Hallux > Index finger > Single digit > Multiple digits
E	Extension to surrounding skin of proximal or lateral nail fold, i.e. Hutchinson's sign
F	Family/Personal history of melanoma

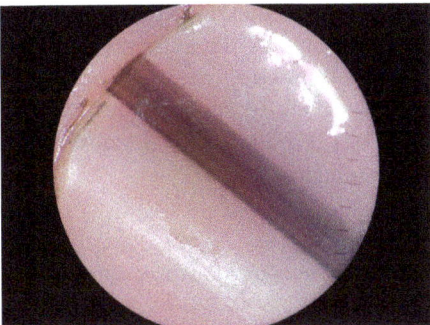

Fig. 12: Longitudinal pigmented band; uniform gray in color with no color variation and parallel edges suggestive of benign melanocyte activation.

Dermoscopy provides better visualization of these features such as band regularity and spacing (Fig. 12) included in the ABC rule. It can help in early detection of the Hutchinson's sign, which is called micro-Hutchinson's sign.[2,32] A melanotic tumor of the nail unit which accounts for about one-fourth of the cases, is more difficult to diagnose. It may present with absence of nail plate, nail bed hyperkeratosis, ulceration with occasional small pigmented tints to a pink or a granulomatous mass which can be better appreciated on dermoscopy.[2]

Prognosis depends on the Breslow and Clark's level of invasion, presence of ulceration and absence of pigment. However, treatment of choice remains excision of the tumor.[2,30]

CONCLUSION

A high index of suspicion is important on clinical examination. Histopathology is the gold standard for the diagnosis of nail tumors. However, a combination of radiological investigations like X-ray, high-resolution ultrasonography, color Doppler and MRI, and onychoscopy permits better diagnosis and management, especially when correlated with clinical and pathologic findings. Intraoperative dermoscopy adds a new dimension to the diagnosis.

REFERENCES

1. Baran R, Richert B. Common nails tumors. Dermatol Clin. 2006;24(3):297-311.
2. Seibert NR, Meehan RE. Nail Disorders. Essential Orthopaedics. Philadelphia, PA: Elsevier Health Sciences; 2010. pp. 803-5.
3. Grover C, Khurana A. Nail Tumors. In: Sacchidanand S, Savitha AS (Eds). Nail and Its Disorders. New Delhi: Jaypee Brothers Medical Publishers (P) Ltd.; 2013.
4. Alessandrini A, Starace M, Piraccini BM. Dermoscopy in the evaluation of nail disorders. Skin Appendage Disord. 2017;3(2):70-82.
5. Herschthal J, McLeod MP, Zaiac M. Management of ungual warts. Dermatol Ther. 2012;25(6):545-50.
6. Piraccini BM, Bellavista S, Misciali C, et al. Periungual and subungual pyogenic granuloma. Br J Dermatol. 2010;163(5):941-53.
7. Zaballos P, Carulla M, Ozdemir F, et al. Dermoscopy of pyogenic granuloma: a morphological study. Br J Dermatol. 2010;163(6):1229-37.
8. Alessandrini A, Bruni F, Starace M, et al. Periungual Pyogenic Granuloma: The Importance of the Medical History. Skin appendage disorders. 2015;1(4):175-8.
9. Girisha BS, Shenoy MM, Mathias M, et al. Glomus tumor of the nail unit. Indian J Dermatol. 2011;56(5):583.

10. Sena L De, Maehara N. Diagnosis of glomus tumor by nail bed and matrix dermoscopy. An Bras Dermatol. 2010;85(2):236-8.
11. Joo HJ, Kim MR, Cho BK, et al. Onychomatricoma: A rare tumor of nail matrix. Ann Dermatol. 2016;28(2):237-41.
12. Lesort C, Debarbieux S, Duru G, et al. Dermoscopic Features of Onychomatricoma: A Study of 34 Cases. Dermatology. 2015;231(2):177-83.
13. Ginoux E, Perier Muzet M, Poulalhon N, et al. Intraoperative dermoscopic features of onychomatricoma: a review of 10 cases. Clin Exp Dermatol. 2017;42(4):395-9.
14. Sobjanek M, Michajlowski I, Peksa R, et al. Onychopapilloma—a rare tumour of the nail apparatus. Przegląd Dermatologiczny. 2013;100(6):374.
15. Tosti A, Schneider SL, Ramirez-Quizon MN, et al. Clinical, dermoscopic, and pathologic features of onychopapilloma: A review of 47 cases. J Am Acad Dermatol. 2016;74(3):521-6.
16. Kim YS, Lee JH, Park YM, et al. Multiple Acquired Periungual Fibrokeratoma. Ann Dermatol. 2016;28(4):513-4.
17. Rubegni P, Poggiali S, Lamberti A, et al. Dermoscopy of acquired digital fibrokeratoma. Australasian J Dermatol. 2012;53(1):47-8.
18. Devi B, Dash B, Behera MRP. Multiple Koenen Tumors: An Uncommon Presentation. Indian J Dermatol. 2011;56(6):772.
19. Piccolo V, Argenziano G, Alessandrini AM, et al. Dermoscopy of Subungual Exostosis: A Retrospective Study of 10 Patients. Dermatology. 2017;233(1):80-5.
20. Salerni G, González R, Alonso C. Dermatoscopic pattern of digital mucous cyst: report of three cases. Dermatol Pract Concept. 2014;4(4):65-7.
21. Chae JB, Ohn J, Mun JH. Dermoscopic features of digital mucous cysts: A study of 23 cases. J Dermatol. 2017;44(11):1309-12.
22. Perruchoud DL, Varonier C, Haneke E, et al. Bowen disease of the nail unit: a retrospective study of 12 cases and their association

with human papillomaviruses. J Eur Acad Dermatology Venereol. 2016;30(9):1503-6.
23. Nakayama C, Hata H, Homma E, et al. Dermoscopy of periungual pigmented Bowen's disease: its usefulness in differentiation from malignant melanoma. J Eur Acad Dermatol Venereol. 2016;30(3):552-4.
24. Haneke E. Important malignant and new nail tumors. JDDG: J Deutschen Dermatol Gesellschaft. 2017;15(4):367-86.
25. Kok WL, Lee JSS, Chio MT. Subungual Squamous Cell Carcinoma: The Diagnostic Challenge and Clinical Pearls. Case Rep Dermatol. 2016;8(3):272-7.
26. Teysseire S, Dalle S, Duru G, et al. Dermoscopic Features of Subungual Squamous Cell Carcinoma: A Study of 44 Cases. Dermatology. 2017;233(2-3):184-91.
27. Spencer JM. Malignant tumors of the nail unit. Dermatol Ther. 2002;15(2):126-30.
28. Sen S, Bandyopadhyay D. Periungual basal cell carcinoma: A case report with review of literature. Indian J Dermatol. 2011;56(2):212.
29. Forman SB, Ferringer TC, Garrett AB. Basal cell carcinoma of the nail unit. J Am Acad Dermatol. 2007;56(5):811-4.
30. Haneke E. Ungual melanoma—Controversies in diagnosis and treatment. Dermatol Ther. 2012;25(6):510-24.
31. Levit EK, Kagen MH, Scher RK, et al. The ABC rule for clinical detection of subungual melanoma. J Am Acad Dermatol. 2000;42(2 Pt 1):269-74.
32. Chiacchio ND, Farias DC, Piraccini BM, et al. Consensus on melanonychia nail plate dermoscopy. An Bras de Dermatol. 2013;88(2):309-13.

CHAPTER 21

Nail Psoriasis versus Onychomycosis

Tulika Yadav, Uday S Khopkar

DERMOSCOPY OF NAIL PSORIASIS

Psoriasis affecting the nails is a significant cause of morbidity in these patients. It affects approximately 50% of psoriasis patients.[1] Dermoscopy can help us to identify nail involvement in psoriasis. Also, dermoscopy is useful as a tool in detecting improvement in nail psoriasis after treatment with biologics.[2] Two common patterns of nail changes observed in nail psoriasis are:

1. *Nail matrix involvement*: Leukonychia, pitting (punctate or cupuliform depressions) (Fig. 1), red spots in the lunula and crumbling.
2. *Nail bed involvement*: Onycholysis, salmon or oil-drop patches, subungual hyperkeratosis, and splinter hemorrhages.[3]

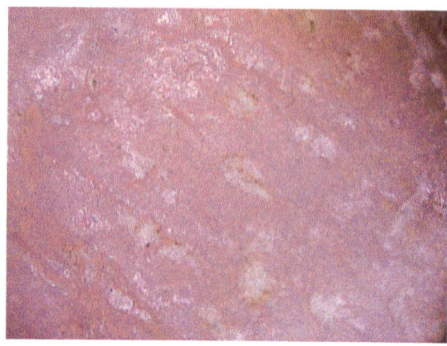

Fig. 1: Psoriasis: Coarse, irregular pits over the nail plate in psoriasis through video dermoscope. (40× white light)

Clinical findings seen on the nail plate are better appreciated through white light of a video dermoscope, whereas polarized light is more useful in distinguishing subungual features. Distinctive features seen on dermoscopy of the nail includes coarse irregular depressions of various sizes and shapes corresponding to pitting of the nail seen clinically. They can be distinguished from pitting seen in alopecia areata (Fig. 2) by the fact that pits in alopecia areata are smooth, regular, shallow, and rounded. On examining the nail bed in psoriasis, dilated globose vessels (Figs. 3 and 4), red in color with a prominent halo, are seen arranged in parallel rows at the onychodermal band.[4] They correspond to dilated vessels in the skin in a psoriasis patient (Fig. 4).[5] In contrast, splinter hemorrhages (Fig. 5) on dermoscopy appear as elongated streak of purple to black stain on the nail plate. Onycholysis appears as yellowish

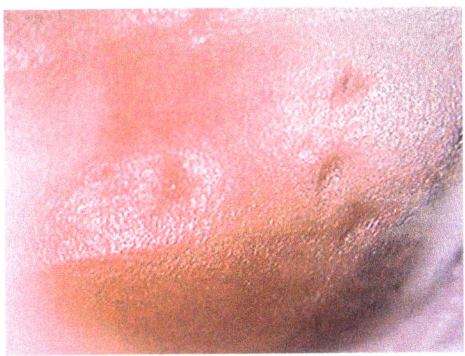

Fig. 2: Alopecia areata: In contrast, smooth, rounded, regular pits of alopecia areata seen on a video dermoscope. (40× white light)

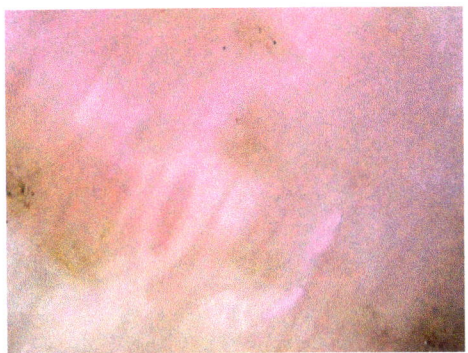

Fig. 3: Psoriasis: Dilated, globose vessels with a prominent halo at the onychodermal band in psoriasis. (40× polarized light)

316 SECTION 5: Nail Disorders

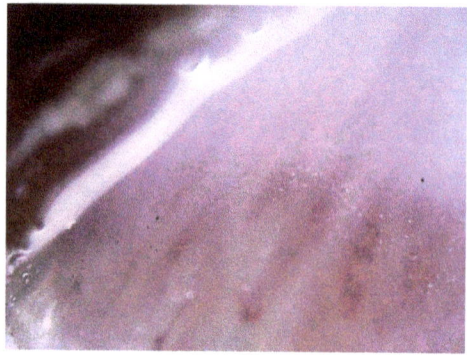

Fig. 4: Psoriasis: Similar dilated vessels with prominent halo seen in psoriasis. (40× polarized light)

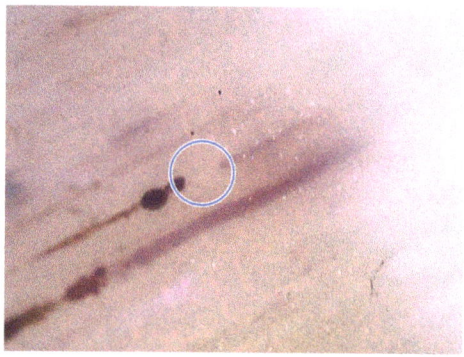

Fig. 5: Psoriasis: Splinter hemorrhages appearing as purple to black linear streaks over the nail plate in psoriasis. (40× polarized light)

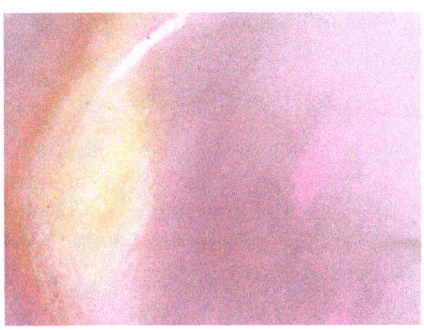

Fig. 6: Psoriasis: Onycholysis appears as yellowish orange stain with an ill-defined margin with the normal nail. (40× video dermoscope using polarized light)

Table 1: Summary of dermoscopic features of nail psoriasis and their correlation with histopathology.

Clinical features	Dermoscopic features	Histopathological features
Pits over nail plate	Coarse irregular depressions	Grouped parakeratosis
Onychodermal vessels	Dilated red globose vessels with a prominent halo	—
Splinter hemorrhages (rarely seen with naked eyes)	Streak of purple to black stain	Red blood cells or hemosiderin within nail plate
Onycholysis	Yellowish orange stain with an ill-defined margin	Clefts in nail plate, next to parakeratotic cells
Leukonychia	White and yellow irregular areas	Parakeratosis with plasma

orange stain with an ill-defined margin with the normal nail (Fig. 6; Table 1).

ONYCHOMYCOSIS

Onychomycosis is a common disease affecting the nail. It occurs due to dermatophytic as well as nondermatophytic infection of the nail. The prevalence of onychomycosis in India is around 54% by culture and/or direct examination.[6] Onychomycosis is classified into four types with distal lateral subungual onychomycosis (DLSO) being the most common.[7] Other types include proximal subungual onychomycosis, white superficial and total dystrophic onychomycosis. Through a dermoscope, onychomycosis cases demonstrated jagged edges with longitudinal streaks with a sharp demarcated edge while lesions diagnosed as traumatic onycholysis had linear edges without spikes.[8] This is helpful in distinguishing distal lateral onychomycosis from traumatic onycholysis (Table 2 and Fig. 7).[9]

Table 2: Differentiating features between dermoscopy of onycholysis and distal lateral onychomycosis.

Onycholysis including due to psoriasis	Distal lateral onychomycosis
Ill-defined margins between the separated part of the nail and the normal nail	Sharply demarcated margins between the affected areas and the normal nail
Margins of separation have smooth edges	Affected nail plate shows jagged edges with longitudinal streaks invading the normal nail
Appears yellow to orange in color	Can occur in any color depending upon the fungus (multicolored streaks resembling Aurora Borealis)

CHAPTER 21: Nail Psoriasis versus Onychomycosis

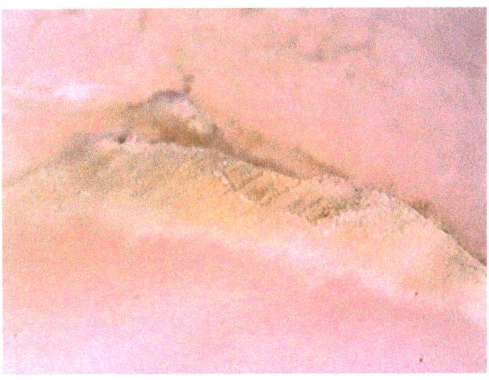

Fig. 7: Onychomycosis: In contrast, jagged edges of distal lateral onychomycosis seen with longitudinal streaks. (40× video dermoscope with polarized light)

Differentiating nail psoriasis from onychomycosis is a common challenge in a dermatology clinic. Clinical features of both the conditions overlap with nail plate discoloration and thickening and subungual hyperkeratosis being common to both the conditions. Potassium hydroxide (KOH) mount and culture certainly add to the clinical acumen but are time-consuming. Hence, onychoscopy can come to the help of clinicians only if one is familiar with the dermoscopic signs of both.

Affection of toenail due to psoriasis or onychomycosis is on increase, use of dermoscopy in some of these clinical conditions may save some time and money for our patients.

REFERENCES

1. Armesto S, Esteve A, Coto-Segura P, et al. Nail psoriasis in individuals with psoriasis vulgaris: a study of 661 patients. Actas Dermosifiliogr. 2011;102:365-72.
2. Hashimoto Y, Uyama M, Takada Y, et al. Dermoscopic features of nail psoriasis treated with biologics. J Dermatol. 2017;44:538-41.
3. Schons KRR, Knob CF, Murussi N, et al. Nail psoriasis: a review of the literature. Anais Brasileiros de Dermatologia. 2014;89(2): 312-7.
4. Yadav TA, Khopkar US. Dermoscopy to Detect Signs of Subclinical Nail Involvement in Chronic Plaque Psoriasis: A Study of 68 Patients. Indian J Dermatol. 2015;60(3):272-5.
5. Heidenreich R, Röcken M, Ghoreschi K. Angiogenesis drives psoriasis pathogenesis. Int J Experiment Pathol. 2009;90(3): 232-48.
6. Kaur R, Kashyap B, Bhalla P. A five-year survey of onychomycosis in New Delhi, India: Epidemiological and laboratory aspects. Indian J Dermatol. 2007;52:39-42.
7. Elewski BE. Onychomycosis: Pathogenesis, Diagnosis, and Management. Clin Microbiol Rev. 1998;11(3):415-29.
8. Yadav TA, Khopkar US. White streaks: Dermoscopic sign of distal lateral subungual onychomycosis. Indian J Dermatol. 2016;61:123.
9. Piraccini BM, Balestri R, Starace M, et al. Nail digital dermoscopy (onychoscopy) in the diagnosis of onychomycosis. J Eur Acad Dermatol Venereol. 2013;27(4):509-13.

CHAPTER 22

Nailfold Capillaroscopy in Connective Tissue Diseases

Pinanky Jadhav, Uday S Khopkar

HISTORICAL BACKGROUND

Giovanni Rasori (1766–1837), an Italian physician, was the first one to describe the close relationship between conjunctival inflammation and presence of an "inextricable knot of capillary loop" using a magnifying lens. Maricq and LeRoy in 1973, for the first time, described capillaroscopic patterns in systemic sclerosis (SSc). They also described the changes in the capillary blood flow that occurs during cold exposure in both primary and secondary Raynaud's phenomenon (RP).[1] Cutolo et al. first described three major patterns in nailfold capillaroscopy (NC) of SSc in year 2000.[2]

NEED FOR NAILFOLD CAPILLAROSCOPY IN CONNECTIVE TISSUE DISEASES

Raynaud's phenomenon may be primary (without an underlying disease) or secondary (with underlying connective tissue disease–CTD) and is frequently the presenting symptom of SSc. Primary and secondary RP are diagnosed on the basis of clinical criteria (i.e. the patient's history and a general physical examination), laboratory criteria (increase in erythrocyte sedimentation rate and the presence of antinuclear antibodies), and NC findings.[3] Presence of this scleroderma pattern in adults with RP indicates potential for development of a CTD even in the absence of other disease symptoms.

PATHOGENESIS

Vascular abnormalities in patients with RP may be purely functional (primary RP) or both functional and structural (secondary RP as in SSc). Functional abnormalities occur due to involvement of the endothelium while structural vascular abnormalities occur in both the microcirculation and the digital arteries of patients with SSc. This causes reduction in the number of capillaries as well as dilatation of capillaries.[4]

CAPILLAROSCOPIC MICROVASCULAR MORPHOLOGY IN RAYNAUD'S PHENOMENON

Normal individuals or patients with primary RP show hairpin-shaped capillary loops, regular capillary diameters, and density without any dystrophy arranged along the nailbed (Figs. 1A and B).

CHAPTER 22: Nailfold Capillaroscopy in Connective Tissue Diseases

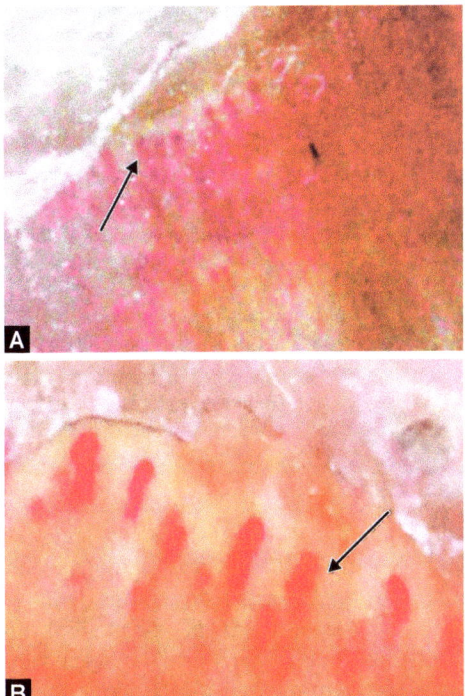

Figs. 1A and B: Normal nailfold videocapillaroscopy pattern: Regular diameter and density, linear 30 capillaries per 5 mm, no architectural derangement.

In patients with secondary RP, presence of the following capillaroscopic findings indicates the possibility of a CTD not yet detected[5] (Table 1).

Table 1: Significance of capillaroscopic findings.

Capillaroscopic morphology	Significance
Giant capillaries	They result from abnormal angiogenic response to peripheral ischemia. Enlarged capillaries are specific for SSc and DMS
Local microhemorrhages	They result from direct injury to capillaries by ischemia/reperfusion
Avascular areas	The severity reflects the peripheral circulatory disturbance. Patients with severe capillary loss frequently develop intractable skin ulcers
Ramified/bushy capillaries	Patients having advanced vascular damage often develop ramification around avascular areas. They occur due to abnormal angiogenic response to peripheral ischemia

(SSc: systemic sclerosis; DMS: dermatomyositis)

- The earliest and most striking changes include presence of giant (enlarged) capillaries, homogeneous, and/or irregularly enlarged microvascular loops.
- Architectural derangement of the nailfold microvasculature—represents an early morphological feature.
- Angiogenesis—tortuous and arborized, capillary loop clusters with a pronounced shape heterogeneity including thin or large meandering and bushy capillaries commonly surrounded by capillary loop dropouts indicate angiogenesis.
- One of the most specific signs includes loss of capillaries with or without presence of avascular areas. A reduction in number of loops (<30 over 5 mm in the distal row of the nailfold).

- Local microhemorrhages—vertically oriented microhemorrhages are associated with the early vascular damage.

SCLERODERMA PATTERN

These capillaroscopic alterations as detected by NC in patients with SSc have been reclassified in three different patterns.[2] The patterns include:
- *"Early" NC pattern*: Few enlarged/giant capillaries, few capillary hemorrhages, relatively well-preserved capillary distribution, no evident loss of capillaries (Figs. 2A to C).
- *"Active" NC pattern*: frequent giant capillaries, frequent capillary hemorrhages, moderate loss of capillaries, mild disorganization of the capillary architecture, absent or mild ramified capillaries (Figs. 3A to D).
- *"Late" NC pattern*: Irregular enlargement of the capillaries, few or absent giant capillaries and hemorrhages, severe loss of capillaries with extensive avascular areas, disorganization of the normal capillary array, ramified/bushy capillaries (Figs. 4A and B).

CAPILLAROSCOPY PATTERN IN VARIOUS CONNECTIVE TISSUE DISEASES

- *Systemic sclerosis*: More than 95% of the patients with SSc present with architectural disorganization, giant capillaries, hemorrhages, loss of capillaries, avascular areas, and neovascularization as main microvascular abnormalities. It can be found in more than 87% of patients with diffuse SS and 61% of patients with limited cutaneous SS.[6]
- *Dermatomyositis (DMS)*: The distinctive microvascular pattern observed in SSc is also present in 27–83% of patients with DMS.

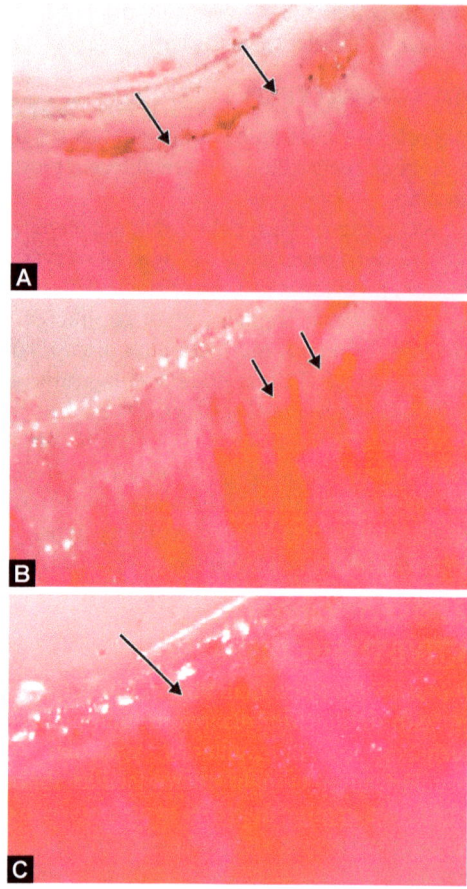

Figs. 2A to C: "Early" scleroderma pattern: Well-preserved capillary architecture and density, presence of enlarged capillaries and hemorrhages.

CHAPTER 22: Nailfold Capillaroscopy in Connective Tissue Diseases

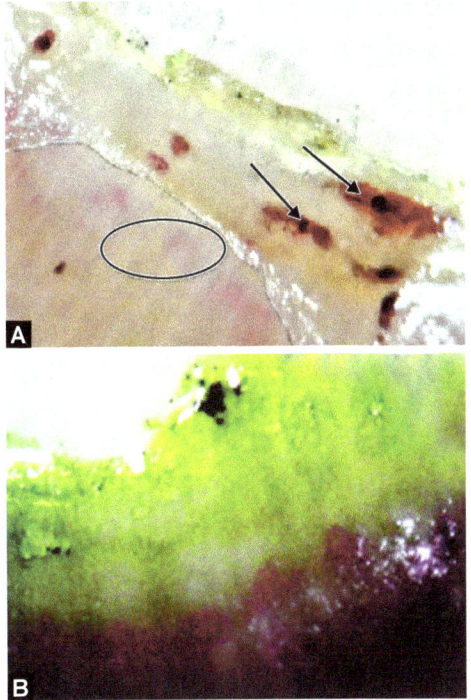

Figs. 3A and B

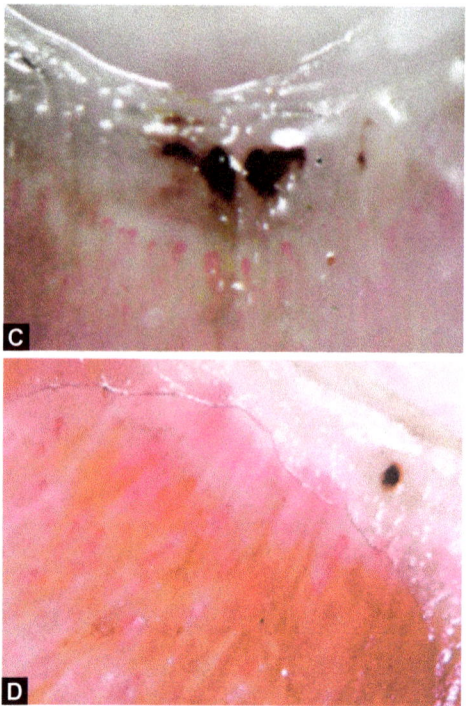

Figs. 3C and D

Figs. 3A to D: Active scleroderma pattern. (A) Loss of capillaries indicated by circle and hemorrhages shown by arrows; (B) Absent or mild ramified capillaries, occasional hemorrhage; (C and D) Frequent giant capillaries and hemorrhages, focal loss of capillaries and disturbed capillary architecture.

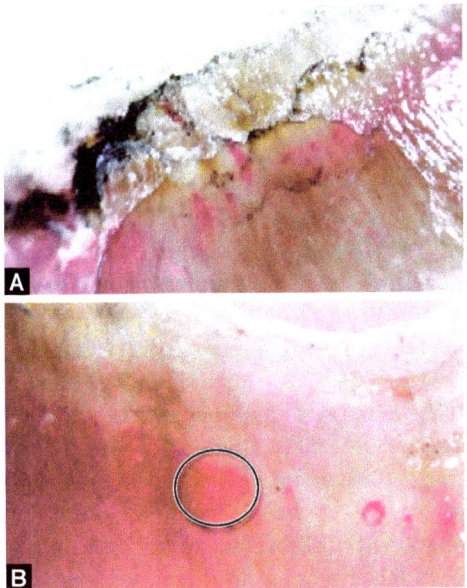

Figs. 4A and B: Late scleroderma pattern: Severe capillary architecture disorganization with loss of capillaries, presence of ramified capillaries, absence of giant capillaries, few or no hemorrhages.

- *Systemic lupus erythematosus*: Though typical scleroderma findings are rarely observed, enlarged capillaries and capillary loss can be observed sometimes. The capillary loss is considered as an indication of pulmonary capillary damage.[7,8]

    The presence of a typical scleroderma capillary pattern seems to be a rare finding seen in only 2–4.8% of patients.[8]

- *Mixed CTD*: The scleroderma capillary pattern and bushy capillary loops can be seen in this disease. About 64% of patients with mixed CTD have been found to have scleroderma-like changes.[8]

CONCLUSION

In a patient clinically suggestive of primary RP, even a single abnormality such as a megacapillary or an irregularly enlarged loop is highly indicative of an underlying CTD. The negative predictive value of NC for CTD is more than 90% in subjects with RP, whereas its positive predictive value is about 50% only, but this is higher than any other single screening test, more than a positive antinuclear antibody test.[9]

This method helps for adjuvant diagnosis of rheumatic diseases, for the follow-up of disease process and to assess disease severity. It has been recommended that 6 monthly capillaroscopic screening of cases with RP is a must to rule out underlying connective tissue disorder.

In 2001, addition of NC as additional minor criteria improved the sensitivity of the ACR criteria in identifying patients with limited disease from 34% to 89%.[10] Changes in nailfold capillaroscopic pattern may be able to predict the risk of pulmonary hypertension in SSc.[11]

REFERENCES

1. Maricq HR, LeRoy EC. Patterns of finger capillary abnormalities in connective tissue disease by Widefield microscopy. Arthritis Rheum. 1973;16:619-28.

2. Cutolo M, Sulli A, Pizzorni C, et al. Nailfold videocapillaroscopy assessment of microvascular damage in systemic sclerosis. J Rheumatol. 2000;27:155-60.
3. LeRoy EC, Medsger TA Jr. Raynaud's phenomenon: a proposal for classification. Clin Exp Rheumatol. 1992;10:485-8.
4. Herrick AL. Pathogenesis of Raynaud's phenomenon. Rheumatology (Oxford). 2005;44:587-96.
5. Cutolo M, Pizzorni C, Sulli A. Nailfold videocapillaroscopy in systemic sclerosis. Z Rheumatol. 2004;63:457-62.
6. Nagy Z, Czirjak L. Nailfold digital capillaroscopy in 447 patients with connective tissue disease and Raynaud's disease. J Eur Acad Dermatol Venereol. 2004;18:62-8.
7. Pallis M, Hopkinson N, Powell R. Nailfold capillary density as a possible indicator of pulmonary capillary loss in systemic lupus erythematosus but not in mixed connective tissue disease. J Rheumatol. 1991;18(10):1532-6.
8. Bergman R, Sharony L, Schapira D, et al. The handheld dermatoscope as a nailfold capillaroscopic instrument. Arch Dermatol. 2003;139(8):1027-30.
9. Luggen M, Belhorn L, Evans T, et al. The evolution of Raynaud's phenomenon: a long-term prospective study. J Rheum. 1995;22(12):2226-32.
10. Lonzetti LS, Joyal F, Raynauld JP, et al. Updating the American College of Rheumatology preliminary classification criteria for systemic sclerosis: addition of severe nailfold capillaroscopy abnormalities markedly increases the sensitivity for limited scleroderma [letter]. Arthritis Rheum. 2001;44(3):735-6.
11. Xia Z, Wang G, Xiao H, et al. Diagnostic value of nailfold videocapillaroscopy in systemic sclerosis secondary pulmonary arterial hypertension: a meta-analysis. Intern Med J. 2018;48(11):1355-9.

Section 6: Trichoscopy

CHAPTER 23

An Overview of Trichoscopy

Vidya Kharkar, Bhagyashri Abak

INTRODUCTION AND DEFINITION

Skin surface microscopy (dermoscopy) when done on scalp is termed as trichoscopy. Trichoscopy is a technique of evaluation of hair and scalp disorders and is used for establishing diagnosis in hair and scalp diseases.[1] It can also be utilized to visualize hair at magnifications ranging from 20-fold to 70-fold, and sometimes still higher.[2,3]

Trichoscopy is a rapid, simple, invaluable, innovative, effective, and a noninvasive method, which can save time and money to accomplish a precise diagnosis and correct treatment.[3] It assists visualization of the surface and subsurface structures.[4] It also helps in deciding prognosis of the disease and obviates the need for biopsy.

HISTORY

Trichoscopy was first used by Saitoh et al. to document the growth of hair in 1970.[5] The method was established by distinguished individuals directed by Lidia Rudnicka in Poland, Antonella Tosti and Giuseppe Micali in Italy, and Shigeki Inui in Japan. In 2005 Malgorzata Olszewska and Lidia Rudnicka first used videodermoscopy for evaluation of disease severity in androgenic alopecia and for monitoring treatment efficacy.[6] The term "trichoscopy" was first introduced by Lidia Rudnicka and Malgorzata Olszewska in 2006.[1]

TRICHOSCOPY EQUIPMENT

Trichoscopy may be done with either handheld dermatoscope or videodermatoscope. Handheld dermatoscopes allow 10-20 times magnification while 20-100 times magnification is common with digital dermatoscopes. Digital dermatoscopes provide the convenience of recording and storage of images and having higher magnifications.[7]

TRICHOSCOPY TERMINOLOGIES, STRUCTURES, AND PATTERNS

Structures which may be visualized by trichoscopy include hair shafts, hair follicle openings, perifollicular epidermis, and cutaneous microvessels.
- *Hair shafts*: Abnormalities in structure of the hair shaft can deliver essential diagnostic clues for several assimilated and inherited causes of hair loss. Normal hair shafts are even in contour and color with continuous, interrupted,

fragmented, or absent medulla.[8] Vellus hair constitute about 10% of normal human scalp hairs which are short, hypopigmented vellus hairs. In androgenic alopecia, an increased in proportion of vellus hairs is observed androgenic alopecia. Acquired hair shaft abnormalities, include micro-exclamation mark hairs, tapered hairs and tulip hairs [in alopecia areata (AA) and trichotillomania (TTM)], regrowing upright or pigtail hairs (in AA), and comma hair or corkscrew hairs (in tinea capitis). Trichoscopy also plays an important role in diagnosing many genetic hair shaft dystrophies, such as monilethrix, trichorrhexis nodosa, trichorrhexis invaginata, pili torti, or pili annulati.

- *Hair follicle openings*: "Dots" are a term applied to follicular openings seen by trichoscopy.[7] Trichoscopy assists in differentiating the status of follicular openings whether they are normal, empty, fibrotic, or having biological material in it, such as keratotic plug or hair residues.

Yellow dots (YDs) are follicular infundibula containing keratotic material and/or sebum. They vary in color, shape, and size. YDs (Fig. 1) are present in AA,[9] discoid lupus erythematosus (DLE), and androgenic alopecia.[3] YD can be observed in 60% of patients of AA and reflects the disease severity and prognosis. YDs are also be observed in cases of patterned hair loss. The preponderance in frontal area of YDs as compared to the occipital area favors the diagnosis of (female) androgenic alopecia.[3] YDs, looking like large "three-dimensional (3D)" soap bubbles located over dark

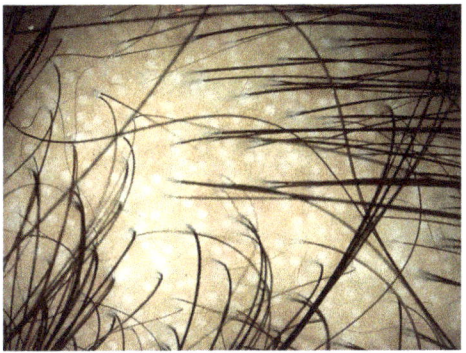

Fig. 1: Yellow dots.

dystrophic hairs, are specific for dissecting cellulitis (DC) of scalp.

Black dots (BDs) (formerly "cadaverized hairs"), characterize pigmented hair shafts which are damaged or destroyed at the level of scalp (Fig. 2).[7] They are detected in AA,[9] DC, tinea capitis, chemotherapy-induced alopecia (CIA), and TTM. Normal scalp or scalp with patterned alopecia does not show BDs.

White dots (WDs)—These correspond to perifollicular fibrosis and most frequently observed in (Fig. 3) late stages of androgenetic alopecia (AGA), follicles may be replaced by collagen tissue, causing permanent follicular loss. These empty follicular ostia can be observed as small and regular WD as compared to larger and irregular WD of lichen planopilaris (LPP). WDs have also been documented in the

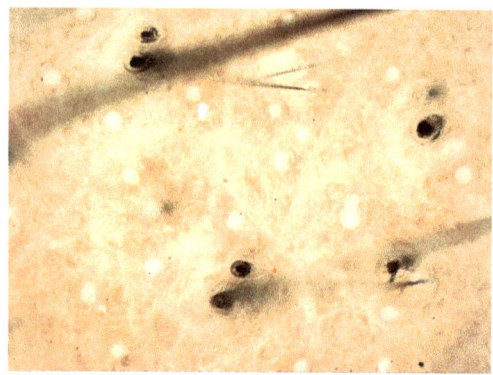

Fig. 2: Black dots.

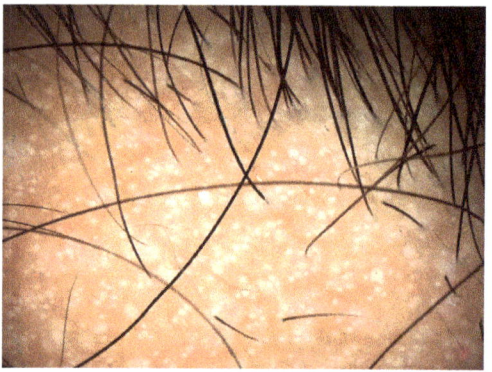

Fig. 3: White dots.

form of small, regular pinpoint white-colored dots that can be visualized in sun-exposed areas as well as in dark skin types regardless of hair loss.[10,11] They correspond to empty hair follicles or to the eccrine sweat duct openings.

Brown dots—Uniformly distributed brown-gray dots over eyebrow region is a better prognostic sign in patients with frontal fibrosing alopecia (FFA). Perifollicular brown areas (peripilar halo) are seen in AGA and TE and even on healthy scalp.

Red dots—Patchy distribution of brown-gray dots is seen in follicular lichen planus. Similar but irregular and larger dots are seen in discoid lupus in association with red dots and telangiectasia (Fig. 4).[12]

Gray dots—Pink gray and gray dots have been observed in the eyebrow area of patients with FFA.[13]

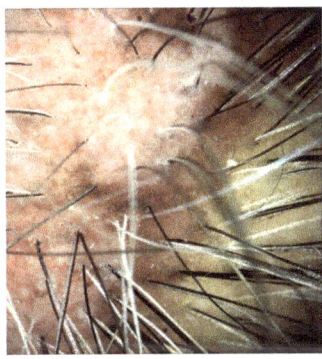

Fig. 4: Red dots.

Black-dotted pigmentation—In asymptomatic individuals, such pigmentation has been associated with *Demodex* infestation.[14] In another study on healthy children, such as tiny BDs were found to be due to nonmicrobial environmental particles on scalp (Fig. 5).[15]

- *Perifollicular and interfollicular epidermis*: Abnormalities of scalp skin color/structure may be divided into peripilar hyperpigmentation mainly seen in AGA and peripilar fibrosis mainly seen in fibrosing alopecias.[16] Perifollicular brown coloration (peripilar sign) (Fig. 6) and peripilar halo correlates with the histopathologic sign of perifollicular inflammation in AGA.[17] Up to 10% of healthy persons also show a positive peripilar halo on trichoscopy.[2]

Interfollicular epidermis shows reticulate hyperpigmentation (Fig. 7) in honeycomb pattern in normal skin in Fitzpatrick skin types IV, V, and VI especially over

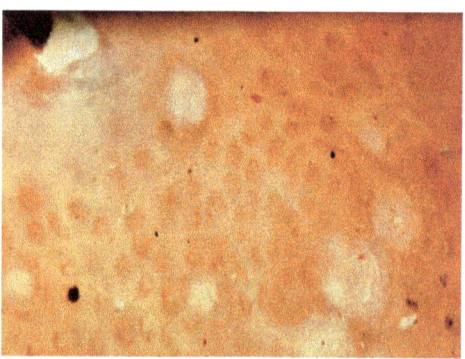

Fig. 5: Black dotted pigmentation (environmental dust).

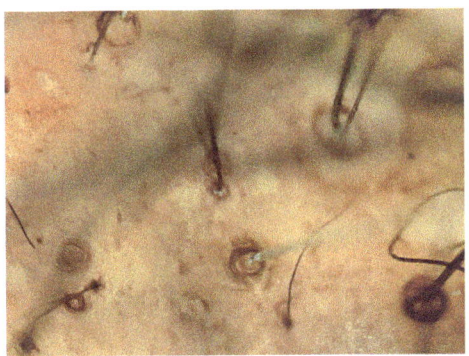

Fig. 6: Peripilar sign.

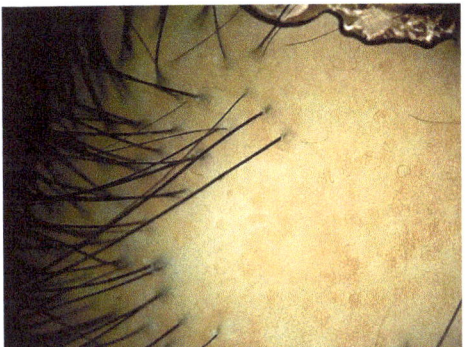

Fig. 7: Honeycomb pigmentation.

sun-exposed regions. Scattered brown discoloration is characteristic of DLE.[18]

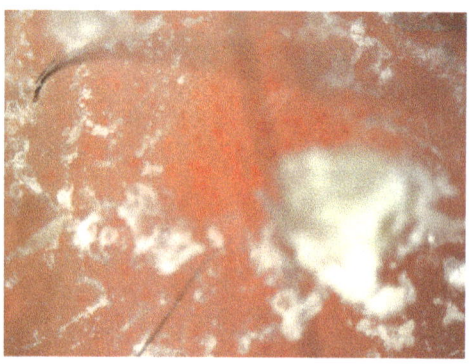

Fig. 8: Glomerular vessels.

- *Blood vessels*: The form of cutaneous microvessels that are observed on trichoscopy can differ depending on the type and number as well as on the disease and activity of the process. Vascular patterns in alopecia include linear telangiectasia in LPP, thick branching linear arborizing telangiectasia in discoid lupus and seborrheic dermatitis. Scalp seborrheic dermatitis also shows twisted red loops or comma vessels. Psoriasis shows twisted red loops, structureless red areas, signet ring vessels, atypical vessels, and coiled vessels in linear or circular alignment (Fig. 8).[3,13,18-20]

Other Structures

Other structures—Other trichoscopic signs are starburst pattern hyperplasia in folliculitis decalvans and yellow-red discharge in folliculitis decalvans, bacterial folliculitis, DC, and tinea capitis.[13,18]

TRICHOSCOPY OF NORMAL SCALP

Healthy scalp shows hairs arranged in follicular units each with two to four terminal hairs of uniform thickness and color and one to two vellus hair. Average thickness of terminal hair shafts is 0.06 mm^3. About 10% of normal scalp hair are of vellus type without any medulla.[2,16] The normal terminal hair display uniform thickness and coloration all throughout its length, the vellus hair can be lightly pigmented.[2] The red fine loops of capillaries observed in dermal papillae, can be observed on trichoscopy as linear arborizing vessels. A perifollicular pigment network can be observed in scalp of dark-skinned people. The sun-exposed areas display a typical honeycomb pattern. WDs are also observed which represent follicular openings and eccrine ducts.

NONCICATRICIAL ALOPECIA

It is characterized by the presence of empty follicular units.

ANDROGENETIC ALOPECIA/FEMALE PATTERN HAIR LOSS

The trichoscopic features of male and female pattern hair loss are similar. They can be observed mainly in the frontal region of the scalp.[2,3]

An increased ratio of vellus hairs to all hairs in androgen-dependent scalp regions is characteristic of AGA.[3,21-23] As per recent recommendation, female cases with more than six vellus hairs in the frontal region of scalp would suggest initial female AGA.[24] In early AGA, there are more multihair follicular unit than the single hair follicular units.[23]

The most important finding of AGA is the hair diameter variability (anisotrichosis) (Fig. 9) which reflects hair miniaturization. Hair miniaturization does not equally affect all hair follicles of the same area, resulting in the simultaneous presence of terminal, intermediate, and vellus hairs. When the hair diameter variability is more than 20%, of all the hairs in the same view, is considered as a hallmark of AGA in previous reports.[21,22,25]

- In addition to this, Rakowska A. formulated following three major diagnostic criteria for diagnosis of female AGA which gave 98% specificity 3.

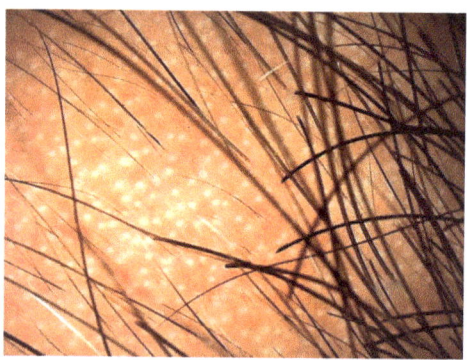

Fig. 9: Anisotrichosis in androgenetic alopecia (AGA).

CHAPTER 23: An Overview of Trichoscopy

- More than four YDs in four images (70-fold magnification) of the frontal area
- A lower than average hair thickness in the frontal area compared to the occipital area
- Vellus hairs (<0.03 mm) comprising more than 10% of hairs in the frontal area.[3]

The other features include YDs, pinpoint WDs, honeycomb pigmentation, focal atrichia, epidermal scaling, arborizing red lines, perifollicular brown and white discoloration (peripilar sign), an increased proportion of vellus hairs, and an increased proportion of follicular units with only one emerging hair shaft instead of two to four hair shafts.[3,13,23,25]

Trichoscopy of severe and advanced stages of AGA, display empty follicular ostia with yellow and brown dots along with honeycomb-like pigmented network in sun-exposed, bald areas.[7,22,23,26]

TELOGEN EFFLUVIUM (FIG. 10)

Telogen effluvium (TE) is a diagnosis of exclusion. It is characterized by:
- Presence of empty hair follicles
- Decreased hair density
- Increased single follicular hair units
- Perifollicular discoloration (peripilar sign)
- Short, dark, and multiple upright regrowing hairs of normal thickness[4,27]
- In absence of the characteristic features of other scalp disorders.

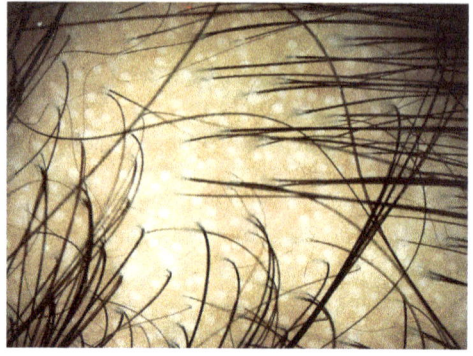

Fig. 10: Telogen effluvium showing empty hair follicle (yellow dots) with decreased hair density.

ALOPECIA AREATA

The most distinctive trichoscopic features include presence of BDs, exclamation mark hairs (Fig. 11), tapered hairs, broken hairs, coudability hairs (hairs of normal length with a narrowed proximal shaft and are mostly found in the scalp surrounding the alopecic patch), coiled hairs, YD, hypopigmented vellus hairs, trichorrhexis nodosa, monilethrix-like hairs (constrictions in the hair shaft), and Pohle–Pinkus constrictions.[7,9,13,21,22,28,29]

Coudability sign: The coudability hair which kinks when bent or pushed inward. This is considered as a sign of disease activity.

The indicators of status of the disease *activity* in AA are BDs (Fig. 12), exclamation marks, broken hairs, trichoptilosis, pig tail, short vellus hairs, and upright regrowing hair (Fig. 13).[30]

CHAPTER 23: An Overview of Trichoscopy

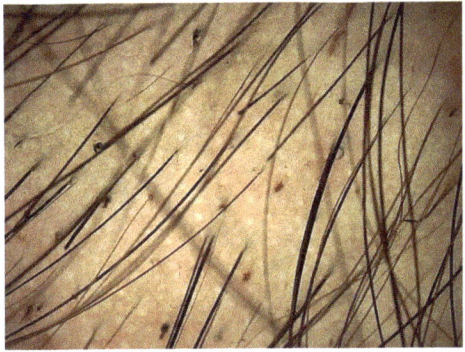

Fig. 11: Alopecia areata showing numerous broken hair shafts, yellow dots with regrowing tapered hair.

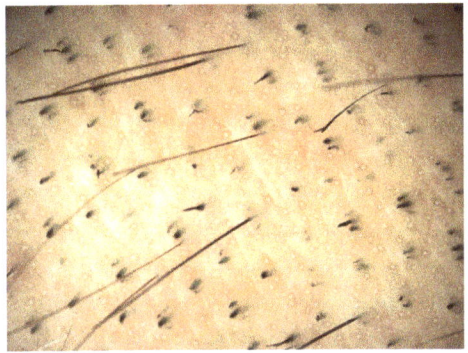

Fig. 12: Alopecia areata showing black dots and exclamation mark hair.

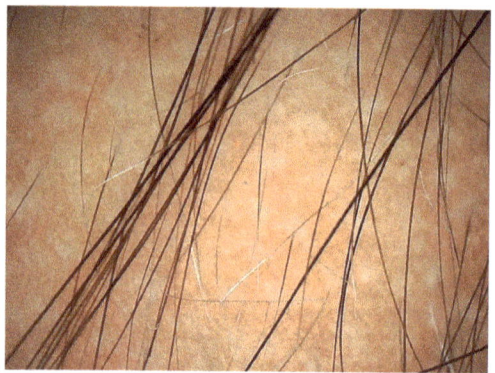

Fig. 13: Alopecia areata showing regrowing vellus hair.

Markers of disease *severity* and *inactive late stage* disease are YD, WD, honeycomb pigmentation, black-dotted pigmentation, and vellus hairs.[9,14,27]

Early features of *hair regrowth* (Fig. 13) are pigmented, upright, regrowing hairs,[9] *vellus hairs*, and pigtail hairs.[23]

TINEA CAPITIS (FIG. 14)

Tinea capitis is a kind of superficial fungal infection of the scalp, most commonly observed among children. Primarily causative agents include *Trichophyton* and *Microsporum* that invade the hair shafts. Comma hairs are comma-like structures that are associated with both ectothrix and endothrix types of fungal invasion.

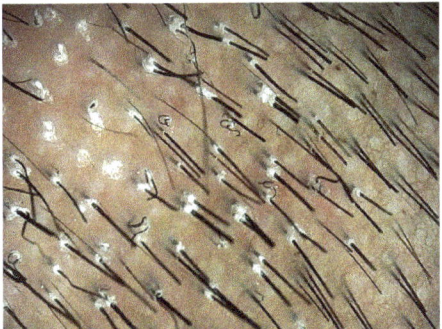

Fig. 14: Tinea capitis—comma hair, broken hair, and corkscrew hair.

Diagnostic trichoscopic features include the followings namely:
- Comma-shaped hairs, corkscrew hairs, BDs, short-broken hairs, and zigzag-shaped hairs.[31]
- Zigzag-shaped hairs or corkscrew (twisting-coiled) hairs are a variant of the comma hair.
- Also seen are the interrupted (morse code-like) hairs.

TRICHOTILLOMANIA (FIGS. 15A AND B)

Characteristic trichoscopic findings are:
- Broken/fractured hair shafts of different lengths (Fig. 15A).
- Short hair with trichoptilosis "split ends".
- Follicular microhemorrhages are characteristic sign of TTM. They appear as red dots next to or around follicular openings due to blood clot formed by traumatic forceful hair plucking.

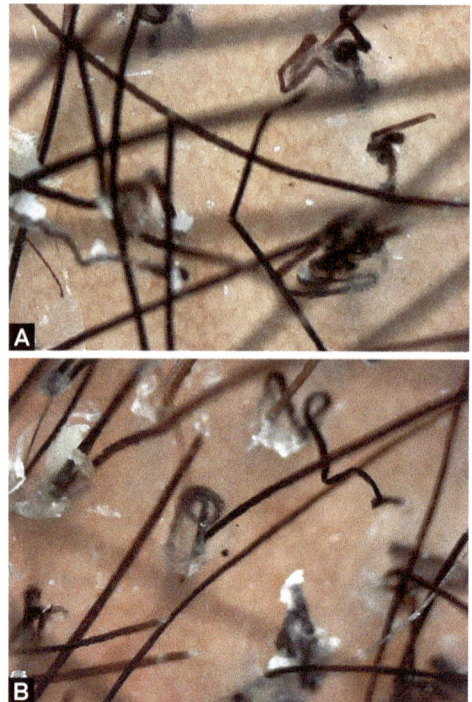

Figs. 15A and B: Trichotillomania. (A) Fractured hair shaft; (B) Irregular coiled hair.

- Hair breakage is visible on trichoscopy in various signs.
- Irregular coiled or twisted hairs are common as also scattered BDs.[32]
- Coiled hairs (Fig. 15B).

- *Flame hairs*: The term flame hairs refer to semitransparent, cone-shaped, and wavy hair residues that are left on the surface after pulling out of anagen hair.
- *V-sign*: Two or more broken hairs of same length coming out from one follicular opening have been termed as the V-sign.
- Tulip hair is used for diagonally broken shafts with tulip leaf-like pigmentation at the distal end.
- Exclamation mark hair or upright regrowing hair may be sometimes seen making distinction from AA difficult.[32,33]
- *Sprinkled hair*: Uncommonly "hair powder" (sprinkled hair) may result from extensive hair trauma.[32,33]
- *Exclamation mark hair*: The exclamation hair in AA has frayed distal ends and in TTM, it has blunt distal ends.[34]

TRACTION ALOPECIA

- *Early stage*: Hair casts are seen around the hair shafts at the periphery of the lesion (Fig. 16).[35]
- *Late stage*: Decreased hair density, predominance of single hair follicular units, and WDs without follicular opening (Fig. 17).[35]

Temporal Triangular Alopecia (TTA)/ Congenital Triangular Alopecia

Common trichoscopic findings include white hairs, vellus hairs, and hairs of diverse diameters. Others include empty follicles, white dots, yellow dots and arboriform vascular pattern. Less commonly seen are epidermal scale, broken hair,

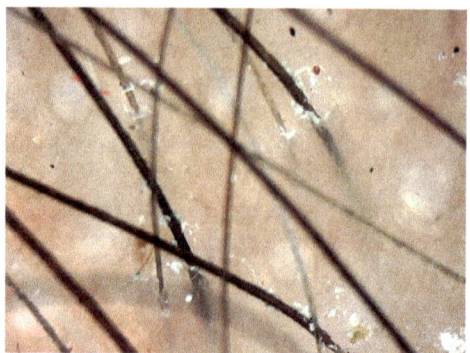

Fig. 16: Traction alopecia (early) hair cast.

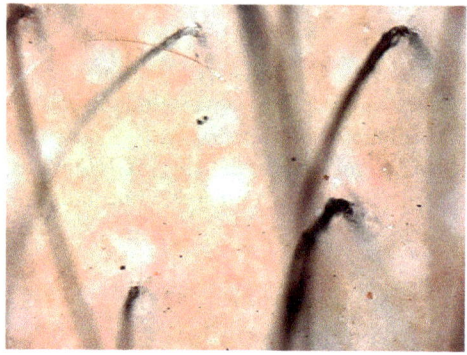

Fig. 17: Traction alopecia (late) white dots with decreased hair density.

black dot.[36] Exclamation hair is not seen. This differentiates it from alopecia areata.

CHEMOTHERAPY-INDUCED ALOPECIA

Trichoscopy of CIA displays BDs, YDs, acute constrictions and color changes along the hair shaft, tapering hairs (Fig. 18A) that is exclamation hairs, and coudability hairs.[37]

Two main alterations in the hair shafts of chemotherapy patients are (1) proximal tapering of the hair shaft (Fig. 18B)

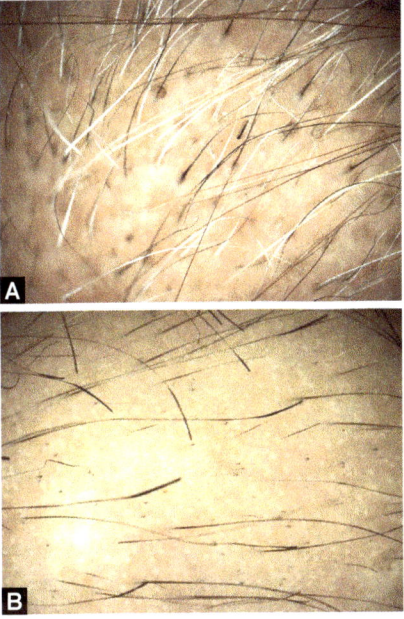

Figs. 18A and B: (A) Chemotherapy-induced alopecia. (A) Tapering hair shaft; (B) Acute constrictions and tapering.

and (2) acute constrictions, consistent to the consecutive courses of chemotherapy.
- Yellow dots, which develop due to accumulation of keratin and sebum within the follicular infundibulum, are sparsely observed in CIA.

SEBORRHEIC ALOPECIA AND SCALP PSORIASIS

Though it is difficult to differentiate seborrheic alopecia and scalp psoriasis clinically, involvement of the frontal hairline is characteristic of scalp psoriasis. Perifollicular scale (Fig. 19), possibly mixed with sebum in absence of YDs, BDs, or broken hairs, is a clue to diagnose seborrheic alopecia.[17]
- Psoriasis rarely causes hair loss, but when it does, it becomes difficult to ascertain the two diseases.

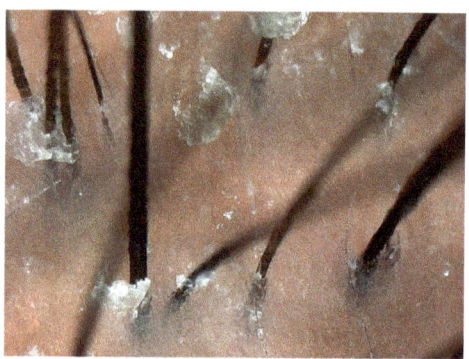

Fig. 19: Seborrhea—perifollicular scales.

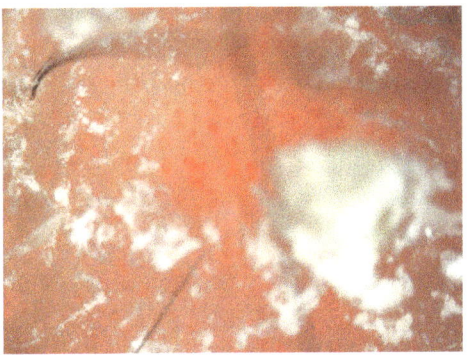

Fig. 20: Psoriasis scales with glomerular vessels.

- The red dots and globules, twisted red loops, and glomerular vessels that correspond to dilated capillaries of the dermal papillae, are typical of scalp psoriasis (Fig. 20).

In seborrheic alopecia, the significant findings are arborizing vessels and atypical red vessels.[20]

COMMON TRICHOSCOPIC DIFFERENCE OF PSORIASIS AND SEBORRHEIC DERMATITIS

The common trichoscopic difference of psoriasis and seborrheic dermatitis is given in Table 1.

CICATRICIAL ALOPECIAS

Lichen planopilaris, DLE, FFA, folliculitis decalvans and tufted folliculitis, pseudopelade of Brocq, central centrifugal alopecia,

Table 1: The common trichoscopic difference of psoriasis and seborrheic dermatitis.

Trichoscopic findings	Scalp psoriasis	Seborrheic dermatitis
Atypical red vessels	++	+
Red dots and globules	++	+
Signet ring vessels	++	+
Structureless red areas	++	+
Glomerular vessels	+	–
Twisted red loops	++	++
Perifollicular pigmentation	+	–
Hidden hair	+	+
Comma vessels	–	++
Arborizing red lines	–	+

and DC are some of the causes of cicatricial alopecia where dermoscopy may be contributory to diagnosis.

Lichen Planopilaris

Depending on disease stage and activity, trichoscopy features of LPP differ.

In active LPP—there is silvery-white perifollicular scaling with scales entangling hair shafts up to few millimeters above scalp surface. It is the most characteristic feature. The somewhat thicker scales stick to the proximal hair shafts emerging at surface and even migrate along the shaft and form tubular perifollicular scales (tubular casts) (Fig. 21).[18]

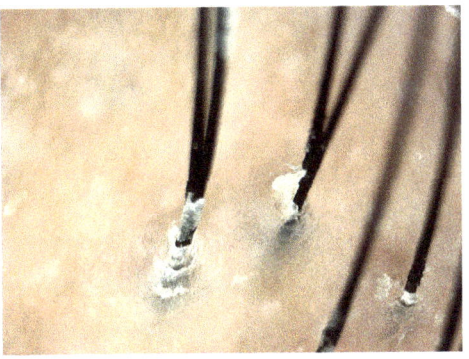

Fig. 21: Lichen planopilaris—tubular perifollicular scaling.

Presence of a group of two or three hairs surrounded by peripilar casts is suspicious of LPP.

Trichoscopy reveals the absence of follicular openings.

There is perifollicular inflammation and elongated, concentrically oriented blood vessels.

After the active phase, violaceous-blue interfollicular areas are seen which corresponds to pigment incontinence (Fig. 22).

In dark skin, LPP shows pinpoint WDs in the background of honeycomb pigment network forming a "starry sky pattern".

In the late fibrotic stage of LPP, important features are big, irregular (classic) WDs. These merge into milky-red (strawberry ice cream color) or white areas.[38] The milky red areas are fibrosis of recent origin and it fades eventually and changes to white patches.

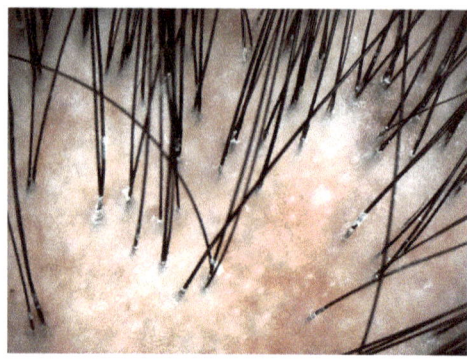

Fig. 22: Tubular perifollicular scaling with violaceous brown pigmentation.

Discoid Lupus Erythematosus

The large YDs are one of the most characteristic findings of active lesion of DLE, the large YDs observed in DLE are much larger and darker, and yellowish brown as compared to AA which are smaller and more yellowish.[18,38,39]

In chronic DLE, thin and radial arborizing vessels emerge from these dots ("red spider in YD" appearance) which is characteristic of DLE.[18,21]

Thick arborizing vessels (giant irregular capillaries) are commonly present at the periphery of the lesion.

Follicular red dots, described by Tosti et al.,[12] are characteristic features of active DLE and are a good prognostic factor for hair regrowth.

Long lasting, inactive DLE lesions show presence of structureless milky-red areas, and lack of follicular orifices.

Per- and interfollicular blue gray dots.
Honeycomb pigment pattern is lost.

Frontal Fibrosing Alopecia

Frontal fibrosing alopecia is a clinical variant of LPP, and is distinguished by the recession of the frontotemporal hairline.

- In *active* FFA, there is almost universal distribution of follicular ostia with only occasional "lonely hair" spared by the process.
- Frontal fibrosing alopecia can be differentiated from LPP by sharply demarcated interruption of the hairline in FFA and near absence of peripilar scaling in FFA.
- The lonely hair surrounded by WDs and lack of vellus hair are helpful clues to the diagnosis of FFA.
- In the *early fibrotic phase* of disease, the background color on dermoscopy is ivory white in FFA while it is milky red in LPP.[40,41] In contrast to classic LPP, where the background may be milky red.
- *Late* FFA is characterized by lack of follicular ostia.
- In the eyebrow area, trichoscopy shows regularly distributed red or gray dots throughout the course disease with some tendency to loss of follicular openings in very late and/or advanced disease.

Pseudopelade of Brocq

This is diagnosis by exclusion by trichoscopy as there is loss of follicular ostia, scattered terminal or dystrophic hair on patchy ivory-white background.

Central Centrifugal Alopecia

- Increased hair shaft variability and reduction in hair density
- Peripilar white halos and WDs that are pinpoint.
- Presence of asterisk-shaped pigmented macules with scant terminal and vellus-like hairs.
- The residual terminal hairs may emerge as a single hair or as a group of two hairs and are generally surrounded by a characteristic, peripilar gray-white halo.[22]

Folliculitis Decalvans and Tufted Folliculitis

- The hallmark sign of folliculitis is emergence of 15–20 hair shafts from a single dilated follicular opening.[42]
- Other features include starburst pattern displaying follicular hyperplasia, yellowish tubular scaling (with a collar-like widening at the distal end), crusting, and follicular pustules.
- Chronic lesions display white and milky red areas displaying lack of follicular openings.

Dissecting Cellulitis of Scalp

- In DC (dissecting folliculitis, perifolliculitis capitis abscedens et suffodiens), the most characteristic finding in trichoscopy is yellow, structureless areas and YDs with "3D" structure imposed over dystrophic hair shafts.
- Early stages display features similar to those observed in AA.
- Black dots are occasionally present.

- Pinpoint-like vessels with whitish halo.
- End-stage disease with scarring lesions display trichoscopic features similar to those of other scarring alopecia with confluent ivory-white areas lacking follicular ostia.

TRICHOSCOPY IN GENETIC HAIR SHAFT ABNORMALITIES

Normal hair is uniform in appearance and structure along the entire length of the hair shaft.

Monilethrix (Beaded Hair) (Fig. 23)

In monilethrix, trichoscopy shows identical elliptical nodes and alternating constrictions of the hair shaft, leading to variation in thickness of the hair shaft, giving a characteristic beaded appearance. Internodes are regularly distributed in

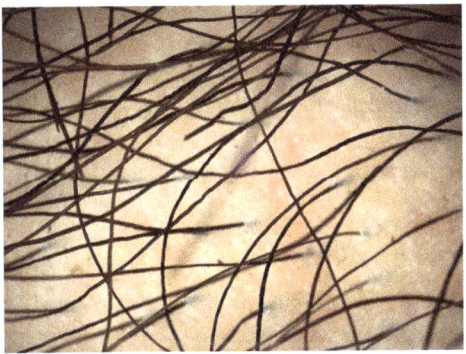

Fig. 23: Monilethrix showing beaded appearance.

constant intervals. Hairs shafts display regular bends and have a tendency to fracture at site of constriction.[43] "Regularly bended ribbon sign" is a term which differentiates monilethrix from pseudomonilethrix and other causes of hair loss.

Pili Annulati

Trichoscopy shows hair shafts with regular light bands. These features were visible in patients with dark and light hairs. In pili annulati, the medulla displays light-colored areas which constitute less than 50% of the hair shaft width. In normal thick hair shafts, "intermittent medulla" is observed, which can be wrongly diagnosed as pili annulati. Subtle glittering, shimmering appearance with alternating light and black areas. Regular width, white bands with misty appearance is also present occasionally.[44,45]

Pili Torti

Trichoscopy of in a case of pili torti displays regular twists of the hair shaft along the long axis. Other features include bending of the hair shafts at different angles and at irregular intervals. On microscopy, regularly spaced twists are seen at irregular intervals along the shaft. Changes will be seen only in few hairs and in only a part of the hair length.

Trichothiodystrophy

Trichoscopy in trichothiodystrophy is nonspecific. At a higher magnification, hairs showed a nonhomogeneous structure reassembling grains of sand within the hair shaft and a slightly wavy contour. On light microscopy, hair shafts with irregular, undulating contour and trichoschisis, i.e. transverse fractures through the hair shaft can be observed. Polarized light microscopy shows bright and dark bands (tiger-tail banding).

Trichorrhexis Nodosa

In trichorrhexis nodosa, the hair shaft displays longitudinal splits into numerous small fibers with a high tendency to break, giving an appearance reminiscent of the ends of two brushes aligned in opposition. Eventually, the hair shaft breaks at these points leaving hair shafts with brush-like ends.

Trichorrhexis Invaginata (Bamboo Hair)

Ball and socket type nodes are seen along hair shafts that resemble bamboos. The shaft break at the nodes formed due to invagination of the distal portion of the shaft into the proximal shaft. Broken hair shows cupped proximal end (golf-tee hair).

Netherton Syndrome

Trichoscopy of trichorrhexis invaginata at higher magnifications displays shows golf tee-like end.

Woolly Hair Syndrome

Trichoscopy of woolly hair syndrome shows hair shafts with a "crawling snake" appearance, with short wave cycles along with broken hair shafts. Light microscopy shows ovoid cross-sections, 180° longitudinal twisting, trichorrhexis nodosa and pili annulati.

INFESTATIONS

Pediculosis Capitis (Fig. 24)

Pediculosis capitis is reliably diagnosed using trichoscopy. It shows the presence of lice nits (empty or full of nymphs).[46] It helps in treatment monitoring of pediculosis capitis. It is a proof of the infestation that can be provided to the patients or their parents.

Trichoscopy is a simple, innocuous, and trustworthy technique which can be instrumental in detecting lice eggs containing nymphs displaying the closed operculum from empty cases of hatched parasites with free plane free ending with displaying open operculum and from amorphous pseudonits and hair casts.

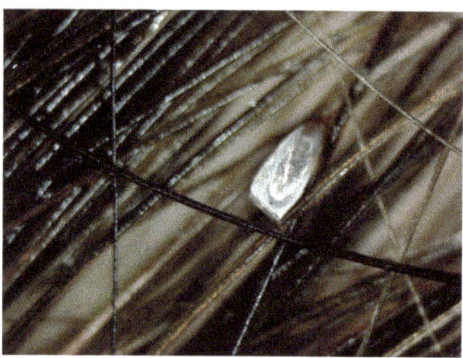

Fig. 24: Lice nits—Note flat free end indicating opened operculum.

CHAPTER 23: An Overview of Trichoscopy

Follicular Orifice (Flowchart 1)

- Look at the orifice on the scalp
- If it is lost, it is suggestive of cicatricial alopecia
- If preserved, it is noncicatricial alopecia.

Black Dots or Broken Hair (Flowchart 2)

- Look at the broken hairs
- Tapering hair or short vellus hair is s/o Alopecia areata
- Curled hair is s/o Trichotillomania

Flowchart 1: Algorithm of follicular orifices.

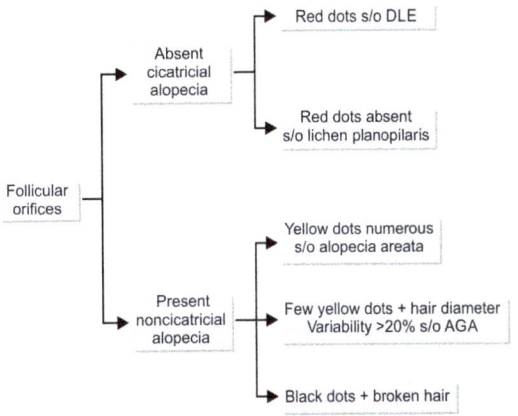

(AGA: androgenetic alopecia; DLE: discoid lupus erythematosus; s/o: signs and symptoms of)

Flowchart 2: Algorithm of black dots and/or broken hair.

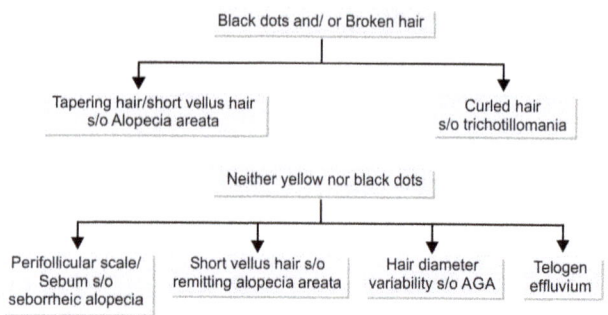

(AGA: androgenetic alopecia; s/o: signs and symptoms of)

REFERENCES

1. Rudnicka L, Olszewska M, Rakowska A, et al. Trichoscopy: a new method for diagnosing hair loss. J Drugs Dermatol. 2008;7(7):651-4.
2. Rakowska A. Trichoscopy (hair and scalp videodermoscopy) in the healthy female. Method standardization and norms for measurable parameters. J Dermatol Case Rep. 2009;3(1):14-9.
3. Rakowska A, Slowinska M, Kowalska-Oledzka E, et al. Dermoscopy in female androgenic alopecia: method standardization and diagnostic criteria. Int J Trichology. 2009;1(2):123-30.
4. Pedrosa AF, Morais P, Lisboa C, et al. The importance of trichoscopy in clinical practice. Dermatol Res Pract. 2013;2013:986970.
5. Saitoh M, Uzuka M, Sakamoto M. Human hair cycle. J Invest Dermatol. 1970;54(1):65-81.
6. Olszewska M, Rudnicka L. Effective treatment of female androgenic alopecia with dutasteride. J Drugs Dermatol. 2005;4(5):637-40.

7. Ross EK, Vincenzi C, Tosti A. Videodermoscopy in the evaluation of hair and scalp disorders. J Am Acad Dermatol. 2006;55(5):799-806.
8. Wagner R, Joekes I. Hair medulla morphology and mechanical properties—Abstract. J Soc Cosmet Chem. 2007;58(4):359-68.
9. Inui S, Nakajima T, Nakagawa K, et al. Clinical significance of dermoscopy in alopecia areata: analysis of 300 cases. Int J Dermatol. 2008;47(7):688-93.
10. de Moura LH, Duque-Estrada B, Abraham LS, et al. Dermoscopy findings of alopecia areata in an African-American patient. J Dermatol Case Rep. 2008;2(4):52-4.
11. Abraham LS, Piñeiro-Maceira J, Duque-Estrada B, et al. Pinpoint white dots in the scalp: dermoscopic and histopathologic correlation. J Am Acad Dermatol. 2010;63(4):721-2.
12. Tosti A, Torres F, Misciali C, et al. Follicular red dots. Arch Dermatol. 2009;145(12):1406-9.
13. Rudnicka L, Olszewska M, Rakowska A, et al. Hair follicle openings: Dots. In: Rudnicka L, Olszewska M (Eds). Atlas of Trichoscopy. London: Springer; 2012. pp. 47-71.
14. Kibar M, Aktan Ş, Lebe B, et al. Trichoscopic findings in alopecia areata and their relation to disease activity, severity and clinical subtype in Turkish patients. Australas J Dermatol. 2015;56(1): e1-6.
15. Fu JM, Starace M, Tosti A. A new dermoscopic finding in healthy children. Arch Dermatol. 2009;145(5):596-7.
16. Van Neste D. Natural scalp hair regression in preclinical stages of male androgenetic alopecia and its reversal by finasteride. Skin Pharmacol Physiol. 2006;19(3):168-76.
17. Inui S. Trichoscopy for common hair loss diseases: algorithmic method for diagnosis. J Dermatol. 2011;38(1):71-5.
18. Rakowska A, Slowinska M, Kowalska-Oledzka E, et al. Trichoscopy of cicatricial alopecia. J Drugs Dermatol. 2012;11(6):753-8.

19. Kibar M, Aktan Ş, Bilgin M. Dermoscopic findings in scalp psoriasis and seborrheic dermatitis; two new signs; signet ring vessel and hidden hair. Indian J Dermatol. 2015;60(1):41-5.
20. Kim GW, Jung HJ, Ko HC, et al. Dermoscopy can be useful in differentiating scalp psoriasis from seborrhoeic dermatitis. Br J Dermatol. 2011;164(3):652-6.
21. Rudnicka L, Olszewska M, Rakowska A, et al. Trichoscopy update 2011. J Dermatol Case Rep. 2011;5(4):82-8.
22. Miteva M, Tosti A. Hair and scalp dermatoscopy. J Am Acad Dermatol. 2012;67(5):1040-8.
23. Kibar M, Aktan S, Bilgin M. Scalp dermatoscopic findings in androgenetic alopecia and their relations with disease severity. Ann Dermatol. 2014;26(4):478-84.
24. Herskovitz I, de Sousa IC, Tosti A. Vellus hairs in the frontal scalp in early female pattern hair loss. Int J Trichology. 2013;5(3):118-20.
25. Inui S, Nakajima T, Itami S. Scalp dermoscopy of androgenetic alopecia in Asian people. J Dermatol. 2009;36(2):82-5.
26. Hu R, Xu F, Han Y, et al. Trichoscopic findings of androgenetic alopecia and their association with disease severity. J Dermatol. 2015;42(6):602-7.
27. Jain N, Doshi B, Khopkar U. Trichoscopy in alopecias: diagnosis simplified. Int J Trichology. 2013;5(4):170-8.
28. Tosti A, Duque-Estrada B. (2017). Dermoscopy in Hair Disorders. [online] Available from http://www.jewds.eg.net/pdf/vol_7_1/1.pdf. [Last accessed January, 2019].
29. Rudnicka L, Rakowska A, Olszewska M. Trichoscopy. Dermatol Clin. 2013;31(1):29-41.
30. Torres F, Tosti A. Trichoscopy: an update. G Ital Dermatol Venereol. 2014;149(1):83-91.

31. El-Taweel AE, El-Esawy F, Abdel-Salam O. Different trichoscopic features of tinea capitis and alopecia areata in pediatric patients. Dermatol Res Pract. 2014;2014:848763.
32. Rakowska A, Slowinska M, Olszewska M, et al. New trichoscopy findings in trichotillomania: flame hairs, V-sign, hook hairs, hair powder, tulip hairs. Acta Derm Venereol. 2014;94(3):303-6.
33. Abraham LS, Torres FN, Azulay-Abulafia L. Dermoscopic clues to distinguish trichotillomania from patchy alopecia areata. An Bras Dermatol. 2010;85(5):723-6.
34. Polat M. Evaluation of clinical signs and early and late trichoscopy findings in traction alopecia patients with Fitzpatrick skin type II and III: a single-center, clinical study. Int J Dermatol. 2017;56(8):850-5.
35. Fernández-Crehuet P, Vaño-Galván S, Martorell-Calatayud A, et al. Clinical and trichoscopic characteristics of temporal triangular alopecia: a multicenter study. J Am Acad Dermatol. 2016;75(3):634-7.
36. Ye Y, Zhang X, Zhao Y, et al. The clinical and trichoscopic features of syphilitic alopecia. J Dermatol Case Rep. 2014;8(3):78-80.
37. Pirmez R, Piñeiro-Maceira J, Sodré CT. Exclamation marks and other trichoscopic signs of chemotherapy-induced alopecia. Australas J Dermatol. 2013;54(2):129-32.
38. Duque-Estrada B, Tamler C, Sodŕe CT, et al. Dermoscopy patterns of cicatricial alopecia resulting from discoid lupus erythematosus and lichen planopilaris. An Bras Dermatol. 2010;85(2):179-83.
39. Lanuti E, Miteva M, Romanelli P, et al. Trichoscopy and histopathology of follicular keratotic plugs in scalp discoid lupus erythematosus. Int J Trichology. 2012;4(1):36-8.
40. Inui S, Nakajima T, Shono F, et al. Dermoscopic findings in frontal fibrosing alopecia: report of four cases. Int J Dermatol. 2008;47(8):796-9.

41. Rubegni P, Mandato F, Fimiani M. Frontal fibrosing alopecia: role of dermoscopy in differential diagnosis. Case Rep Dermatol. 2010;2(1):40-5.
42. Kang H, Alzolibani AA, Otberg N, et al. Lichen planopilaris. Dermatol Ther. 2008;21(4):249-56.
43. Rakowska A, Slowinska M, Czuwara J, et al. Dermoscopy as a tool for rapid diagnosis of monilethrix. J Drugs Dermatol. 2007;6(2):222-4.
44. Rakowska A, Slowinska M, Kowalska-Oledzka E, et al. Trichoscopy in genetic hair shaft abnormalities. J Dermatol Case Rep. 2008;2(2):14-20.
45. Wallace MP, De Berker DA. Hair diagnoses and signs: the use of dermatoscopy. Clin Exp Dermatol. 2010;35(1):41-6.
46. Bakos RM, Bakos L. Dermoscopy for diagnosis of pediculosis capitis. J Am Acad Dermatol. 2007;57(4):727-8.

CHAPTER 24

Trichoscopy of Patchy Alopecia

Viral Thakkar, Shekhar S Haldar

PATCHY NONSCARRING ALOPECIAS

Alopecia Areata

Alopecia areata (AA) is a common, autoimmune, and inflammatory disease involving hair follicles leading to patchy hair loss.[1] Dermoscopy shows many peculiar findings in AA and these differ according to the activity of the disease.

Purpose of Dermoscopy for Patchy Alopecia

Alopecia areata is usually diagnosed clinically. Sometimes, the clinical diagnosis may not be straightforward, and in such cases, biopsy is required for establishing diagnosis. Recent reports have indicated that AA shows upon dermoscopy certain distinctive findings, such as cadaverized hairs (black dots) (Figs. 1 and 2), exclamation mark hairs (tapering hairs), broken hairs, yellow dots, and clustered short vellus hairs in the hair loss areas.[2] Those findings taken together allow fairly reliable differentiation of AA from lichen planopilaris (LPP), pseudopelade, and tinea capitis.

Dermoscopic Findings of Alopecia Areata

Yellow dots: They are considered to be the most sensitive dermoscopic feature of AA. These are characterized by yellow round or polycyclic dots that vary in size and are uniform in color (Fig. 3). These represent distension of affected follicular infundibulum with keratinous material and sebum.[3]

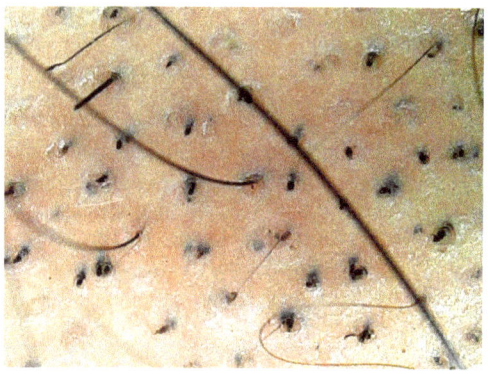

Fig. 1: Dermoscopic image of alopecia areata showing black dots: Black dots represent hair shafts that broke as soon as they reach surface, it is a marker of disease activity.

CHAPTER 24: Trichoscopy of Patchy Alopecia

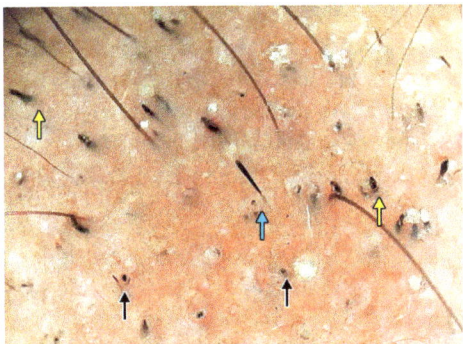

Fig. 2: Active alopecia areata showing black dots (black arrows), exclamation mark hair (blue arrows) and broken hair shafts (yellow arrows).

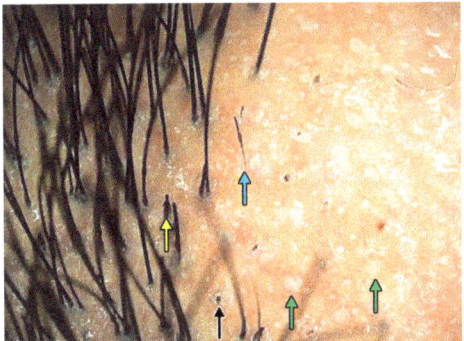

Fig. 3: Active border of alopecia areata showing exclamation mark hair (blue arrows), black dots (black arrows), broken hair (yellow arrow) and yellow dot (green arrow). Yellow dots represent distention of affected follicular infundibulum with keratinous material.

Short vellus hair: These are commonly seen and do have prognostic significance (indicates the potential for regrowth in AA). The regrowth of short vellus hairs, after treatment, can be quickly appreciated on dermoscopy, even when the regrowing hairs are difficult to make out by naked eye alone. These are seen as new, thin, and unpigmented hairs within the patch (Figs. 2 and 4).

Exclamation hair (tapering hair) and black dot and broken hair shaft: These are considered as a marker of disease activity and are known to reflect exacerbation of disease.[2] Exclamation mark hairs are short broken hairs that taper toward the root and are also lighter in color in their lowermost part (Fig. 5).

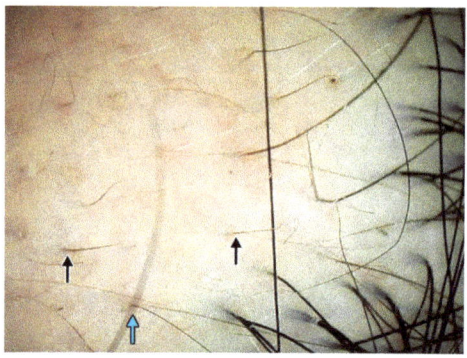

Fig. 4: Stable patch of alopecia areata showing several long depigmented hair (spared white hair, blue arrow) and shorter regrowing vellus hair (black arrows). Regrowing hair are lighter towards the tip and get progressively darker towards their roots.

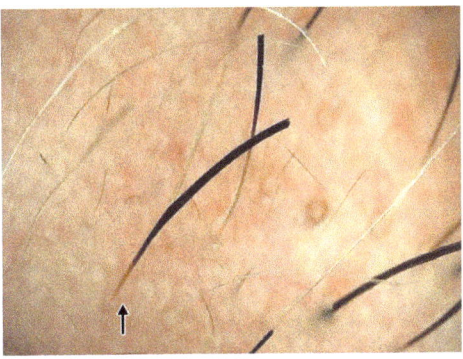

Fig. 5: Dermoscopic signs of activity and regrowth may at times be seen together in alopecia areata. This picture shows exclamation mark hair (black arrow) as well as regrowing vellus hair.

Black dots represent hair shafts that break as soon as they reach surface due to the weakness in shaft structure secondary to the affection of anagen matrix in AA. Break in the hair shafts seen a short distance from the scalp surface with a sharp angular cut are observed when the activity of the disease is high (Fig. 2). Multiple depressed follicular ostia may also be observed under dermoscopy (Figs. 2 and 6). It has been suggested that these represent abnormal hair follicles containing incompletely differentiated hair shafts.[3,4]

These dermoscopic findings are helpful for prognostication and judging the activity of disease in patients with AA. Broken hair, exclamation mark hair, and black dots (cadaverized hairs) all indicate active disease. The yellow dots and short vellus hairs enable AA to be differentiated from other hair loss disorders.

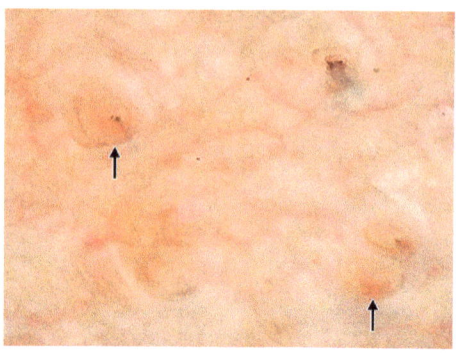

Fig. 6: Depressed follicular ostia (black arrows) in stable alopecia areata. These represent affected hair follicles containing incomplete differentiated hair shafts.

In addition, black dots, tapering hairs, and broken hairs are usually seen only in AA (except for trichotillomania). Hence, while a single dermoscopic feature may not be enough to reach a diagnosis of AA, the constellation of above findings are diagnostic for AA.

Tinea Capitis

Tinea capitis is the most common dermatophyte infection of childhood and has an increasing incidence worldwide. It may be inflammatory or noninflammatory in nature.[1]

Purpose of Dermoscopy for Tinea Capitis

Culture is usually considered as the gold standard to establish the diagnosis. The absence of a rapid, reliable, confirmatory test, coupled with a nonspecific presentation, means that patients often wait several weeks for a fungal culture result before commencing appropriate systemic therapy. Dermoscopy can be a quick, noninvasive, reliable, and reproducible method for diagnosing tinea capitis. It can be of diagnostic and prognostic importance.

Dermoscopy Findings in Tinea Capitis

Broken hair shaft: Shafts break at a short distance from the surface or at the surface (black dots) due to weakening of the shaft due to destruction by the fungal elements (Fig. 7).

Comma hair:[5] These short stubs of hair, seen near surface, are considered to be a specific finding of tinea capitis[2] (Fig. 7).

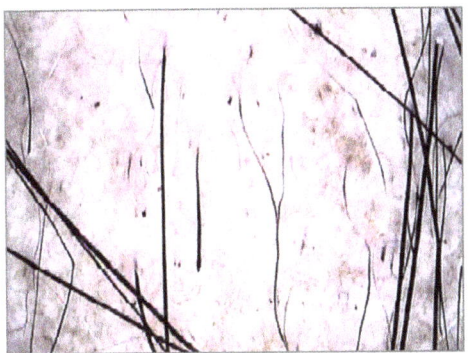

Fig. 7: Dermoscopic image of tinea capitis: Black dots, decreased hair density, and comma hair are seen.

Blotchy pigmentation: It is rarely seen with most of the hair loss disorder apart from LPP and discoid lupus erythematosus (DLE) (Figs. 8 and 9).

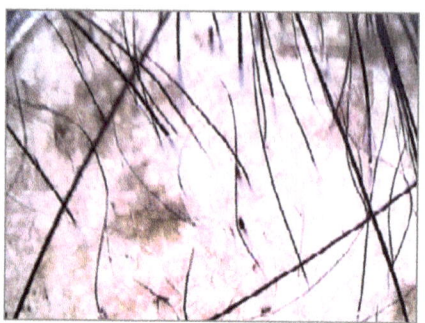

Fig. 8: Dermoscopic image of tinea capitis: Broken shafts, microscales, blotchy erythema and pigmentation.

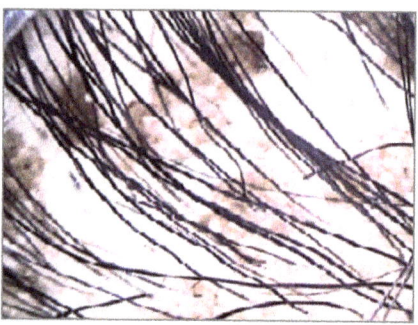

Fig. 9: Dermoscopic image of tinea capitis is showing distorted hair shafts along with blotchy pigmentation.

Other features of inflammation like erythema, scaling, micropustules, and follicular scale-crust may be seen in tinea capitis. Fluorescence can be demonstrated on use of ultraviolet (UV) light source in a videodermoscope.

Differential diagnosis should include AA, LPP, DLE, and trichotillomania.

Trichotillomania (Hair Pulling Tic)

Trichotillomania can be defined as an irresistible urge to pull one's own hair, accompanied by a sense of relief once the hair has been plucked. This compulsive disorder most commonly affects preschool children and adolescents; majority of the adolescents being females. The most common area of the scalp that is involved is the vertex. Clinically, trichotillomania usually presents as irregular patch(es) of incomplete nonscarring alopecia.

Purpose of Dermoscopy for Trichotillomania

Trichotillomania can resemble AA or noninflammatory tinea capitis, as these conditions present with patchy nonscarring alopecia and also affect patients of similar age group. History of hair pulling is difficult to elicit in children and may be unreliable. Dermoscopy would be very useful for differentiating between these conditions, probably obviating the need for an invasive procedure like biopsy in children and which, at times, can be inconclusive.

Dermoscopic Findings in Trichotillomania[6]

Majority of the dermoscopic findings in trichotillomania are due to traumatic stretch of the hair shafts, accordingly the findings are as follows:

Fractured hair shafts of varying lengths: The hair shafts are broken at variable distances from the surface resulting in black dots, if they are fractured very close to the follicle or hair shafts of varying lengths, and if they are broken at different distances from the follicle (Fig. 10).

Frayed hair shafts with split ends: The distal ends of the fractured hair shafts are frayed and, at times, show longitudinally split ends (trichoptilosis).

Coiled hair shafts: Sometimes, the distal ends of the fractured hair shafts may be coiled. This is due to the alteration in the protein structure of the hair shaft as a result of stretching.

Other Dermoscopic Findings

These include sparse hair, empty follicular ostia, and some yellow dots. Short vellus hair can be seen in both AA and trichotillomania. However, unlike in AA, they are never white (Fig. 10). "Exclamation hairs" pathognomonic of AA are not seen in trichotillomania.

Microscales especially around follicles, perifollicular erythema, perifollicular hyperpigmentation, or perifollicular hemorrhages may be sometimes seen.

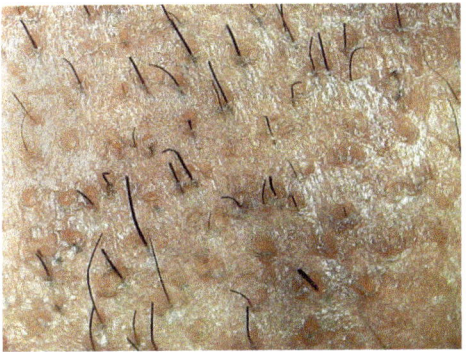

Fig. 10: Dermoscopic image of trichotillomania: Variable length of broken hair shafts, some of them fractured or frayed. Some regrowing vellus hairs are also seen. Skin shows microscaling and pigmentary changes.

Conclusion

Dermoscopy has the potential to become a quick diagnostic aid for differentiating the various patchy nonscarring alopecias. However, more experience and wider usage are needed to validate the above findings.

PATCHY SCARRING ALOPECIAS

Lichen Planopilaris

Lichen planopilaris is the most common cause of cicatricial alopecia that frequently affects middle-aged women. Clinical examination reveals irregular patches of hair loss, which become confluent, affecting most frequently the parietal and vertex regions.

Purpose of Dermoscopy in LPP

Scarring alopecia due to LPP may not be associated with overt signs of inflammation and therefore, especially in its early phase, needs to be differentiated from nonscarring alopecia due to AA. Most of the times, a scalp biopsy is needed to establish the diagnosis. Dermoscopy can aid in the diagnosis of LPP and differentiate it from AA without the need to perform a biopsy.

Dermoscopic Features of LPP

The primary finding in scarring alopecias is loss of follicular ostia and this can be very well appreciated with a dermoscope. Before complete loss of follicle occurs, other signs of microscopic inflammation in LPP are evident as follows:

Peripilar cast and follicular plugging: Dermoscopy reveals presence of characteristic perifollicular scales (peripilar casts) at the periphery of the patch (Figs. 11A and B). Follicular plugging may be observed with prominent scaling (Fig. 12).

Perifollicular pigmentation and pigment network in interfollicular area: Perifollicular pigmentation in the form of dark brown to blue gray granular deposits encircling the follicular opening can be appreciated. This finding is very specific for LPP. Also the pigment network in-between the follicles is preserved as LPP spares the interfollicular dermis.

White dots: After complete destruction of the follicles, the site of the lost follicle is marked by a white dot, which is surrounded by honeycombed hyperpigmentation (Figs. 11A and B).

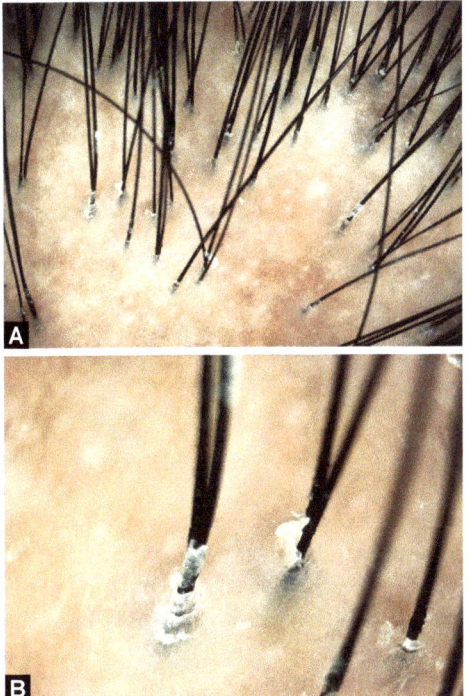

Figs. 11A and B: Dermoscopic image of lichen planopilaris: Peripilar casts a very characteristic feature of lichen planopilaris.

Discoid Lupus Erythematosus

Discoid lupus erythematosus of the scalp also presents clinically as single or multiple patches of scarring alopecia.

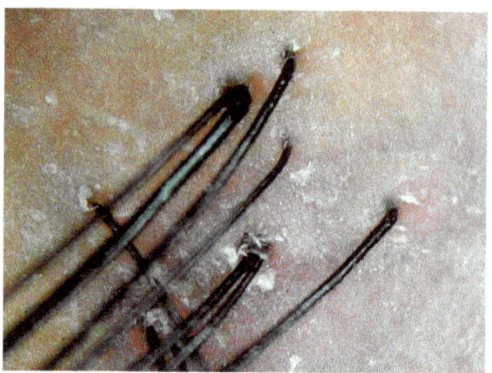

Fig. 12: Dermoscopic image of lichen planopilaris: Perifollicular erythema and scaling.

Purpose of Dermoscopy in DLE

Though cicatricial in nature diagnosing a lesion at an early stage and prompt treatment sometimes results in regrowth of hair. Dermoscopy can serve as a quick method of establishing the diagnosis of early lesions with subtle findings.

Dermoscopic Features of DLE

Loss of pigment network (Fig. 13): The reticular pigmentation is lost because of atrophy of the epidermis and consequently the scalp appears pale in color.

Increased vascularization (Fig. 13): Arborizing and tortuous vessels are commonly seen inside DLE plaques. These are not seen so commonly in LPP.

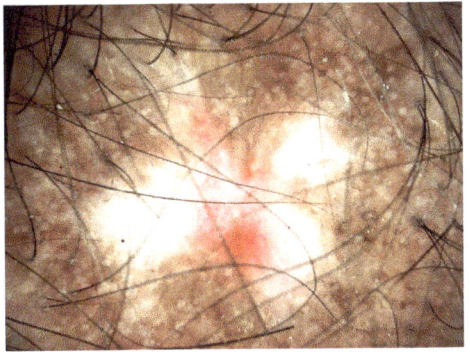

Fig. 13: Dermoscopic image of discoid lupus erythematosus: Pale white areas lacking any pigment network. Also note the increase in the vasculature of the scalp in the form of tortuous vessels.

Hyperkeratotic follicular plugging (Fig. 14): Prominent follicular plugging is seen at the periphery.

Brown dots in the interfollicular area: Dark brown to blue-gray granular pigmentation is seen in the interfollicular areas (Fig. 15). This is because DLE involves the interfollicular dermis as well. This is in contrast to LPP where these granular pigment deposits are situated around the follicles sparing the interfollicular region.

Thus, alopecias presenting with cicatricial patches can be reliably and quickly differentiated with the help of a dermoscope.

However, more experience and consistency in findings would be required to validate it as an easier and quicker

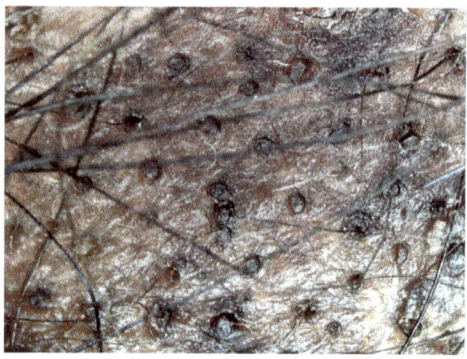

Fig. 14: Multiple follicular plugs in a plaque of discoid lupus erythematosus.

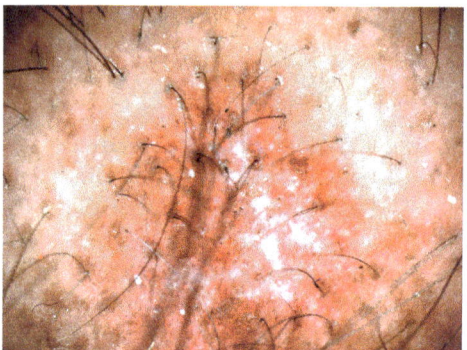

Fig. 15: Dermoscopic image of discoid lupus erythematosus: Brown to blue–gray dots and pigment granules in the interfollicular area indicating pathologic involvement of the interfollicular area in discoid lupus erythematosus.

alternative to biopsy in patients presenting with patchy scarring alopecia.

REFERENCES

1. Wasserman D, Guzman-Sanchez DA, Scott K, et al. Alopecia areata. Int J Dermatol. 2007;46(2):121-31.
2. Inui S, Nakajima T, Itami S. Significance of dermoscopy in acute diffuse and total alopecia of the female scalp: Review of twenty cases. Dermatology. 2008;217(4):333-6.
3. Tosti A, Whiting D, Iorizzo M, et al. The role of scalp dermoscopy in the diagnosis of alopecia areata incognita. J Am Acad Dermatol. 2008;59(1):64-7.
4. Tosti A. Dermoscopy of Hair and Scalp Disorders with Clinical and Pathological Correlations. London, England: Informa Healthcare Books; 2007.
5. Slowinska M, Rudnicka L, Schwartz RA, et al. Comma hairs: a dermatoscopic marker for tinea capitis: a rapid diagnostic method. J Am Acad Dermatol. 2008;59(5 Suppl):S77-9.
6. Spagnol AL, Nogueira TF, Luna AA. Dermoscopic clues to distinguish trichotillomania from patchy alopecia areata. An Bras Dermatol. 2010;85(5):723-6.

CHAPTER 25

Phototrichogram and TrichoScan®

Punit Saraogi, Rachita Dhurat

INTRODUCTION

Phototrichogram and TrichoScan® are two investigations useful in the assessment of hair loss as well as measuring the effects of therapies promising hair growth promoting benefits. Both these involve taking dermoscopic pictures of the target scalp area as the initial step.

PHOTOTRICHOGRAM

The term phototrichogram was introduced by Saitoh in 1970.[1] It is a non-invasive technique to study the hair cycle in vivo and can be used to measure various parameters of hair namely hair density, thickness, length, and vertical growth rate.

The parameters for phototrichogram are calculated by demarcating an area of 1 cm² over scalp over 48 hours. Thus, it helps in measuring the density of the hair, in calculating the anagen (growing) and the telogen (nongrowing) hair and thus, measuring the anagen–telogen ratio, grossly measuring the hair diameter and in monitoring of treatment.

Procedure

Clipping of Hair

Day 0: A particular site is selected in the scalp and demarcated using a stencil into 1 cm² (Fig. 1). Then, hairs in the marked area are to be shaved or cut using a curved scissor (Figs. 2 and 3).

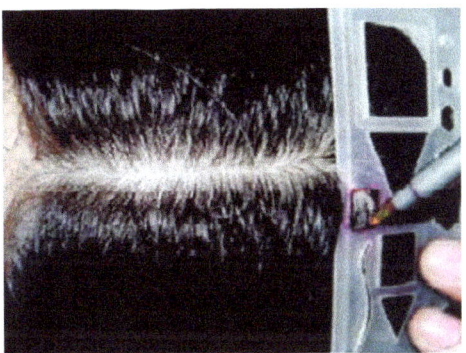

Fig. 1: The selected site is being marked with the permanent marker using a 1 cm² stencil.

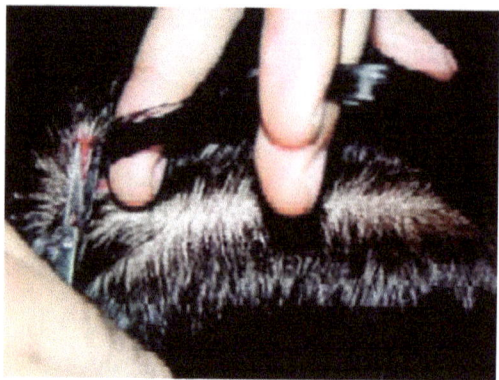

Fig. 2: Hairs in the marked area are cut as close as possible to the scalp surface using a curved surgical scissor.

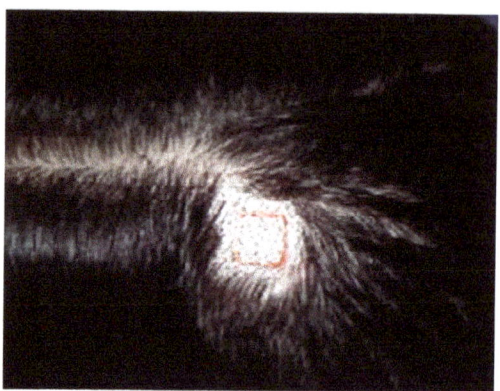

Fig. 3: The marked area after the hairs has been cut.

Hair Diameter Measurement

The clipped hairs are spread on a glass slide (Fig. 4) and dry mounted with a transparent adhesive tape to measure their diameter under the microscope using 40X magnifications. A calibrated micrometer scale having a least measurement of 0.01 mm is used. The diameter of hairs is measured close to their bases using the measuring eyepiece.

Image Recording

Day 0 (t0): The marked area is then photographed using a digital camera, under fixed light conditions, from a fixed distance, using a fixed distance adapter specially designed for this purpose (Fig. 5A).

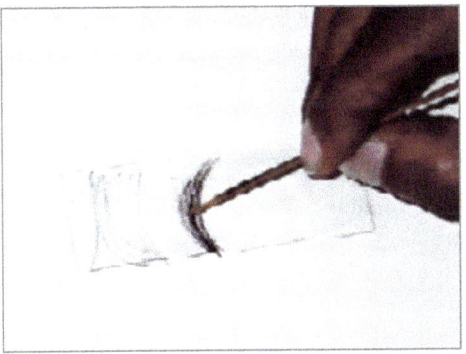

Fig. 4: Clipped hairs are spread on a glass slide and dry mounted with a transparent adhesive tape to measure their diameter.

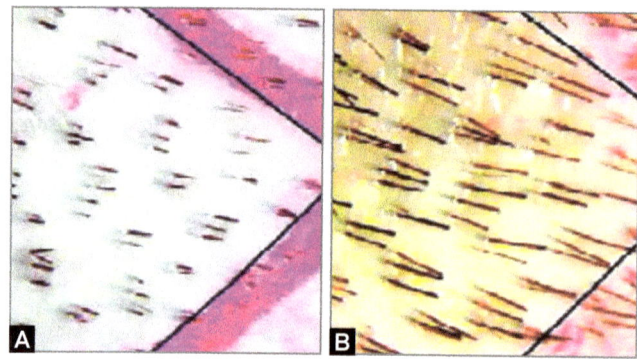

Figs. 5A and B: (A) On day 0 (t0), marked area is photographed using a digital camera, under fixed light conditions, from a fixed distance, using a fixed distance; (B) On day 2 (t2), second photograph is taken in a similar manner as for Figure A from the specified site.

Day 2 (t2): The patient is advised not to wash his/her hair for the next 2 days (to keep the permanent mark on the scalp intact) and then, exactly after 48 hours, the second photograph was taken in a similar manner from the specified site (Fig. 5B).

Hair Variables at t0 (Fig. 6A)

The following variables are evaluated from the first photograph taken at t0:
- Density of hair in the specified area
- Length of hairs at t0 (L1).

Hair Variables at t2 (Fig. 6B)

The following variables are evaluated from the second photograph (t2):

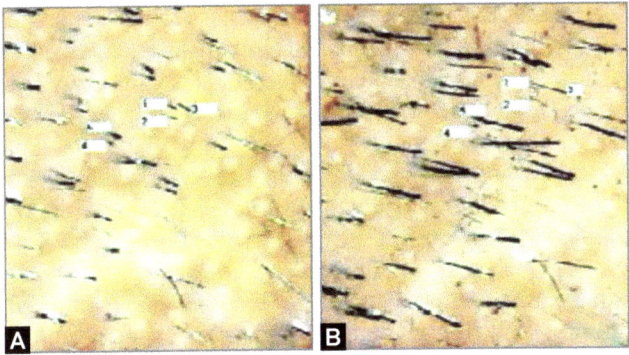

Figs. 6A and B: (A) The following variables are evaluated from the first photograph taken at t0: (1) Density of hair in the specified area, (2) Length of hairs at t0 (L1); (B) The following variables are evaluated from the second photograph (t2): (1) The length of hairs at t2 (L2), (2) Hair growth in mm/day (L2–L1)/2, (3) Number of hairs showing hair growth in t2 (anagen hairs), (4) Number of hairs not grown in t2 (telogen hairs), and (5) Anagen and telogen percentage.

- The length of hairs at t2 (L2)
- Hair growth in mm/day (L2–L1)/2
- Number of hairs showing hair growth in t2 (anagen hairs)
- Number of hairs not grown in t2 (telogen hairs)
- Anagen and telogen percentage.

Contrast-enhanced Phototrichogram

Contrast-enhanced phototrichogram procedure involves coloring hair with black-colored dye immediately before starting the procedure.[2,3] These temporarily colored hairs give a better contrast against the white scalp, making this method more sensitive for less-pigmented and thin hairs. This contrast enhancement is not required in the Indian setting as we have usually darkly pigmented hairs, thus making the procedure still simpler for us to carry out.

The phototrichogram is a noninvasive procedure that is well tolerated by the patient. It is also possible to repeat the examination on the same area of the scalp at regular intervals, allowing evaluation of progress or reversion of pathology with treatment. This method has been validated with scalp biopsies. However, it is not diagnostic, is time-consuming, somewhat subjective, and requires expertise. The necessary equipment and image analysis software are not easily available commercially.

TRICHOSCAN® (TRICHOLOG GmbH)

TrichoScan® can be viewed as on automated phototrichogram. It combines standard epiluminescence microscopy with automatic digital image analysis for the measurement of human hair. The software quantifies the number of hairs and the anagen–telogen ratio within one operation. The use of TrichoScan® initially involves shaving a scalp area (approximately 1.8 cm^2) (Fig. 7A).

After 3 days, hairs in the shaven area are dyed and a digital photograph is taken at 20-fold magnification and saved (Fig. 7B). The TrichoScan® software works on the basis that telogen hairs do not grow. The software uses this as a basis for calculation of the anagen–telogen ratio (Fig. 8). Thus, the basic procedure is quite similar to that of the classical phototrichogram.

CHAPTER 25: Phototrichogram and TrichoScan®

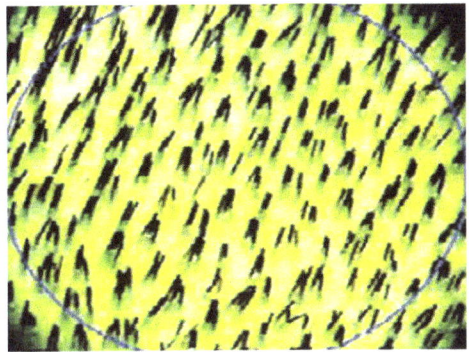

Fig. 7A: The use of TrichoScan® initially involves shaving a scalp area (approximately 1.8 cm²).

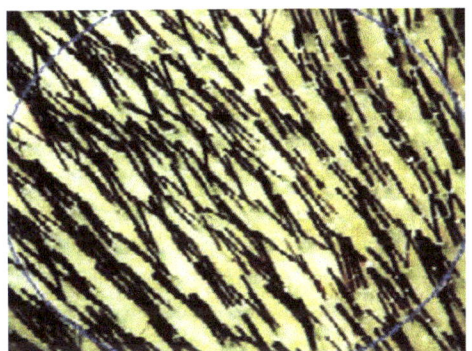

Fig. 7B: After 3 days, hairs in the shaven area are dyed and a digital photograph is taken at 20-fold magnification and saved.

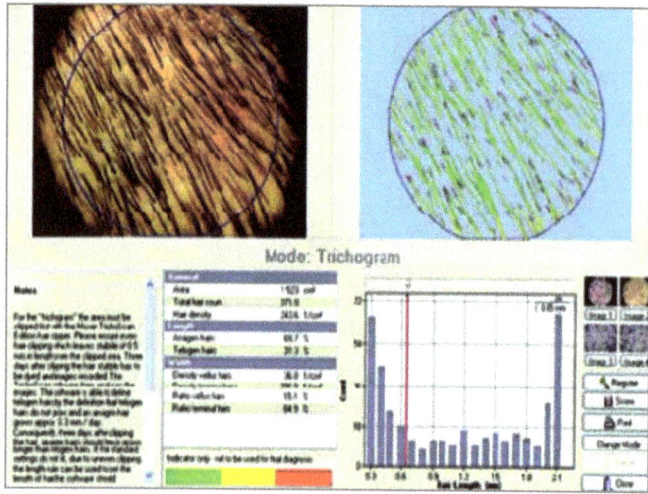

Fig. 8: Screenshot of the layout of the result that is displayed on the computer screen after the software has completed the hair analysis.

The claimed advantage of this procedure lies in its simple and speedy photographic processing and the painlessness of the procedure with the reproducibility of results. The software is extremely easy to run and time saving, thereby reducing the manual time and effort spent in measuring each single hair as in the classical phototrichogram. However, in our experience, the software is error prone in terms of determining proportion of telogen hair as well as vellus hair and we do not recommend it for clinical trials.[4] Moreover, the software does not have facility for measurement of hair growth rate.

To conclude, phototrichogram is the most precise method available for the assessment of hair growth. However, since it is tedious to perform, it is better reserved for detailed clinical trials. TrichoScan®, on the other hand, needs further refinement to improve the accuracy of its analysis.

REFERENCES

1. Saitoh M, Uzuka M, Sakamoto M. Human hair cycle. J Invest Dermatol 1970;54:65-81.
2. Dhurat R. Phototrichogram. Indian J Dermatol Venereol Leprol. 2006;72:242-4.
3. Van Neste DJ. Contrast enhanced phototrichogram (CE-PTG): an improved non-invasive technique for measurement of scalp hair dynamics in androgenetic alopecia—validation study with histology after transverse sectioning of scalp biopsies. Eur J Dermatol. 2001;11:326-31.
4. Saraogi P, Dhurat R. Automated digital image analysis (TrichoScan®) for human hair growth analysis: ease versus errors. Int J Trich. 2010;2:5-13.

Section 7: Miscellaneous Dermoscopy Application

CHAPTER 26

Dermoscopy of Granulomatous Skin Diseases

Shubhangi Mahajan, Uday S Khopkar

INTRODUCTION

Dermatoscope is a noninvasive diagnostic tool useful for evaluation of morphologic structures of the layers of skin, which are not visible to the naked eye. Traditionally, it is used for the evaluation of skin tumors,[1] pigmented and nonpigmented skin lesions[2,3] but more recently, its use has been expanded to diagnose and differentiate common inflammatory or infectious skin diseases.[4] However, existing data on the dermoscopic patterns of granulomatous dermatoses are limited.

Granulomatous disorders, especially of infective etiology, pose a diagnostic challenge to a dermatologist. Histopathology aids in confirmation of diagnosis; however, a noninvasive tool like dermoscopy may have an edge over histopathology.

The dermoscopic hallmark of granulomatous skin disease is the structureless orange–yellowish patches, which is highly suggestive of an underlying dermal granuloma.[5-7] These orange–yellowish patches are commonly associated with focused linear or branching vessels. Other possible findings include milia-like cysts, erythema, reticular streaks, follicular plugs, dilated follicles, pigmentation structures, and white and/or yellow scales.[8-15]

LUPUS VULGARIS

Lupus vulgaris is the most common form of cutaneous tuberculosis. Sometimes, unusual clinical manifestations like atypical features and atypical sites make the clinical diagnosis difficult. Dermoscopy and diascopy of the reddish plaque of cutaneous lupus vulgaris showed yellowish–orange discoloration ("apple-jelly" sign) along with few milia-like cysts, white reticular streaks (Fig. 1),[5,8] erosions, and scaling (Fig. 2). Different vascular patterns observed were linear branching vessels,[6] fine focused telangiectasia (Fig. 3)[8] and arborizing telangiectasia.[16]

LICHEN SCROFULOSORUM

Lichen scrofulosorum, also known as "tuberculosis cutis lichenoides", is a rare form of tuberculid that clinically presents as tiny lichenoid papules. These lesions make the diagnosis of lichen scrofulosorum difficult as they resemble many other dermatological conditions. Dermoscopic features of lichen scrofulosorum such as milia-like cysts with perifollicular halo (Fig. 4) and a starburst-like pattern in old healed lesion (Fig. 5) help differentiate it from other papular dermatoses.

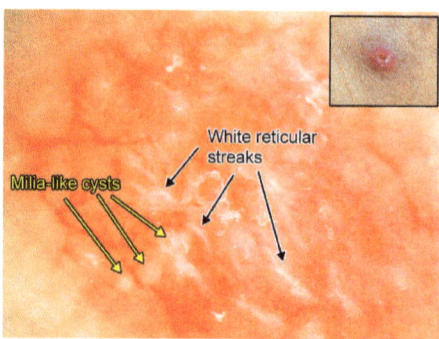

Fig. 1: Dermoscopy of the reddish plaque of lupus vulgaris showing yellowish orange discoloration in the background along with milia-like cysts and white reticular streaks with numerous broad and long arborizing telangiectasia. Clinical picture of the early plaque is seen in the inset.

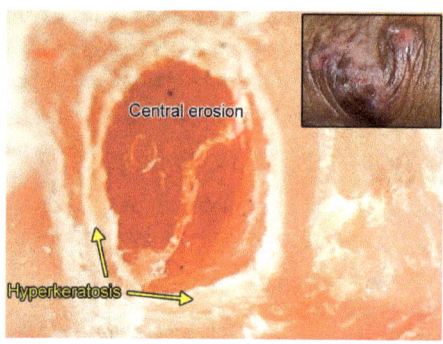

Fig. 2: Dermoscopy of perifollicular erosion (inset) over a plaque of lupus vulgaris showing concentric lamellae of hyperkeratosis with a pool of crimson red blob surround a plugged central erosion and scaling (hyperkeratosis).

CHAPTER 26: Dermoscopy of Granulomatous Skin Diseases

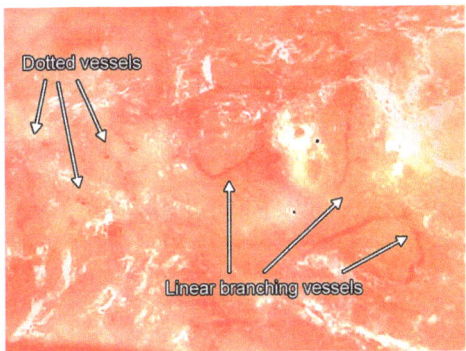

Fig. 3: Dermoscopy of resolving lupus vulgaris lesion with a variety of vascular patterns peripheral telangiectasia.

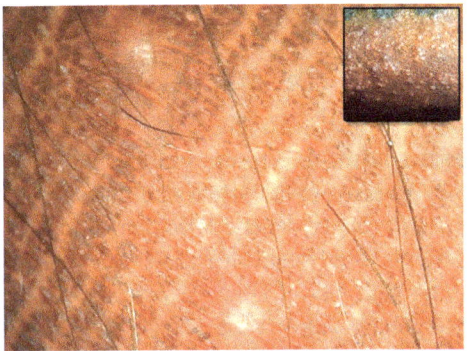

Fig. 4: Dermoscopic image of active papular lesion (top left) and resolving lesion (bottom) of lichen scrofulosorum with active lesion showing disturbed pigmentary pattern, irregular milia-like cysts with perifollicular halo and colored radial streaks.

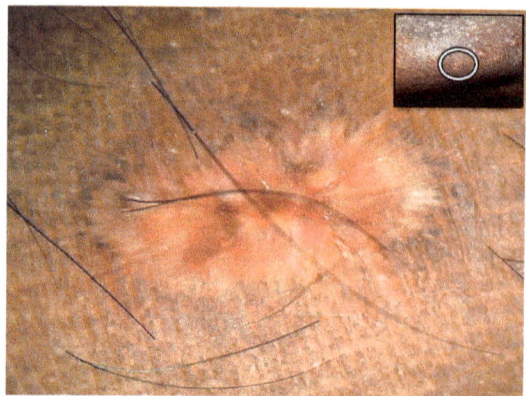

Fig. 5: Resolved lesion of lichen scrofulosorum showing a starburst like pattern on dermoscopy due to accentuated radiating streaks.

POST-KALA-AZAR DERMAL LEISHMANIASIS

Post-kala-azar dermal leishmaniasis (PKDL) is a cutaneous sequel of partially treated or untreated visceral leishmaniasis. Dermoscopy in case of PKDL showed diffuse erythema along with yellow tears shaped structures that correspond to follicular plugs, salmon-colored ovoid structures (Fig. 6), starburst like pattern along with loss of follicular openings, ulcer/erosion, and inflated balloon appearance (Fig. 7).[13,17-19] One of us (USK) has observed that a slightly infiltrated hypopigmented plaque of post-kala-azar dermal leishmaniasis shows closely spaced polygonal whitish globules with central white dots (bubble wrap pattern) (Fig. 8).

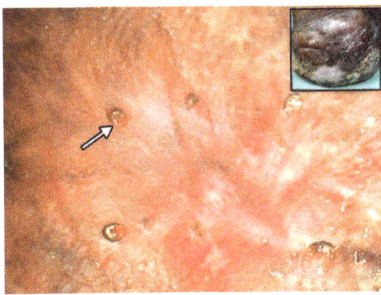

Fig. 6: A plaque of post-kala-azar dermal leishmaniasis (PKDL) over heal (inset) showing loss of dermatoglyphics lines with irregular white areas (scarring) salmon-colored patches (atrophy) ovoid patches (atrophy), surrounding there are acrosyringeal dilatations and plugs with milia-like cyst (arrow) resolving lesion showing crateriform depression with irregular white area surrounding it with peripheral skin-colored radiating streaks on dermoscopy.

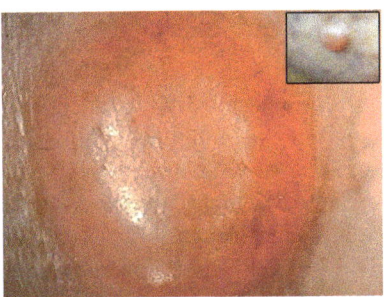

Fig. 7: Dermoscopy of a slightly umbilicated nodule of post-kala-azar dermal leishmaniasis (PKDL) showing inflated balloon appearance along with numerous tortuous telangiectasia. Note the absence of central plugged crater that differentiated it from molluscum, orangish hue is seen at the periphery.

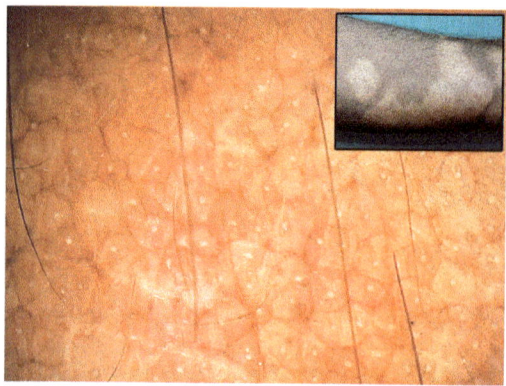

Fig. 8: Hypopigmented patch of PKDL over hand (inset) showing polygonal globular pattern with central white dots (follicular openings) and peripheral reticulate hyperpigmentation.

HISTOPLASMOSIS

Mucocutaneous histoplasmosis is a deep fungal infection frequently reported in immunocompromised patients. Clinically, it presents with numerous skin-colored papules and nodules. Some of them grow in size and ulcerate. Dermoscopy of a shiny papule showed inflated balloon appearance with bigger and stretched (parchment like/patulous) follicular openings, increased vellus hair follicles (white dots) (Fig. 9), and telangiectasia. Dermoscopy of an erythematous plaque revealed lack of skin markings and appendages with linear telangiectasia over orange–pink background (Fig. 10).

CHAPTER 26: Dermoscopy of Granulomatous Skin Diseases

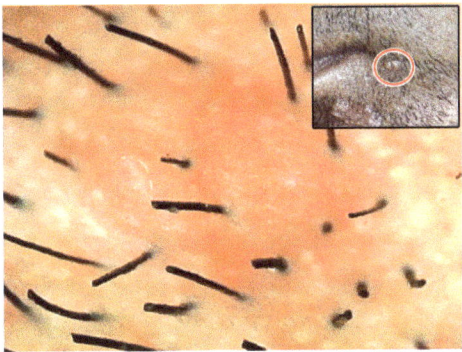

Fig. 9: Dermoscopic image of an umbilicated papule of histoplasmosis showing bigger and stretched (parchment like/patulous) follicular and appendageal openings numerous telangiectasia on an orangish background.

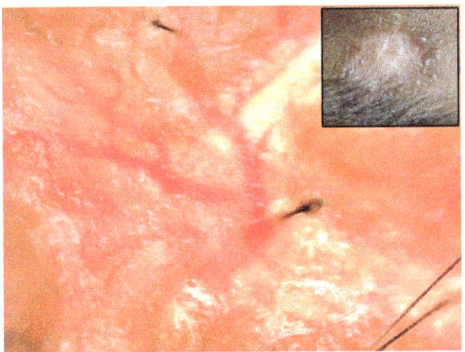

Fig. 10: Dermoscopy of an indurated plaque of histoplasmosis showing arborizing telangiectasia on orangish background.

HANSEN'S DISEASE

Hansen's disease is a chronic granulomatous infection caused by *Mycobacterium leprae*. Borderline lepromatous Hansen's disease is characterized by large number of lesions of variable morphology. Dermoscopy of the ichthyotic lesion of borderline lepromatous leprosy showed diffuse orange area along with linear and globular telangiectasia (Fig. 11). Hypopigmented patch showed linear white streaks and loss of pigment network or reverse skin pigmentary network (Fig. 12). These dermoscopic findings to some extent help differentiate the lepromatous lesions.

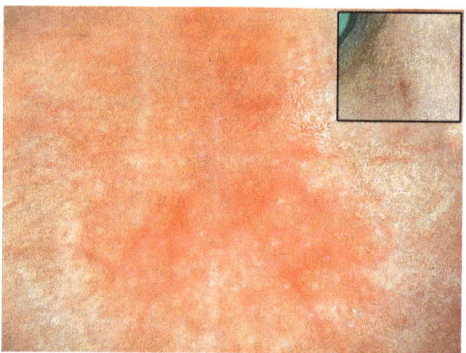

Fig. 11: Dermoscopic image of an ichthyotic patch of borderline lepromatous Hansen's disease with periphery of patch shows accentuated pigment network, broad telangiectasia, and center shows patchy loss of pigment network.

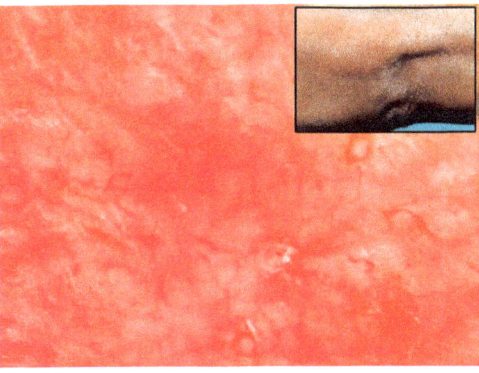

Fig. 12: Hypopigmented patch of borderline lepromatous Hansen's disease on dermoscopy showing linear white streaks and loss of skin pigmentary network except around follicle along with irregular white areas lacking acrosyringeal openings and pigment network (atrophy).

GRANULOMA ANNULARE

Granuloma annulare (GA) clinically presents with skin-colored or violaceous papules coalescing to form annular or roundish plaques. The dermoscopic findings of GA differ from other granulomatous disorders due to lack of specific vascular structures.[9] It shows structureless orange–pink areas distributed focally or diffusely suggestive of underlying granuloma (Fig. 13). Presence of unfocused vessels of varying morphology on the pinkish–reddish background is characteristic feature of GA (Fig. 13).[9,20,21]

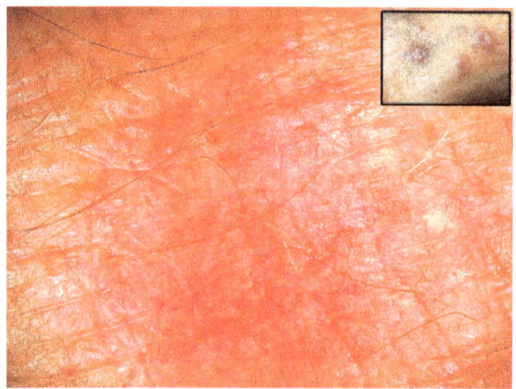

Fig. 13: Dermoscopy of an annular plaque of granuloma annulare (GA) showing structureless orange–pink area along with unfocused vessels.

SARCOIDOSIS

Sarcoidosis is a multisystem disorder characterized by formation of noncaseating granulomas. Clinical diagnosis of sarcoidosis becomes challenging due its variable clinical presentation. Dermoscopically, sarcoidosis is characterized by diffuse translucent yellow to orange globular-like or structureless areas, possibly corresponding to the well-defined sarcoid granulomas and linear or branching vessels.[6,7,11,15,22,23]

NECROBIOSIS LIPOIDICA

Dermoscopy in case of necrobiosis lipoidica is helpful to diagnose the early stage lesions or lesions located at atypical sites. Necrobiosis lipoidica lesions show a characteristic pattern of linear arborizing vessels and a yellow background color, either alone or in combination with white or red areas. Other common features were yellow crusting and ulceration. Incipient lesions of necrobiosis lipoidica showed comma-shaped vessels, more developed lesions showed network-shaped/hairpin-like vessels, and advanced lesions showed elongated, branching and focused serpentine vessels along with the yellowish–orange/whitish–pinkish background as a common finding in all the stages.[9,11,12,14,15]

Dermoscopic examination of necrobiosis lipoidica is also helpful to differentiate it from sarcoidosis. The telangiectasias of necrobiosis lipoidica are longer and more branching, (probably caused by atrophic changes) compared to those present in cutaneous sarcoidosis (short telangiectasia with white dots).[14]

CONCLUSION

Dermoscopic pattern of yellowish–orange patches or structureless erythematous area is characteristically suggestive of dermal granuloma. Different vascular patterns and other dermoscopic findings like reticular streaks, follicular plugs, milia-like cysts, pigmentation structures, and white and/or yellow scales, ulceration help diagnose the different granulomatous disorders. However, because some dermoscopic features of different granulomatous disorders overlap, histopathology, and other laboratory tests become mandatory for confirmation of diagnosis.

REFERENCES

1. Argenziano G, Ferrara G, Francione S, et al. Dermoscopy—The Ultimate Tool for Melanoma Diagnosis. Semin Cutan Med Surg. 2009;28(3):142-8.
2. Lallas A, Argenziano G, Moscarella E, et al. Diagnosis and management of facial pigmented macules. Clin Dermatol. 2014;32(1):94-100.
3. Zalaudek I, Kreusch J, Giacomel J, et al. How to diagnose nonpigmented skin tumors: A review of vascular structures seen with dermoscopy. J Am Acad Dermatol. 2010;63(3):361-74.
4. Russo T, Piccolo V, Lallas A, et al. Recent advances in dermoscopy. F1000Res. 2016;5. pii: F1000 Faculty Rev-184.
5. Lallas A, Giacomel J, Zalaudek I. Dermoscopy in general dermatology: practical tips for the clinician. Br J Dermatol. 2014;170(3):514-26.
6. Lallas A, Argenziano G, Apalla Z, et al. Dermoscopic patterns of common facial inflammatory skin diseases. J Eur Acad Dermatol Venereol. 2014;28(5):609-14.
7. Pellicano R, Tiodorovic-Zivkovic D, Ganrhant JY, et al. Dermoscopy of Cutaneous Sarcoidosis. Dermatology. 2010; 221(1):51-4.
8. Brasiello M, Zalaudek I, Ferrara G, et al. Lupus Vulgaris: A New Look at an Old Symptom—The Lupoma Observed with Dermoscopy. Dermatology. 2008;218(2):172-4.
9. Pellicano R, Caldarola G, Filabozzi P, et al. Dermoscopy of Necrobiosis Lipoidica and Granuloma Annulare. Dermatology. 2013;226(4):319-23.
10. Errichetti E, Stinco G. Dermoscopy in General Dermatology: A Practical Overview. Dermatology and Therapy. Springer Healthcare; 2016.
11. Bombonato C, Argenziano G, Lallas A, et al. Orange color: A dermoscopic clue for the diagnosis of granulomatous skin diseases. J Am Dermatol. 2015;72(1):S60-3.

12. Balestri R, La Placa M, Bardazzi, et al. Dermoscopic subpatterns of granulomatous skin diseases. J Am Dermatol. 2013;69(5): e217-8.
13. Llambrich A, Zaballos P, Terrasa F, et al. Dermoscopy of cutaneous leishmaniasis. 2009;(Table 1):756-61.
14. Dl VE, Mart B. Dermoscopy of Necrobiosis Lipoidica. Dermatoscopia de la necrobiosis lipoídica. 2017;104(6):534-7.
15. Ramadan S, Hossam D, Saleh MA. Dermoscopy could be useful in differentiating sarcoidosis from necrobiotic granulomas even after treatment with systemic steroids. 2016;6(3):17-22.
16. Chatterjee M. Dermoscopy in darker skin. Chapter 12: dermoscopy of granulomatous disorders. New York: Mcgraw-Hill Education; 2017. pp. 67-74.
17. Yu A. Tropical medicine rounds Cutaneous leishmaniasis : new dermoscopic findings. Int J Dermatol. 2013;52(7):831-7.
18. Fernandez-crehuet P. White starburst-like pattern as a dermoscopic clue in Old World cutaneous leishmaniasis. An Bras Dermatol. 2017;92(2):266-7.
19. Cembrero-saralegui H, Pérez MM, Imbernón-moya A. Dermoscopy of acute cutaneous leishmaniasis. Med Clin (Barc). 2017;148(5):e29.
20. Errichetti E, Apalla Z, Stefani D, et al. Dermoscopy of Granuloma Annulare: A Clinical and Histological Correlation. Dermatology. 2017;233(1):74-79.
21. Arribas P, Berbegal L, Dele FJ, et al. Yellow and orange in cutaneous lesions: clinical and dermoscopic data. J Eur Acad Dermatol Venereol. 2015;29(12):2317-25.
22. Hadj I, Mernissi FZ. Dermoscopic features of sarcoidosis. Pan Afr Med J. 2014;18:111.
23. Huet P, Barnéon G, Cribier B. Cutaneous sarcoidosis: correlation between dermatopathology and dermoscopy. Ann Dermatol Venereol. 2016;143:404-6.

CHAPTER 27

Dermoscopy of Benign Skin Tumors

Manas Chatterjee, Ruchi Hemdani

INTRODUCTION

Benign skin tumors are commonly seen by dermatologists. It is necessary to properly diagnose and treat common benign tumors and distinguish them from malignant lesions. Uncertain clinical diagnosis requires confirmation by biopsy, which is invasive, to rule out malignancy. Herein the use of dermoscopy as a noninvasive technique to diagnose and differentiate benign skin tumors comes handy especially in patients who are reluctant for biopsy, children and lesions on face.

CLASSIFICATION

There are multiple benign skin tumors based on their origin: keratinocyte, melanocyte, appendage, vascular, lymphatic, neural, and muscle. We shall be discussing the dermoscopic features of commonly seen benign tumors in this chapter and we have divided them into benign melanocytic and benign nonmelanocytic tumors based on pigmentary alterations (Table 1).

Table 1: Classification of common benign tumors based on pigmentary alterations (benign melanocytic and benign nonmelanocytic tumors).

Benign melanocytic tumors	Benign nonmelanocytic tumors
Congenital melanocytic nevus	Dermatofibroma
Compound melanocytic nevus	Neurofibroma
Dermal melanocytic nevus	Cherry angioma
Junctional melanocytic nevus	Pyogenic granuloma
Spitz nevus	Lymphangioma circumscriptum
Halo nevus	Seborrheic keratosis
Nevus spilus	Sebaceous hyperplasia
	Angiokeratoma
	Angiofibroma
	Milia
	Epidermal cyst
	Apocrine hidrocystoma
	Trichoepithelioma
	Steatocystoma
	Fibrokeratoma
	Syringoma

DERMOSCOPIC FEATURES OF INDIVIDUAL CONDITIONS

Congenital Melanocytic Nevus

In congenital melanocytic nevus (CMN), two main dermoscopic patterns are seen: (1) reticular and (2) globular. CMNs with prominent globular pattern tend to occur over the scalp, face, neck and trunk and those with prominent net-like pattern are commonly visualized on the lower limbs. This "reticular or netlike pattern" is a honeycomb-like arrangement of dark pigment lines (corresponds to elongated hypermelanotic rete ridges)[1] and "globular" pattern refers to well-defined rounded or ovoid dark aggregates (melanocyte nests within the upper dermis). Similarly sized and shaped dark brown to black globules are distributed uniformly (Figs. 1A and B) throughout the nevus.[2]

Hypertrichosis, perifollicular hyperpigmentation and milia-like cysts are other dermoscopic features that are common to CMNs. Additionally, few CMNs may reveal comma, dotted and serpentine vessels under dermoscopy.[3]

Acquired Melanocytic Nevus

Peripheral reticular network (diffuse or patchy) with central hyperpigmentation (darker skin)/hypopigmentation (fair skin types) are seen. At times, globular pattern may also be seen. A subset of growing acquired nevi which show peripheral globules (Figs. 2A and B) on dermoscopy is also mentioned.[4,5]

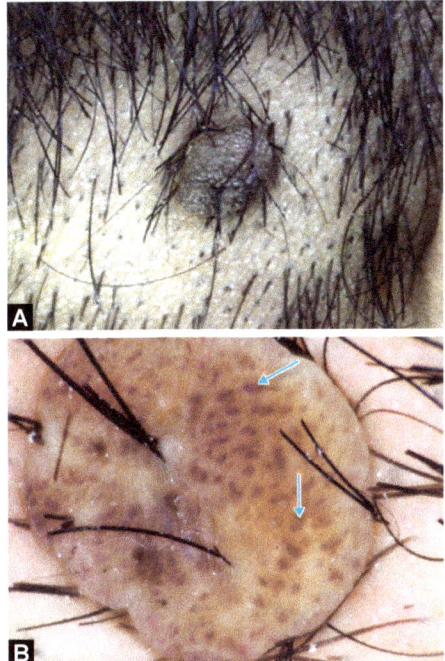

Figs. 1A and B: Congenital melanocytic nevus: (A) Clinical; (B) Dermoscopy images showing multiple globules arranged uniformly (blue arrows).

Halo Nevus

Central region shows dark brown to black globular or homogeneous pattern while the peripheral depigmented area may show lack of pigment network (Figs. 3A and B).[6]

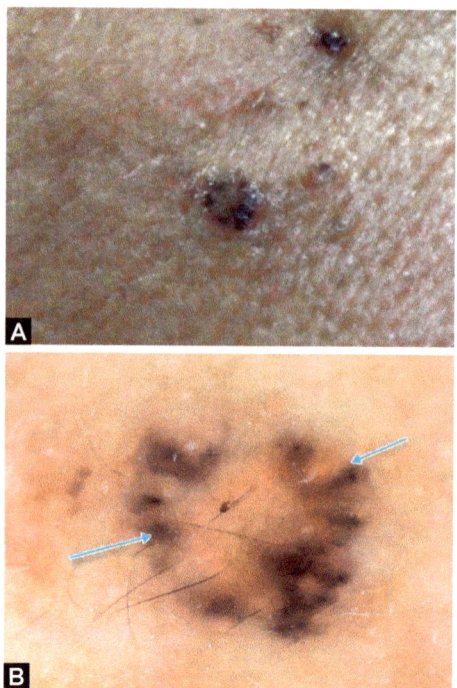

Figs. 2A and B: Acquired melanocytic nevus: (A) Clinical; (B) Dermoscopy images showing peripheral globular pattern (blue arrows) in an actively growing acquired melanocytic nevus.

Nevus Spilus

Homogeneous tan color or faint and delicate networks in the background are observed. On this background there are seen

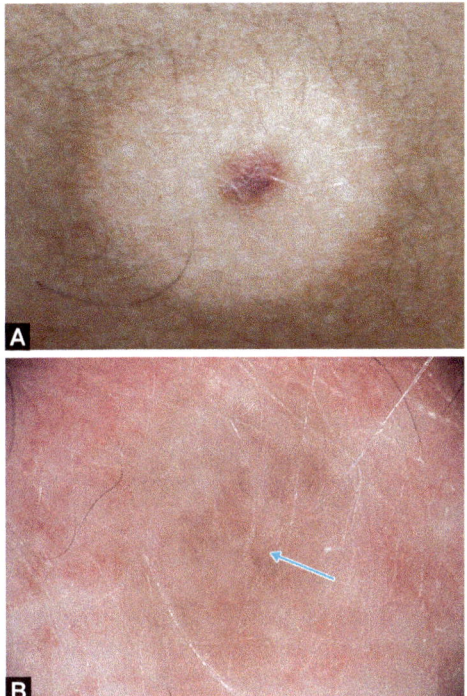

Figs. 3A and B: Halo nevus: (A) Clinical; (B) Dermoscopy images showing peripheral depigmentation with globular nevus in center (blue arrow).

scattered brown or pink macules or papules that show focal features of the type of nevus (usually junctional, spitz, blue nevi, and compound nevi).[7-9]

Spitz Nevus

Dermoscopic patterns include thick (atypical) reticular, atypical globular, typical star-burst (streaks—radial streaming or pseudopods), homogeneous (pink or with a black lamella), negative pigment network, and atypical/multicomponent. Negative network pattern, with or without chrysalis-like structures, is another common pattern. The negative network consists of light areas making up the "grid" of the network and dark areas are the "holes".[10]

Dermatofibroma

Various patterns encountered are total homogeneous area, a uniform homogeneous pattern or a uniform white scar-like patch combination of or a combination of those or an atypical pattern. Delicate peripheral pigment network is hallmark of dermatofibroma (DF).[11]

Neurofibroma

Pink-red homogeneous areas, peripheral pigment network, fingerprint-like structures, fissures (Figs. 4A and B) scar-like white areas and blood vessels are visible.[12]

Cherry Angioma

Numerous, well-demarcated round or oval, red-bluish lacunae (Figs. 5A and B) corresponding histologically to enlarged dilated vascular spaces in the upper dermis, are seen. Thrombosed and involuted hemangioma has dark lacunae and scar-like appearance.[13]

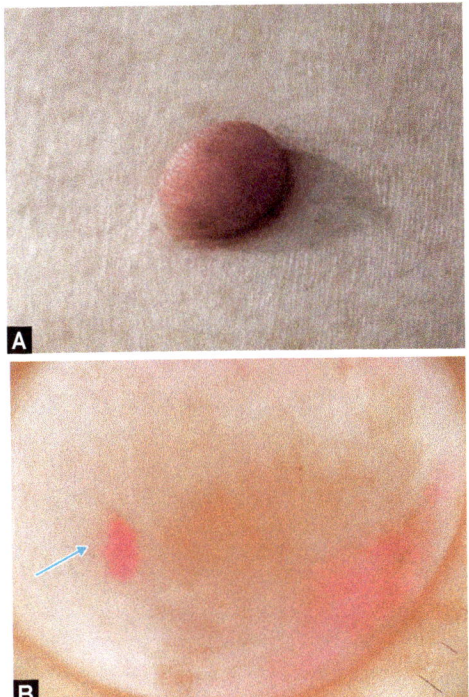

Figs. 4A and B: Neurofibroma: (A) Clinical; (B) Dermoscopy images revealing pink–red homogeneous areas (blue arrow), peripheral pigment network and blood vessels.

Pyogenic Granuloma

The specific dermoscopic features include presence of reddish homogeneous areas wtih white collarette, white rail line and

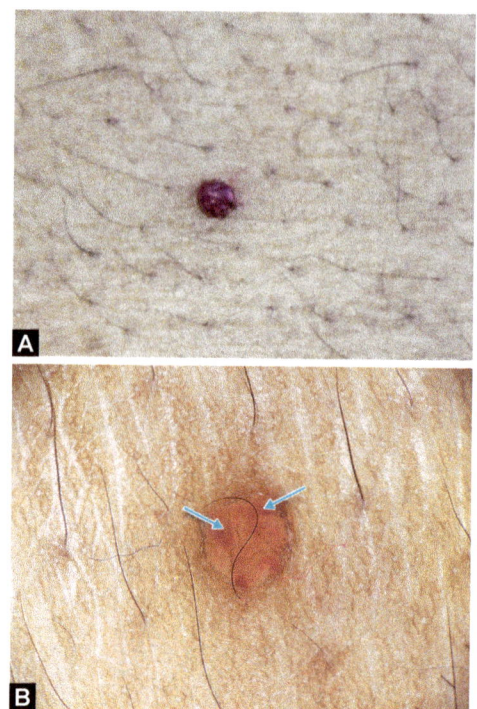

Figs. 5A and B: Cherry angioma: (A) Clinical; (B) Dermoscopy images showing multiple and well-demarcated round or oval red–bluish lacunae (blue arrows).

vascular structures (Figs. 6A and B). Red areas correspond to dilated vessels and white structures suggest collagen bundles separating vascular lobules in the dermis.[14]

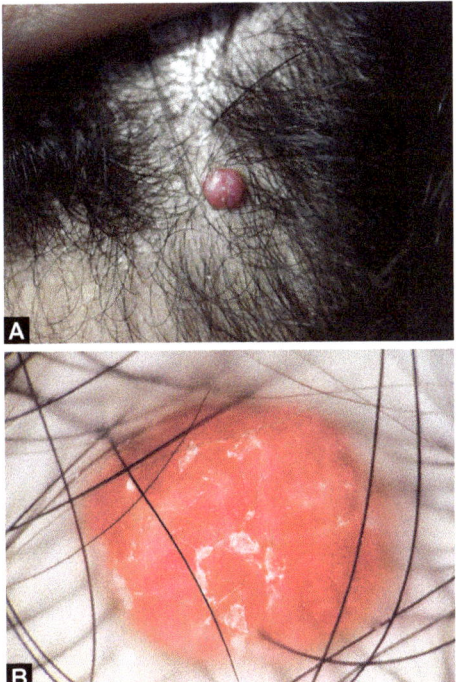

Figs. 6A and B: Pyogenic granuloma: (A) Clinical; (B) Dermoscopy images showing reddish homogeneous areas, white rail-line and vascular structures.

Lymphangioma Circumscriptum

Two patterns are described: Yellow lacunae surrounded by pale septa which do not contain blood and yellow to pink lacunae due to inclusion of blood.[15]

Seborrheic Keratosis

Cerebriform pattern (most commonly seen), moth eaten borders, comedo-like openings, milia-like cysts (MLC), hairpin vessels; fat fingers, and finger print patterns are described and seen (Figs. 7A to F). Recently, pigment network-like structures

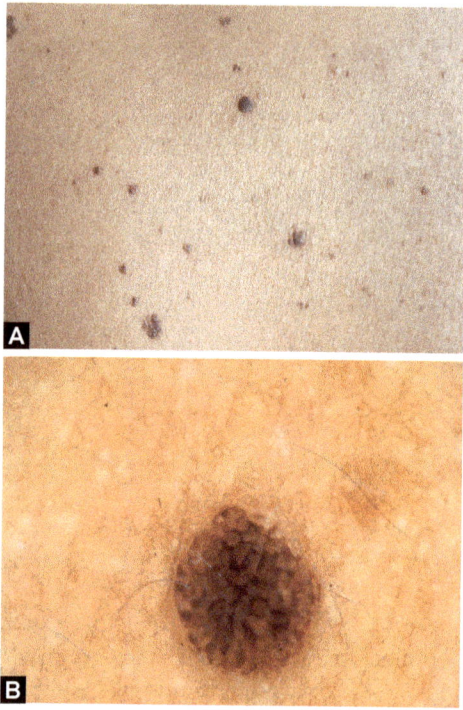

Figs. 7A and B

CHAPTER 27: Dermoscopy of Benign Skin Tumors

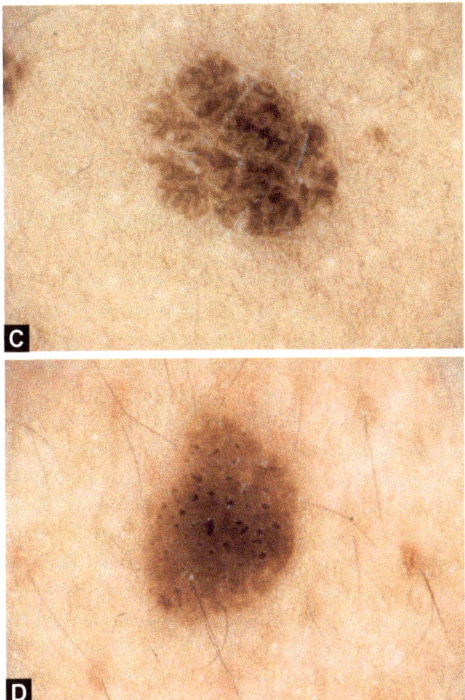

Figs. 7C and D

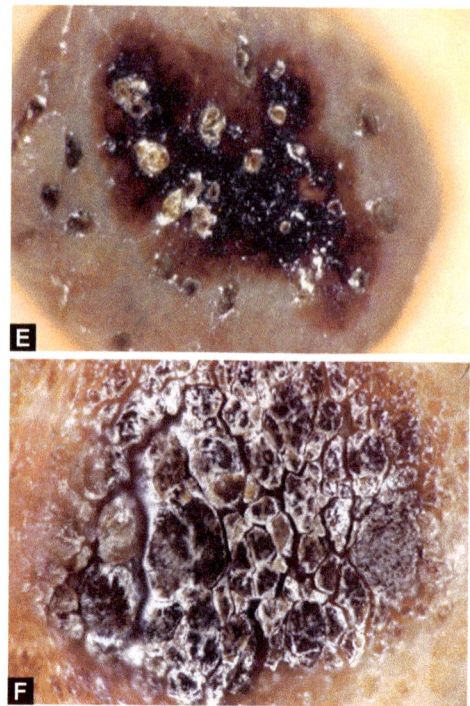

Figs. 7E and F

Figs. 7A to F: Seborrheic keratosis: (A) Clinical; (B) Dermoscopy images showing fingerprint pattern; (C) Cerebriform pattern with moth-eaten borders; (D) Comedo-like openings; (E) Milia-like cysts; (F) Thick crusts.

were described which look like pigment network (melanocytic criteria) but are not actually a pigment network. Thick crusts appear as "parchment-like" pattern.[16]

Sebaceous Hyperplasia

Specific patterns: yellow to white globules occupying whole of the lesion and linear vessels running from periphery to the center are seen. These are called "crown vessels". Vessels are pushed to the periphery due to hyperplastic glands. Yellow globules correspond to sebaceous glands (Figs. 8A and B).[17]

Angiokeratoma

Peripheral erythema, dark blue lagoons, whitish veil appear as ground-glass film that correspond to acanthosis and hyperkeratosis (Figs. 9A and B).[18]

Angiofibroma

White globules on whitish-red or pinkish background are the patterns seen.[19] Bluish-white lacunae and white globules corresponding to proliferative vessels and to fibrosis respectively may also be visible.[14]

Milia

White to yellow homogeneous areas occupy the whole lesion. Brownish peripheral rim are distinctly present (Figs. 10A and B).[20]

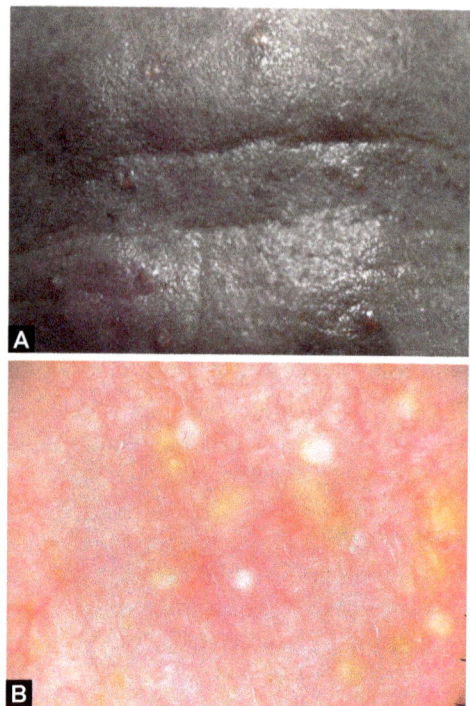

Figs. 8A and B: Sebaceous hyperplasia: (A) Clinical; (B) Dermoscopy images showing yellow-to-white globules.

CHAPTER 27: Dermoscopy of Benign Skin Tumors 425

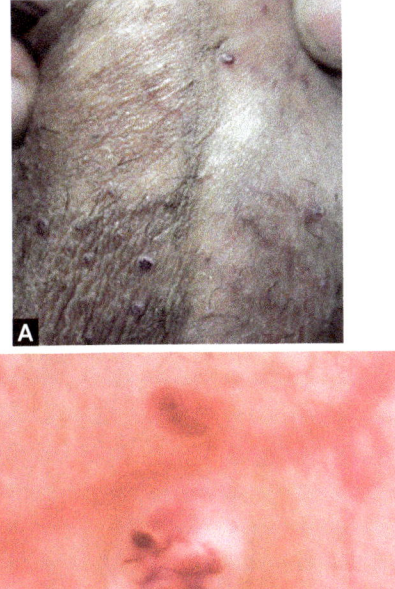

Figs. 9A and B: Angiokeratoma: (A) Clinical; (B) Dermoscopy images showing peripheral erythema, dark blue/purple lagoons.

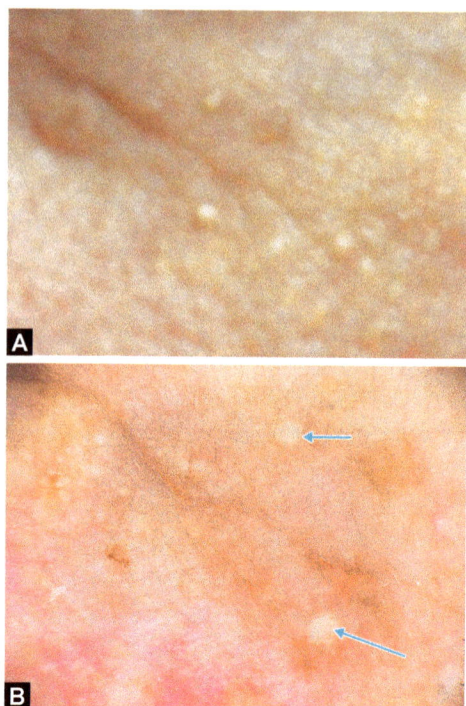

Figs. 10A and B: Milia: (A) Clinical; (B) Dermoscopy images showing white-to-yellow homogeneous area (blue arrows) and brownish peripheral rim.

Epidermal Cyst

Characteristic pore sign (Figs. 11A and B) correspond to central crater and follicular opening. The area of the pore is keratin-

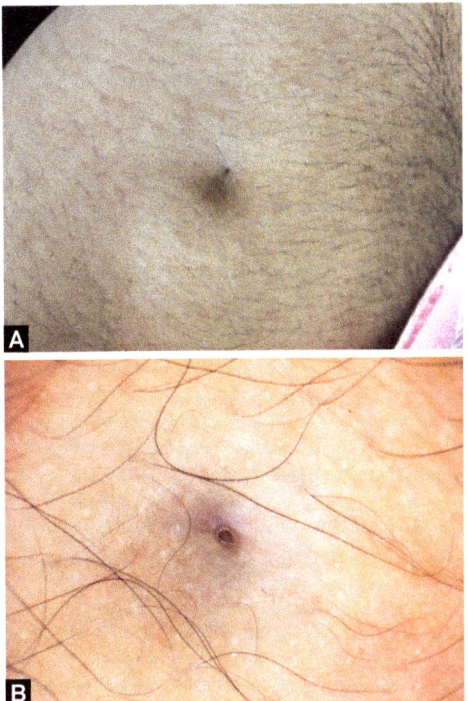

Figs. 11A and B: Epidermal cyst: (A) Clinical; (B) Dermoscopy image showing pore sign.

filled and may appear yellow, white, brown or black colored. Peripheral erythema with linear vessels and ivory white color in the center indicate ruptured cyst.[21] Branching vessels with bluish areas in the center indicate an unruptured cyst. Bright yellow areas in very early lesions and structureless whitish-blue areas in late lesions are other features.[22]

Apocrine Hidrocystoma

Dermoscopic patterns are translucent to opaque homogeneous areas that occupy the entire lesion, brown pigment globules, white areas and arborizing blood vessels.[23] Another study describes yellowish-brown homogeneous area covering whole lesion, linear irregular vessels running across the lesion and white globules.[14]

It mimics nodular basal cell carcinoma (BCC) on dermoscopy but additional presence of blue-gray globules favors nodular BCC.

Trichoepithelioma

Ivory white background with homogeneous brown structures corresponding to pseudo network, white globules and arborizing vessels are dermoscopic features.[24]

Steatocystoma

Yellow homogeneous area covering entire lesion (Figs. 12A and B), linear vessels, and peripheral brown rim are observed. Sweat duct openings are seen as glistening white dots on the tumor.[25]

Fibrokeratoma

Central homogeneous rosy-white areas surrounded by thin dark linear concentric structures with several dotted vessels

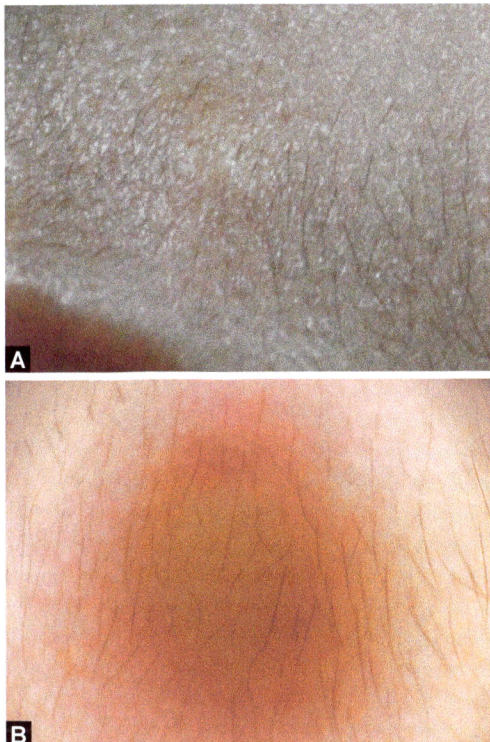

Figs. 12A and B: Steatocystoma: (A) Clinical; (B) Dermoscopy images showing yellow homogeneous area surrounded by peripheral brown rim.

within are seen. White areas correspond to fibrous tissue in the dermis.[26]

Syringoma

Brownish pseudonetwork-occupying whole lesion and tiny white dots representing sweat duct openings are observed (Figs. 13A and B).[27]

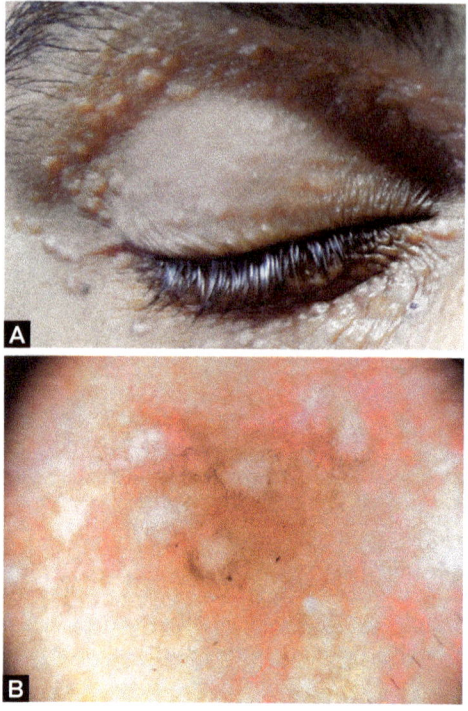

Figs. 13A and B: Syringoma: (A) Clinical; (B) Dermoscopy images showing brownish pseudonetwork-occupying whole lesion and tiny white dots.

CONCLUSION

Dermoscopy is an excellent tool in the hands of dermatologists in the diagnosis of various benign skin tumors with characteristic dermoscopic features. In addition, it supports the diagnosis of several others. Benign skin tumor diagnosis is another area where the increased use of dermoscopy would enable a therapeutic choice to be made in association with the patient.

REFERENCES

1. Changchien L, Dusza SW, Agero AL, et al. Age- and site-specific variation in the dermoscopic patterns of congenital melanocytic nevi: an aid to accurate classification and assessment of melanocytic nevi. Arch Dermatol. 2007;143:1007-14.
2. Argenziano G, Soyer HP, Chimenti S, et al. Dermoscopy of pigmented skin lesions: results of a consensus meeting via the internet. J Am Acad Dermatol. 2003;48:679-93.
3. Marghoob AA, Braun RP, Kopf AW. Atlas of Dermoscopy. Abingdon: Taylor and Francis; 2005.
4. Zalaudek I, Grinschgl S, Argenziano G, et al. Age-related prevalence of dermoscopy patterns in acquired melanocytic naevi. Br J Dermatol. 2006;154:299-304.
5. Zalaudek I, Hofmann-Wellenhof R, Kittler H, et al. A dual concept of nevogenesis: theoretical considerations based on dermoscopic features of melanocytic nevi. J Dtsch Dermatol Ges. 2007;5:985-92.
6. Kolm I, Di Stefani A, Hofmann-Wellenhof R, et al. Dermoscopy patterns of halo nevi. Arch Dermatol. 2006;142:1627-32.
7. Cramer SF. Speckled lentiginous nevus (nevus spilus): the "roots" of the "melanocytic garden". Arch Dermatol. 2011;137:1654-5.

8. Schaffer JV, Orlow SJ, Lazova R, et al. Speckled lentiginous nevus: within the spectrum of congenital melanocytic nevi. Arch Dermatol. 2001;137:172-8.
9. Zalaudek I, Sgambato A, Mordente I, et al. Melanocytic skin lesions in children: dermoscopy patterns and management considerations. G Ital Dermatol Venereol. 2006;141:366-70.
10. Soyer HP, Argenziano G, Hofmann-Wellenhof R, et al. Color Atlas of Melanocytic Lesions of the Skin. New York: Springer-Verlag; 2007.
11. Zaballos P, Puig S, Llambrich A, et al. Dermoscopy of dermatofibromas: A prospective morphological study of 412 cases. Arch Dermatol. 2008;144:75-83.
12. Duman N, Elmas M. Dermoscopy of cutaneous neurofibromas associated with neurofibromatosis type 1. J Am Acad Dermatol. 2015;73:529-31.
13. Wolf IH. Dermoscopic diagnosis of vascular lesions. Clin Dermatol. 2002;20:273-5.
14. Ankad BS, Sakhare PS, Prabhu MH. Dermoscopy of non-melanocytic and pink tumors in brown skin: A descriptive study. Indian J Dermatopathol Diagn Dermatol. 2017;4:41-51.
15. Amini S, Kim NH, Zell DS, et al. Dermoscopic-histopathologic correlation of cutaneous lymphangioma circumscriptum. Arch Dermatol. 2008;144:1671-2.
16. Braun RP, Rabinovitz HS, Krischer J, et al. Dermoscopy of pigmented seborrheic keratosis: A morphological study. Arch Dermatol. 2002;138:1556-60.
17. Zaballos P, Ara M, Puig S, et al. Dermoscopy of sebaceous hyperplasia. Arch Dermatol. 2005;141:808.
18. Zaballos P, Daufı C, Puig S, et al. Dermoscopy of Solitary Angiokeratomas: A Morphological Study. Arch Dermatol. 2007;143:318-25.

19. Ozeki M, Saito R, Tanaka M. Dermoscopic features of pearly penile papules. Dermatology. 2008;217:21-2.
20. Stricklin SM, Stoecker WV, Oliviero MC, et al. Cloudy and starry milia-like cysts: How well do they distinguish seborrheic keratoses from malignant melanomas? J Eur Acad Dermatol Venereol. 2011;25:1222-4.
21. Ghigliotti G, Cinotti E, Parodi A. Usefulness of dermoscopy for the diagnosis of epidermal cyst: The 'pore' sign. Clin Exp Dermatol. 2014;39:649-50.
22. Suh KS, Kang DY, Park JB, et al. Usefulness of Dermoscopy in the Differential Diagnosis of Ruptured and Unruptured Epidermal Cysts. Ann Dermatol. 2017;29:33-8.
23. Zaballos P, Bañuls J, Medina C, et al. Dermoscopy of apocrine hidrocystomas: A morphological study. J Eur Acad Dermatol Venereol. 2014;28:378-81.
24. Ardigo M, Zieff J, Scope A, et al. Dermoscopic and reflectance confocal microscope findings of trichoepithelioma. Dermatology. 2007;215:354-8.
25. Bañuls J, Arribas P, Berbegal L, et al. Yellow and orange in cutaneous lesions: Clinical and dermoscopic data. J Eur Acad Dermatol Venereol. 2015;29:2317-25.
26. Rubegni P, Poggiali S, Lamberti A, et al. Dermoscopy of acquired digital fibrokeratoma. Australas J Dermatol. 2012;53:47-8.
27. Hayashi Y, Tanaka M, Nakajima S, et al. Dermatol Reports. 2011;3:e42.

# CHAPTER 28

Dermoscopy of Malignant Cutaneous Tumors

Laxmisha Chandrashekar

INTRODUCTION

Dermoscopy is a noninvasive outpatient procedure that has been originally used to differentiate benign nevi from malignant melanomas. Its use has expanded to the diagnosis of actinic keratoses, Bowen's disease (BD), and squamous and basal cell carcinomas (BCCs). In this chapter, we will discuss the findings on dermoscopy in various malignant neoplasms.

KERATINIZING SKIN CANCERS

On the basis of dermoscopic findings, these lesions display a spectrum ranging from actinic keratosis (AK) to intraepidermal carcinoma to frank squamous cell carcinoma (SCC). Hence, several features, such as scaling, blood vessels, and erythema, are common among them.

Dermoscopy of Actinic Keratosis

Actinic keratosis is a neoplastic keratinocytic skin lesion that develops commonly over sun-damaged skin in elderly individuals, with a slight preponderance in males. AK develops in form of an ill-defined macule, papule, or plaque with color ranging from skin-colored to pink to red to brown, with dry, adherent scales. Lesions can be single or more commonly multiple, and the singular lesion can vary in size from few millimeters to 1–2 cm.

The clinical variants of AK are enumerated here including hypertrophic AK, lichenoid AK, proliferative AK, pigmented AK (also known as spreading pigmented AK), and actinic cheilitis.

Nonpigmented Actinic Keratoses

The dermoscopic appearance varies with the thickness of the lesion (Table 1). In the slightly palpable variants, it is characterized by an erythematous component and the thicker ones are characterized by keratotic scales (Fig. 1). The sensitivity and specificity of dermoscopy in establishing the diagnosis of actinic keratoses have been reported to be 98% and 95%, respectively.

Pigmented Actinic Keratoses

The pigmented AKs on dermoscopy display multiple slate-gray to dark-brown dots and globules around the follicular ostia, annular-granular pattern, and brown to gray pseudonetwork (Fig. 2).

Table 1: Dermoscopic findings in various grades of actinic keratoses.

Grade of actinic keratoses	Clinical description	Dermoscopic findings
1.	Slightly palpable, felt more than seen	Red pseudonetwork and discrete white scales
2.	Moderately thick. Easily felt and seen	Erythematous background that is intertwined with white to yellow keratotic partially confluent and enlarged follicular openings resembling a strawberry
3.	Thick hyperkeratotic lesions	Keratotic plugs or white or yellow structureless areas

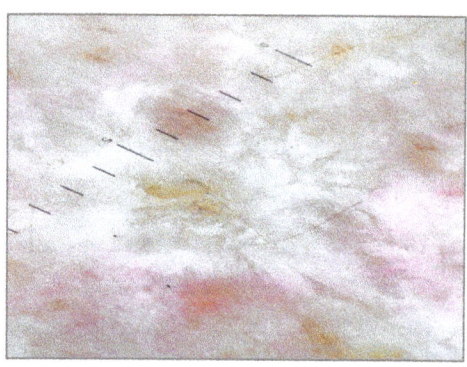

Fig. 1: Hypertrophic actinic keratoses (grade 3) demonstrating yellow keratinous scale in the center surrounded by out of focus linear vessels.

CHAPTER 28: Dermoscopy of Malignant Cutaneous Tumors

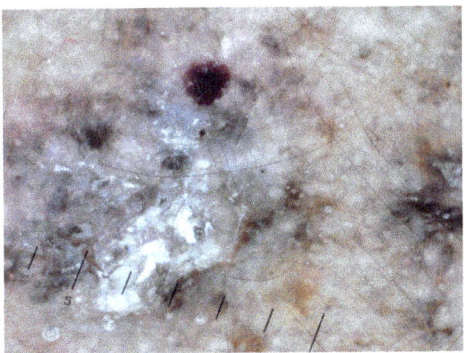

Fig. 2: Pigmented actinic keratoses demonstrating central scale, peripheral pseudonetwork, black dots, and keratotic plugging.

Dermoscopy of Bowen's Disease

Bowen's disease is a type of SCC in situ, that usually presents in form of a slow growing, well-defined red or pink lesion ranging from a patch or plaque with uneven borders with or without scaling or crusting over surface.

Dermoscopic features described among Asian population is typified by the occurrence of a scaly surface (Fig. 3) and vascular structures, out of which glomerular vessels are frequently observed and others being dotted, linear, irregular, atypical, and arborizing vessels. Glomerular vessels are a modified form of dotted vessels and large in size, commonly congregated and regularly organized in clusters, similar to renal glomerular vessels. Fading of these glomerular vessels with treatment has been reported.

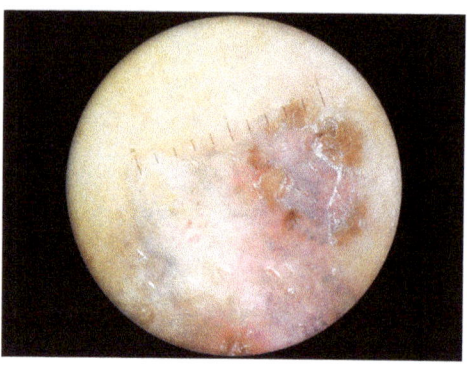

Fig. 3: Clustered glomerular vessels and yellow scale crust noted in Bowen's disease.

Dermoscopy of Squamous Cell Carcinoma

The various dermoscopic features described for SCC are keratin crust/scale, central keratin mass, white circles, white structureless area, blood spots, and polymorphous vessels (Figs. 4 and 5). Bright white-colored circles surrounding the dilated infundibulum are filled with a yellow/orange keratin plug which is also known as white circles. A four-clover leaf pattern consists of a rosette with four bright white clods or dots arranged in a two by two pattern. Polarized light can be used to observe it and it corresponds to keratin filled adnexal openings that are observed mostly in actinically damaged skin, AK, and SCC.

CHAPTER 28: Dermoscopy of Malignant Cutaneous Tumors

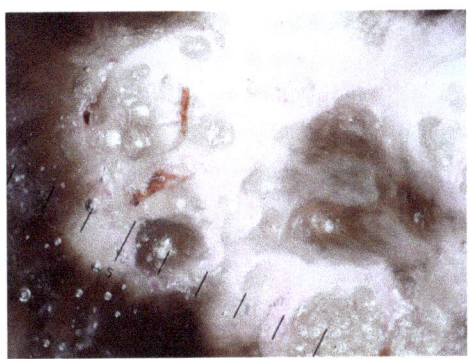

Fig. 4: White clods with central scale with polymorphous vessels (serpentine and dotted) in a case of squamous cell carcinoma.

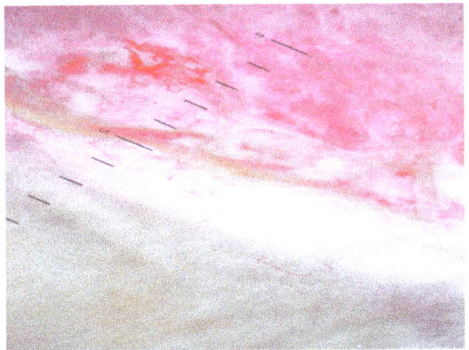

Fig. 5: Predominant vascular component (linear and looped vessels) with white circles and central yellow scale in a case of squamous cell carcinoma.

Dermoscopy of Basal Cell Carcinoma

The dermoscopic features varies depending upon the patient's skin color and histopathological subtype (Table 2). The various dermoscopic features described for BCC are arborizing vessels, superficial fine telangiectasia (Fig. 6), blue-gray ovoid nests (Fig. 7), multiple blue-gray globules (Fig. 8), in-focus dots,

Table 2: Dermoscopic features of basal cell carcinoma.

Dermoscopic features	Corresponding histopathological findings
Arborizing vessels	Dilated vessels in the dermis
Superficial telangiectasia	Telangiectatic vessels in the papillary dermis
Blue-gray ovoid nests	Large well-defined tumor nests invading the dermis
Blue-gray globules	Papillary or reticular dermal located around small, round blue tumor
In-focus dots	Aggregates of pigmented neoplastic cells or free pigment deposition, and/or melanophages
Maple leaf-like areas	Interconnected multifocal tumor nests
Spoke wheel areas	Tumor nests arising and connected to the epidermis
Ulceration	Loss of the epidermis
Shiny white-red structureless areas	Fibrotic tumoral stroma
Short white streaks (chrysalis) (only under polarized dermoscopy)	Collagenous stroma and fibrosis in the dermis

CHAPTER 28: Dermoscopy of Malignant Cutaneous Tumors

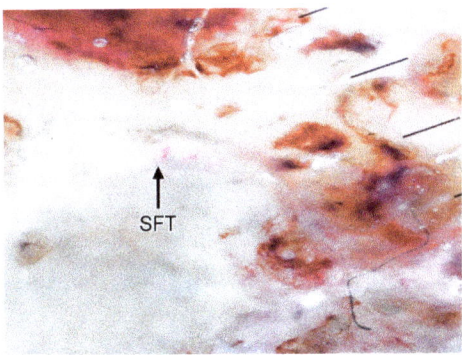

Fig. 6: Ulceration and superficial telangiectasia (SFT) in basal cell carcinoma (BCC) (arrow).

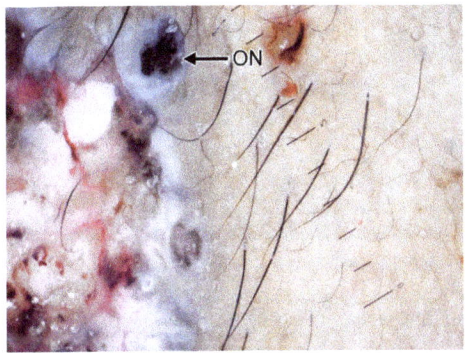

Fig. 7: Blue-gray ovoid nests (ON) in basal cell carcinoma (BCC) (arrow).

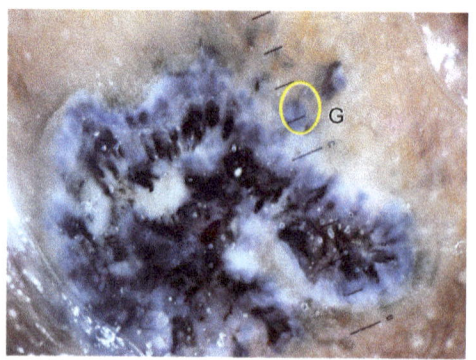

Fig. 8: In-focus blue-gray globules (G) in basal cell carcinoma (BCC).

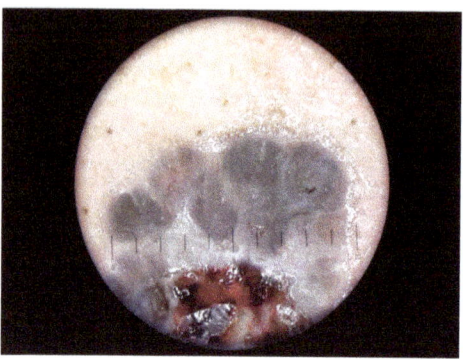

Fig. 9: Maple leaf-like areas in basal cell carcinoma (BCC).

maple leaf-like areas (Fig. 9), spoke wheel areas, concentric structures, ulceration, multiple small erosions, shiny white-red structureless areas (Fig. 10), and short white streaks (chrysalis).

CHAPTER 28: Dermoscopy of Malignant Cutaneous Tumors

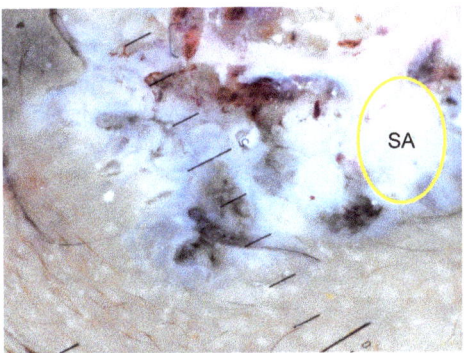

Fig. 10: White structureless areas (SA) in basal cell carcinoma (BCC).

The dermoscopic criteria proposed for BCC is lack of pigment network and occurrence of one of the earlier positive structures (ulceration, multiple blue-gray globules, leaf-like areas, large blue-gray ovoid nests, spoke wheel areas, and arborizing telangiectasia).

Dermoscopy of Malignant Melanoma

Out of various morphological and histological subtypes of malignant melanoma, the acral melanomas (acral lentiginous melanoma and melanoma of nail apparatus) are common in Indian population. The skin of palms and soles lacks follicles (glabrous) and is marked by dermatoglyphic lines that form unique patterns of ridges and furrows. The nevus cells have a tendency to aggregate or form nests near the dermoepidermal junction of the crista limitans (dermatoglyphic furrows) while the melanoma cells in the early phase that aggregate near the crista intermedia (dermatoglyphic ridges).

Hence, if dermoscopy reveals a predominantly lattice-like parallel furrow pattern, then it suggests benign nature of the lesion (Fig. 11) and if it displays a parallel ridge pattern, there is a possibility of melanoma (Figs. 12 and 13). This parallel ridge sign is considered to be the one of the most reliable dermoscopic sign for diagnosing acral melanoma.

The dermoscopic structures described in acral lentiginous melanoma are diffuse asymmetrical pigmentation, and the parallel-ridge pattern (in contrast to parallel furrow pattern that is observed in benign lesions). The dermoscopic features of acral amelanotic melanoma are dominated by retention of microscopic pigmentation, milky-red areas, and polymorphous

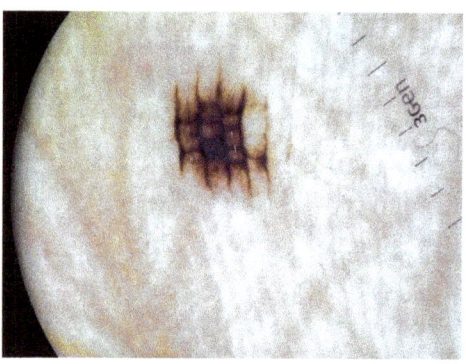

Fig. 11: Lattice pattern of a benign acral nevi.

CHAPTER 28: Dermoscopy of Malignant Cutaneous Tumors

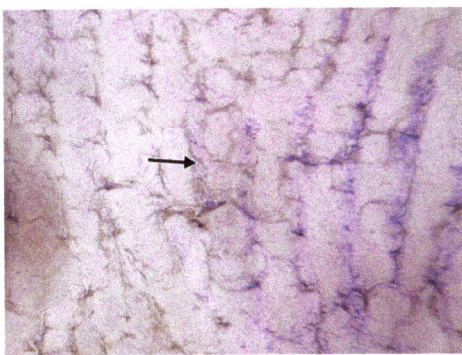

Fig. 12: Ink furrow test demonstrating some pigment in the ridges suggestive of malignancy (arrow).

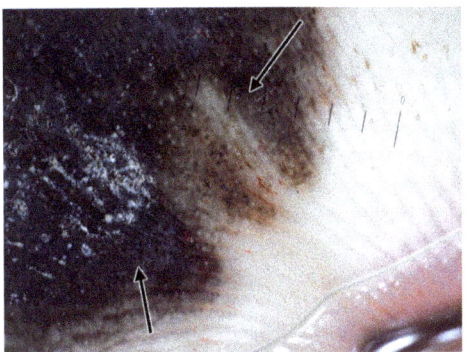

Fig. 13: Acral lentiginous melanoma demonstrating parallel ridge pattern and irregular diffuse pigmentation (arrows).

vascular pattern consisting of linear irregular vessels, dotted vessels, and hairpin vessels.

The ABCD criterion is used to differentiate a benign nevi from a malignant melanoma. The presence of two or three criteria is suggestive of a suspicious lesion, and this lesion must be excised.

These criteria are as follows:
1. Asymmetry (of color and structure in one or two perpendicular axes)
2. Atypical network (pigmented network with irregular holes and thick lines)
3. Blue-white structures (any type of blue and/or white color).

BIBLIOGRAPHY

1. Boyd AS, Stasko TS, Tang YW. Basaloid squamous cell carcinoma of the skin. J Am Acad Dermatol. 2011;64:144-51.
2. Bugatti L, Filosa G, De Angelis R. Dermoscopic observation of Bowen's disease. J Eur Acad Dermatol Venereol. 2004;18:572-4.
3. Chung E, Marchetti MA, Pulitzer MP, et al. Streaks in pigmented squamous cell carcinoma in situ. J Am Acad Dermatol. 2015;72:S64-5.
4. Giacomel J, Lallas A, Argenziano G, et al. Dermoscopic "signature" pattern of pigmented and nonpigmented facial actinic keratoses. J Am Acad Dermatol. 2015;72:e57-9.
5. Lallas A, Apalla Z, Argenziano G, et al. The dermatoscopic universe of basal cell carcinoma. Dermatol Pract Concept. 2014;4:11-24.
6. Lallas A, Argenziano G, Zendri E, et al. Update on non-melanoma skin cancer and the value of dermoscopy in its diagnosis and treatment monitoring. Expert Rev Anticancer Ther. 2013;13: 541-58.

CHAPTER 28: Dermoscopy of Malignant Cutaneous Tumors

7. Lin MJ, Pan Y, Jalilian C, et al. Dermoscopic characteristics of nodular squamous cell carcinoma and keratoacanthoma. Dermatol Pract Concept. 2014;4:9-1.
8. Longo C, Lallas A, Kyrgidis A, et al. Classifying distinct basal cell carcinoma subtype by means of dermatoscopy and reflectance confocal microscopy. J Am Acad Dermatol. 2014;71:716-24.e1.
9. Menzies SW, Westerhoff K, Rabinovitz H, et al. Surface microscopy of pigmented basal cell carcinoma. Arch Dermatol. 2000;136:1012-6.
10. Moscarella E, Rabinovitz H, Zalaudek I, et al. Dermoscopy and reflectance confocal microscopy of pigmented actinic keratoses: a morphological study. J Eur Acad Dermatol Venereol. 2015;29:307-14.
11. Mun JH, Kim SH, Jung DS, et al. Dermoscopic features of Bowen's disease in Asians. J Eur Acad Dermatol Venereol. 2010;24:805-10.
12. Phan A, Dalle S, Touzet S, et al. Dermoscopic features of acral lentiginous melanoma in a large series of 110 cases in a white population. Br J Dermatol. 2010;162:765-71.
13. Saida T, Miyazaki A, Oguchi S, et al. Significance of dermoscopic patterns in detecting malignant melanoma on acral volar skin: results of a multicenter study in Japan. Arch Dermatol. 2004;140:1233-8.
14. Zalaudek I, Kreusch J, Giacomel J, et al. How to diagnose nonpigmented skin tumors: a review of vascular structures seen with dermoscopy: part II. Nonmelanocytic skin tumors. J Am Acad Dermatol. 2010;63:377-88.

CHAPTER 29

Dermoscopy in Keratosis Pilaris

Mary Thomas, Uday S Khopkar

INTRODUCTION

Keratosis pilaris (KP) is an autosomal dominantly inherited trait clinically characterized by keratinous plugs in the follicular orifices and varying degrees of perifollicular erythema (Fig. 1). It affects nearly 50–80% of all adolescents and approximately 40% of adults.[1] Most people with mild KP are otherwise asymptomatic and are frequently unaware of the condition though occasionally it may be cosmetically displeasing.

The sites of predilection are the extensor surfaces of the upper arms (92%), thighs (59%), and buttocks (30%).[2] The classically described histology is distention of the follicular orifice by a keratinous plug that may contain one or more twisted hair. However, this histopathological picture is not frequently seen in skin biopsies.

Known associations of KP include atopy, ichthyosis vulgaris, ichthyosis follicularis, atrichia with papular lesions, ectodermal dysplasia, and keratitis-ichthyosis-deafness (KID) syndrome.[3]

PATHOGENESIS OF KERATOSIS PILARIS

Keratosis pilaris was believed to be a disorder of keratinization caused by a mutation in the filaggrin (FLG) gene. Hyperandrogenism is also known to play a role by causing hyperkeratinization of the pilosebaceous unit of terminal hair, which explains the increased incidence of KP in the pubertal age group.[4] Newer theories hypothesize that it may in fact be a disorder of the hair shaft. Circular hair shafts rupture the follicular epithelium leading to inflammation and abnormal follicular keratinization. The reduction of KP following permanent hair reduction supports this hypothesis.[3,5] More recently, atrophy and absence of sebaceous glands has been identified as an early feature indicating that they might play a role in the pathogenesis of KP.[6]

DERMOSCOPIC FEATURES OF KERATOSIS PILARIS

The pathognomonic dermoscopic finding in KP is a coiled hair shaft that can be visualized emerging from a stellate area with radiating white streaks in the center. These areas correspond to keratinized plugs in the follicular infundibulum (Figs. 2 and 3). The hair shaft may be a semicircle (Fig. 4) or a loop (Fig. 5); and at times, it is coiled and superficially embedded in the uppermost layers of epidermis next to the follicular opening (Fig. 6). With the help of a needle tip, it is possible

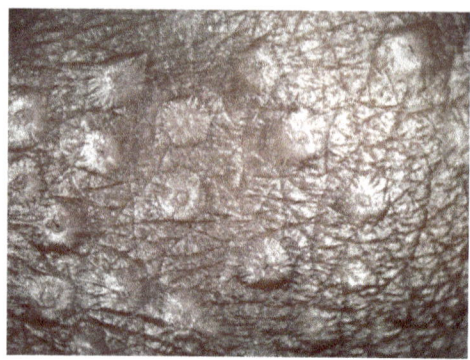

Fig. 1: Dermoscopy of keratosis pilaris, which, on white light dermoscopy, reveals keratinous plugs in follicular openings.

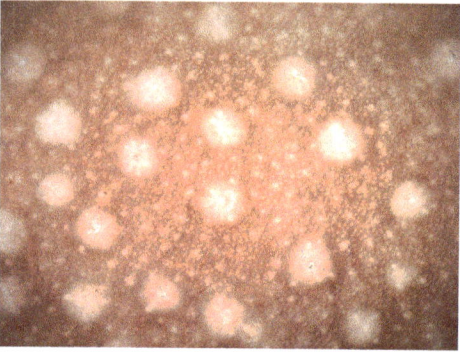

Fig. 2: The same lesion when observed under polarized light displays stellate areas with radiating white streaks with vellus follicle in the center.

CHAPTER 29: Dermoscopy in Keratosis Pilaris

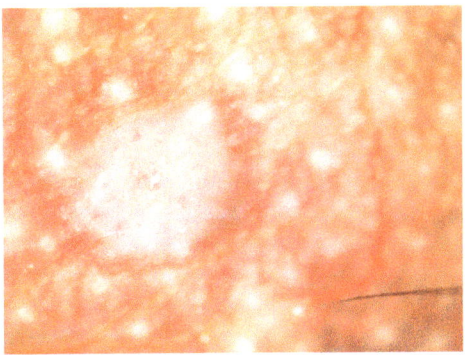

Fig. 3: Keratinous plug in follicular opening.

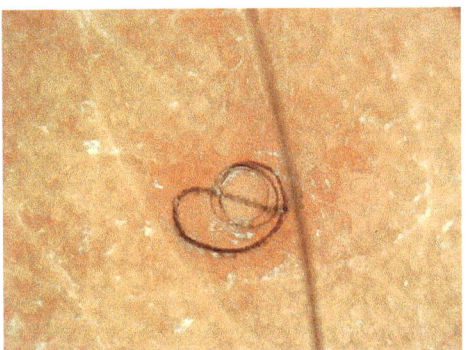

Fig. 4: A semicircular hair shaft emerging from a follicle.

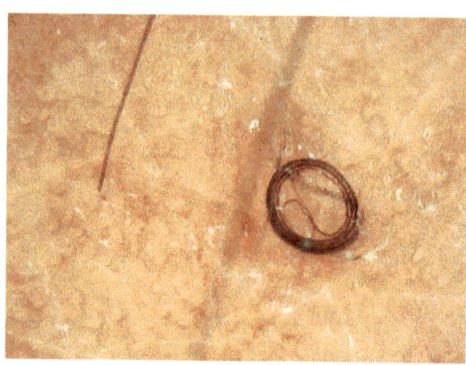

Fig. 5: Keratosis pilaris: coiled hair shaft seen in the follicular opening.

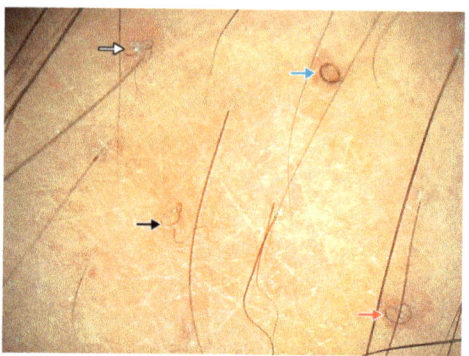

Fig. 6: Keratosis pilaris on polarized light dermoscopy displays coiled hair (white arrow), serpentine hair (black arrow), circular loop (blue arrow), and semicircular hair (red arrow) shaft emerging from a follicle.

to easily dislodge and uncoil the hair shaft from the skin. Follicular plugging may or may not be present in every follicle examined. The plugs are small and lighter in color in lesions that have not been irritated by friction or topical applications. The number of sebaceous glands visualized dermoscopically appears to be decreased in individuals prone to KP and may be a manifestation of concomitant atopy and ichthyosis.

DIFFERENTIAL DIAGNOSIS OF KERATOSIS PILARIS

Conditions presenting as keratotic follicular papules may be considered in the differential diagnosis of KP.

- *Follicular eczema:* This condition is characterized by grouped follicular papules commonly seen on the extremities that have an exacerbating and remitting course. On dermoscopy, we see perifollicular hypopigmentation and scaling (Fig. 7).

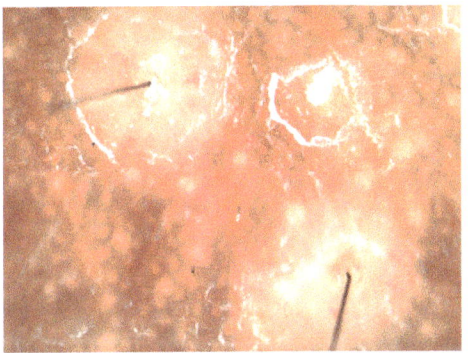

Fig. 7: Follicular eczema: dermoscopy reveals perifollicular scaling.

- *Ingrown hair*: This condition, also referred to as pseudofolliculitis, occurs when curly terminal hairs that emerge at an acute angle grow back toward the surface of the skin after shaving or depilation.[7] It is commonly seen in the beard, pubic region, and axillae.

Clinically, these lesions present as follicular papules. On dermoscopy, we see prominent raised follicular papules with terminal hair emerging from the center. These hairs may be seen as loops. Very often, we see more than one hair shaft emerging from the center of the papule (Fig. 8).

The presence of raised papules and terminal hair differentiate this condition from KP on dermoscopy.

The dermoscopic features of other common clinical differentials of KP are summarized in Table 1.

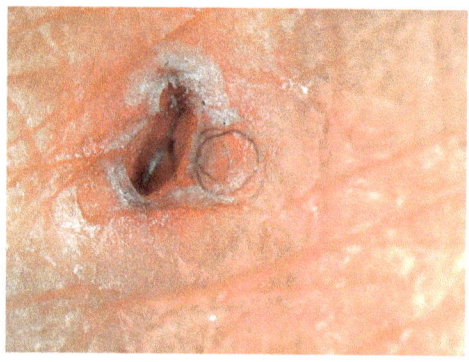

Fig. 8: Pseudofolliculitis: dermoscopy reveals prominent raised follicular papules with 2–3 terminal hair shafts emerging from the center.

Table 1: Dermoscopic features of the differential diagnoses of keratosis pilaris (KP).

Number	Clinical condition	Dermoscopic finding
1.	Follicular lichen planus	Follicular plugging surrounded by violaceous to black clods
2.	Follicular psoriasis	Regularly arranged dotted vessels and white scales
3.	Pityriasis rubra pilaris	Round yellowish areas surrounded by linear and dotted vessels
4.	Acne vulgaris	Brown–yellow hard central plug sparse inflammation
5.	Hypovitaminosis A	Follicular papules with translucent spines and perilesional floret-like structures
6.	Perforating folliculitis	Bright white clods centered in a structureless gray area surrounded by reticular brown lines
7.	Scurvy	Whitish hair follicles with corkscrew hair surrounded by a violaceous halo
8.	Eruptive vellus hair cyst	Nonmelanocytic round structure, central, oval, light–yellow plaque occasionally erythematous-maroon halo, radiating capillaries

REFERENCES

1. Alai NN. (2012). Keratosis pilaris—Emedicine. [online] Available from http://emedicine.medscape.com/article/1070651-overview. [Accessed December, 2018].

2. Judge MR, McLean WH, Munro CS. Disorders of keratinization. In: Burns DA, Breathnach SM, Cox NH, Griffiths CE (Eds). Rook's textbook of dermatology, 7th edition. Oxford, England: Blackwell Publishing; 2004. pp. 34.60-34.62.
3. Thomas M, Khopkar US. Keratosis pilaris revisited: is it more than just a follicular keratosis? Int J Trichology. 2012;4(4):255-8.
4. Mevorah B, Marazzi A, Frenk E. The prevalence of accentuated palmoplantar markings and keratosis pilaris in atopic dermatitis, autosomal dominant ichthyosis and control dermatological patients. Br J Dermatol. 1985;112(6):679-85.
5. Saelim P, Pongprutthipan M, Pootongkam S, et al. Long-pulsed 1064-nm Nd:YAG laser significantly improves keratosis pilaris: a randomized, evaluator-blind study. J Dermatolog Treat. 2013;24(4):318-22.
6. Gruber R, Sugarman JL, Crumrine D, et al. Sebaceous gland, hair shaft, and epidermal barrier abnormalities in keratosis pilaris with and without filaggrin deficiency. Am J Pathol. 2015;185(4):1012-21.
7. Puhan MR, Sahu B. Pseudofolliculitis corporis: a new entity diagnosed by dermoscopy. Int J Trichology. 2015;7(1):30-2.

CHAPTER 30

Porokeratosis

Sarvesh S Thatte, Uday S Khopkar

Porokeratosis is an autosomal dominant disorder of keratinization characterized by overexpression of p53 in epidermal cells. It is clinically characterized by presence of annular plaque with mild atrophy at the center and a raised, keratotic ridge in periphery, at the summit of which, is a gutter-like furrow. Histologically, it is characterized by cornoid lamella, which is an epidermal invagination of parakeratotic column with absence of underlying granular layer.[1,2]

It can be divided into five classical variants, i.e. (1) porokeratosis of Mibelli (Fig. 1), (2) disseminated superficial porokeratosis, (3) disseminated superficial actinic porokeratosis (Fig. 2), (4) porokeratosis palmaris et plantaris disseminata and (5) linear porokeratosis.[3] The distinctive keratotic ridge is usually seen in all the types though it may not be prominently

SECTION 7: Miscellaneous Dermoscopy Application

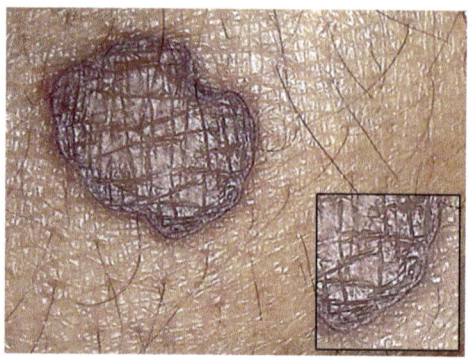

Fig. 1: Classic porokeratosis of Mibelli (keratotic ridge—hallmark of porokeratosis) (this is a clinical photograph).
(*Acknowledgment*: Skin Institute and School of Dermatology, New Delhi)
Picture edited as advised by Dr Khopkar

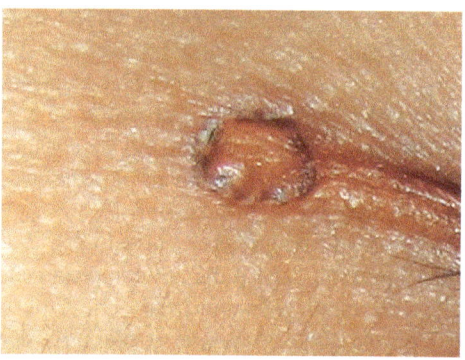

Fig. 2: Disseminated superficial actinic porokeratosis (canon power shot G12 camera) (this is a clinical photograph).

visible to naked eye in superficial variants of porokeratosis. In such instances, characteristic dermoscopic features help in the diagnosis of porokeratosis. Dermoscopy helps in distinguishing porokeratosis from psoriasis and annular lichen planus and also aids in early detection of its transformation into Bowen's disease, basal cell carcinoma (BCC) or squamous cell carcinoma (SCC).[2,4]

In order to visualize characteristic *histopathological features* of porokeratosis, biopsy should be taken from the hyperkeratotic ridge which reveals[5] (Fig. 3):

- *Cornoid lamella*, a thin column of parakeratotic cells that invaginates the epidermis.
- *Absence or reduced granular layer* beneath cornoid lamella.

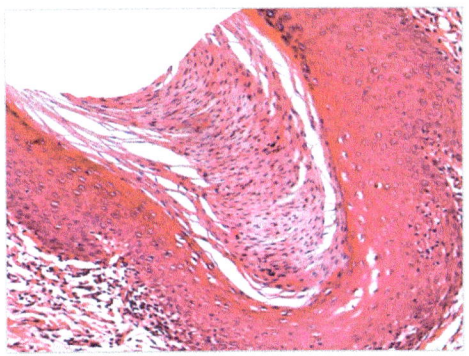

Fig. 3: Histopathology of porokeratosis depicting characteristic cornoid lamella with reduced underlying granular layer along with basal vacuolar change. (Hematoxylin and Eosin, 400×)
(*Acknowledgment*: Skin Institute and School of Dermatology, New Delhi)

- *Vacuolated or dyskeratotic cells in mid spinous layer* along with *basal layer vacuolar change.*
- Dilated capillaries in papillary dermis along with dermal patchy lichenoid infiltrate consisting of lymphocytes.

However, in primary cases of superficial porokeratosis, the cornoid lamella is either too subtle to notice in histopathological examination or may not be included in the section submitted for histopathological examination. During such instances, diagnosis of porokeratosis may be missed. Repeated serial sections and meticulous examination may help to find cornoid lamella in some of these cases.[6] In such instances, dermoscopic features can help to diagnose porokeratosis when the characteristic cornoid lamella is missed on histopathology.

Dermoscopic features seen in porokeratosis are:
- **White light dermoscopy:** Annular structure having raised hyperpigmented border, appearing as *"the outlines of a volcanic crater as observed from a high point"*, having central sharply demarcating flat pink–white scar-like area (Fig. 4), which is better appreciated on polarized light dermoscopy with whitish–yellowish annular structure at periphery[1] (Fig. 5).
- **Polarized light dermoscopy:**
    - Presence of peripheral white rim (*white track*, which corresponds to cornoid lamella) (Fig. 6) in conjunction with multiple *dotted/pinpoint and linear irregular vessels* (corresponds to dilated capillaries)[7,8] (Fig. 7).
    - *Brownish globules or dots* (corresponds to melanin in dermis) on inner side of white track with central homogeneous scar-like area[8,9] (Fig. 6).

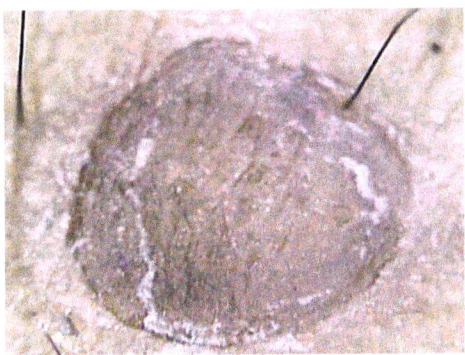

Fig. 4: Porokeratosis appearing as *"the outlines of a volcanic crater as observed from a high point"* with raised hyperpigmented border. (Ultracam TLS, white light, 40×)

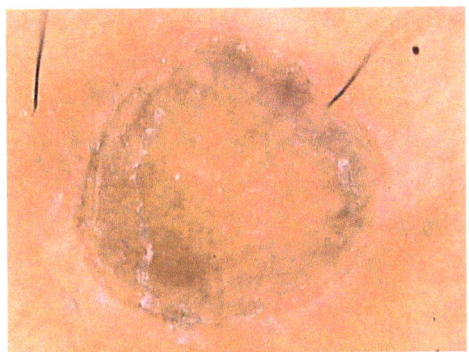

Fig. 5: Porokeratosis appearing as *"the outlines of a volcanic crater as observed from a high point"* with whitish-yellow annular structure at periphery. (Ultracam TLS, polarized light, 40×)

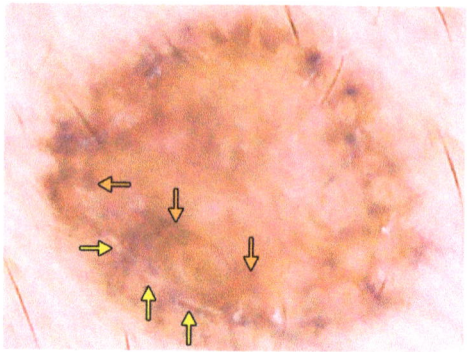

Fig. 6: White track at the periphery (yellow arrows) with brown globules/dots on inner side (orange arrows). (Ultracam TLS, polarized light, 40×)

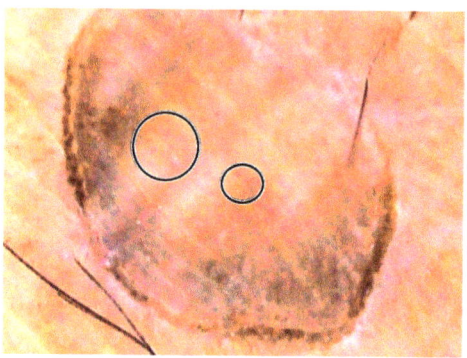

Fig. 7: Dotted/pinpoint (Black large circle) and linear vessel (small circle). (Ultracam TLS, polarized light, 40×)

- Whitish or brownish center that may exhibit *circular and/or linear whitish and/or hyperpigmented tracks, blue-gray dots* (corresponds to acanthotic epidermis)[8] (Fig. 8).
- *Ultraviolet light dermoscopy*: Hyperkeratotic ridge in porokeratosis that glows on ultraviolet light dermoscopy, which resembles *diamond necklace*[10] (Fig. 9).

Dermoscopy, a noninvasive technique, can help to diagnose and distinguish porokeratosis from other close clinical differentials thus obviating the need for biopsy.

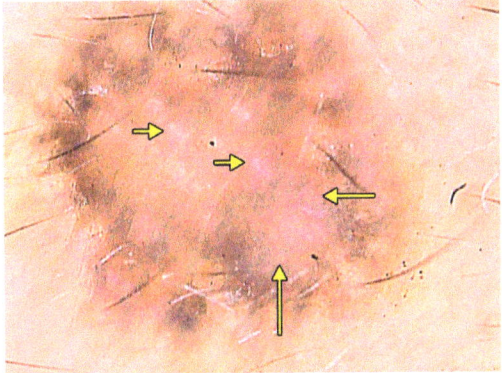

Fig. 8: Circular and/or linear whitish and/or hyperpigmented tracks, blue-gray dots (yellow arrows) corresponding to acanthotic epidermis. (Ultracam TLS, polarized light, 40×)

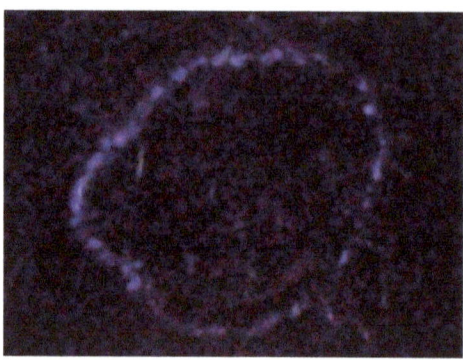

Fig. 9: "Diamond necklace" appearance of hyperkeratotic ridge in porokeratosis on ultraviolet light dermoscopy. (Ultracam TLS, ultraviolet light, 40×)

REFERENCES

1. Delfino M, Argenziano G, Nino M. Dermoscopy for the diagnosis of porokeratosis. J Eur Acad Dermatol Venereol. 2004;18:194-5.
2. Lee HR, Han TY, Son SJ, et al. Squamous Cell Carcinoma Developing within Lesions of Disseminated Superficial Actinic Porokeratosis. Ann Dermatol. 2011;23:536-8.
3. Bhaskar S, Jaiswal AK, Raj N, et al. Porokeratosis—Head to toe: An unusual presentation. Indian Dermatol Online J. 2015;6:101-4.
4. De Simone C, Paradisi A, Massi G, et al. Giant verrucous porokeratosis of Mibelli mimicking psoriasis in a patient with psoriasis. J Am Acad Dermatol. 2007;57:665-8.
5. Weedon D. Disorders of epidermal maturation and keratinization. In: Weedon D (Ed). Skin Pathology, 3rd edition. China: Elsevier; 2010. pp. 262-4.

6. Joshi R, Mesquita L. Interface dermatitis without cornoid lamellae is a pitfall in the diagnosis of porokeratosis: A report of three cases. Indian J Dermatol Venereol Leprol. 2016;82:70-2.
7. Moscarella E, Longo C, Zalaudek I, et al. Dermoscopy and confocal microscopy clues in the diagnosis of psoriasis and porokeratosis. J Am Acad Dermatol. 2013;69:e231-3.
8. Ankad BS, Savitha LB. Dermoscopy Picks Porokeratosis: A Case Report. Austin J Dermatolog. 2016;3:1061.
9. Nicola A, Magliano J. Dermoscopy of Disseminated Superficial Actinic Porokeratosis. Actas Dermosifiliogr. 2017;108:e33-7.
10. Thatte SS, Kharkar VD, Khopkar US. "Diamond necklace" appearance in superficial porokeratosis. J Am Acad Dermatol. 2014;70:e125-6.

CHAPTER 31

Genodermatoses

Atul M Dongre, Uday S Khopkar

INTRODUCTION

In genodermatoses, recognition of cutaneous lesions can be an important clue to the diagnosis. Dermoscopy findings of various pigmentary genodermatoses have not been described in literature.

NEVOID BASAL CELL CARCINOMA SYNDROME

Multiple basal cell carcinomas (BCCs) and palmar/plantar pits are the typical cutaneous findings in nevoid BCC syndrome. Lesions of BCC usually occur at younger age and these early lesions are difficult to diagnose. An early lesion of BCC may present as a small and nondescript papule, which may be difficult to diagnose unless biopsied. Dermatoscopy of such lesions shows telangiectasia, blotchy pigmentation of different colors (blue–gray blotches) (Figs. 1 and 2).

An early lesion of BCC may show only pigmentary network and lacks telangiectasia (Fig. 3). Scaling, ulceration, and

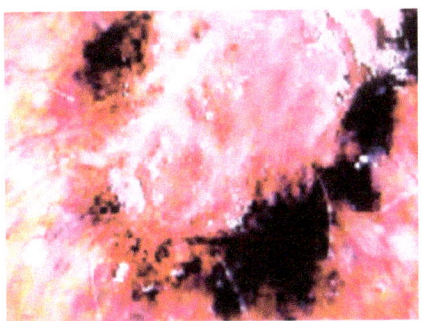

Fig. 1: Early basal cell carcinoma: Telangiectasia with blue–gray dots, globules, and blotches.

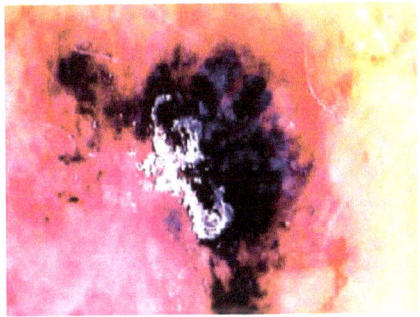

Fig. 2: Blue–gray globules, blotches and leaf like structures and telangiectasia.

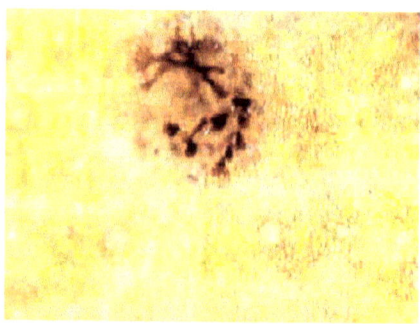

Fig. 3: Spoke-wheel and maple leaf-like pigmented structures in early lesion of nevoid basal cell carcinoma.

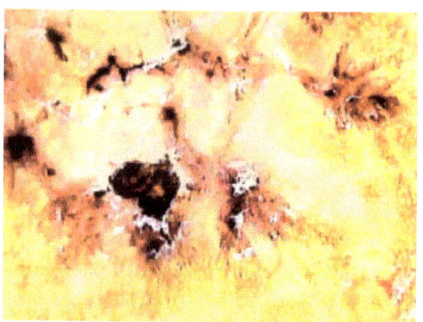

Fig. 4: Superficial spreading pigmented basal cell carcinoma: Pigmented brown black blotches with radiating leaf-like structures, ovoid nests and globules.

blue–gray pigmentation are less obvious in early lesions. In advanced lesion, telangiectasia, scaling, and ulceration are well appreciated (Fig. 4).

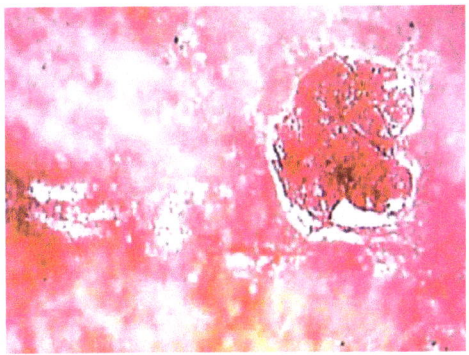

Fig. 5: White light dermoscopic image of palmar pits in nevoid basal cell carcinoma: Pits are seen like craters with brown dots and globules of pigment.

Palmoplantar pits are consistently present in cases of nevoid BCC syndrome. Dermoscopy helps to identify these pits, which may not be obvious to the naked eye. These pits are seen like a crater, which may show focal pigmentation (Fig. 5).

DOWLING–DEGOS DISEASE

Dowling–Degos disease (DDD) is characterized by multiple reticular pigmented macules over the flexors, neck, and occasionally on the dorsa of the hands. Pitted scars, comedones, and cystic lesions can also occur.

Pigmented macules in DDD show fine reticulated network of pigmentation (Fig. 6).

Certain lesions display minute annular pigmented rings with central hypopigmentation (Fig. 7). The annular pattern

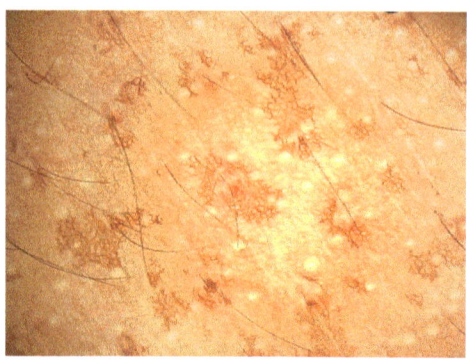

Fig. 6: Dermoscopy of pigmented macules in Dowling-Degos disease shows numerous irregular or polyangulated zones of accentuation of pigment network or pseudonetwork that corresponds with antler like branching seen on histopathology.

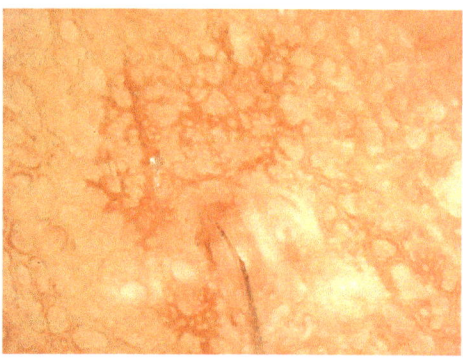

Fig. 7: Higher magnification dermoscopy of a single macule brings out the fine reticular nature of the pigmentation.

correlates with the rete ridges, which display irregular hyperplasia and hyperpigmentation on histopathology, and the central hypopigmented area corresponds to a follicular infundibulum from which these rete ridges are seen to proliferate from microscopically. Older macules show similar pattern but more intense pigmentation (Fig. 8).

The palmar pits display peripheral pigmentation along the margins of depression (Fig. 9). Occasionally, a reticular pigmentation pattern resembling the normal pattern of skin can also be observed on the palms (Fig. 10). In the beginning, the lesions develop short depressed pigmented lines, which join to form the annular pattern with interruptions along the dermatoglyphic lines.

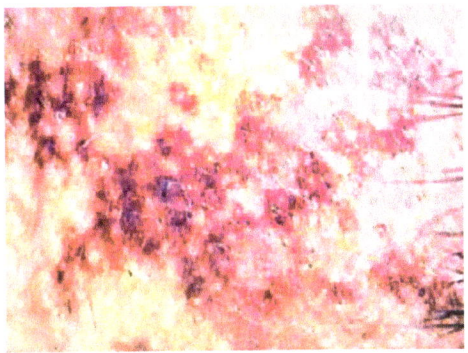

Fig. 8: Dermoscopic image of a late macule of Dowling–Degos disease: A late macule showing intensely dark pigmentation with central white globules forming pseudonetwork.

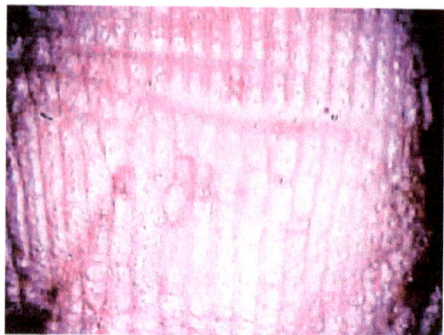

Fig. 9: Dermoscopic image of palmar pits in Dowling–Degos disease: Pits on the palm with pigmentation at the margins.

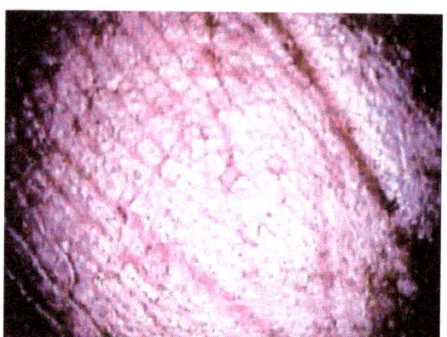

Fig. 10: Dermoscopic image of palm in Dowling–Degos disease: Breaks in the dermatoglyphics by pigmented linear furrows in a reticular pattern along with pits on the palm.

CHAPTER 32

Dermoscopy: Infections and Infestations

Manas Chatterjee, Gopalsing Rajput

INTRODUCTION

Over the last few years, dermoscopy has been proven to be an important tool for diagnosing various conditions without actually doing invasive investigations like biopsy. On a number of occasions, infections and infestations in daily outpatient department (OPD) have altered or atypical morphology, which mimics various unrelated disorders. Dermoscopy may help in diagnosing these conditions with fair accuracy thus obviating the need for biopsy in many cases. The aim of this chapter is to describe the various dermoscopic findings in common infections, which include bacterial infection like impetigo, Hansen's disease, lupus vulgaris, viral infections like verrucae, molluscum contagiosum, hand, foot, mouth disease (HFMD), fungal infections like pityriasis versicolor, tinea capitis and infestations like pediculosis capitis and scabies.

BACTERIAL INFECTIONS

Impetigo

It is a self-limited condition characterized by honey-colored crust clinically (Fig. 1); early diagnosis in important to avoid complications.[1] Dermoscopy of lesion reveals thick honey-colored crust-scale with some irregular vessels at base as occasional finding (Fig. 2).

Lupus Vulgaris

Lupus vulgaris (LV) is a form of high-resistance cutaneous tuberculosis, which can occur after direct inoculation of

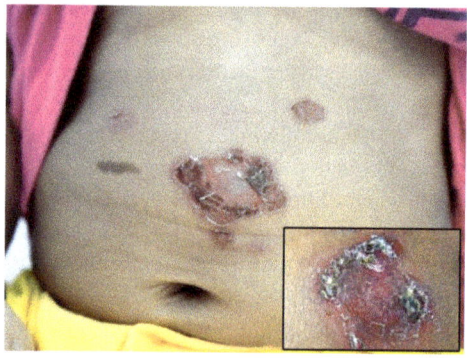

Fig. 1: Impetigo with honey-colored crusts clinically with close-up at inset.

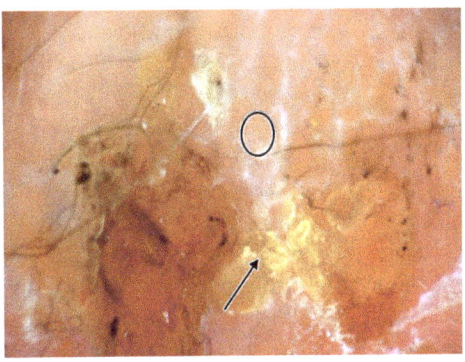

Fig. 2: Thick honey color crust-scale (black arrow) with some irregular vessels (black circle).

Mycobacterium tuberculosis bacilli or from hematogenous and lymphatic spread from internal tuberculous foci. The earliest lesion is a red brown soft papule, which grows by peripheral extension with central clearing (Fig. 3) and thighs and buttocks are most commonly affected sites. Dermoscopy of LV lesion shows golden-yellow or orange-yellow background with fine long telangiectasias (Fig. 4). Yellowish background is also seen in some other granulomatous conditions. Less frequent findings are milia-like cysts and white reticular streaks.[2,3]

Hansen's Disease

Leprosy is an endemic disease in India and has varied manifestations as evidenced by spectral classification by Ridley and Jopling and has hypopigmented, hypoesthetic lesion as a characteristic finding (Fig. 5). Dermoscopy of these lesions,

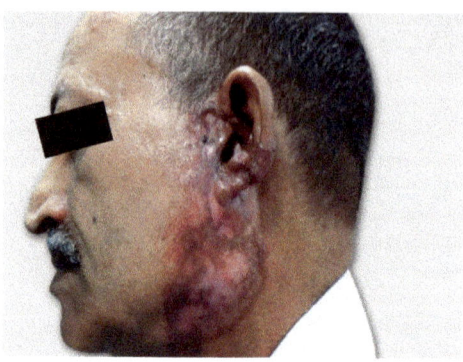

Fig. 3: Well-defined hyperpigmented plaque with central clearing.

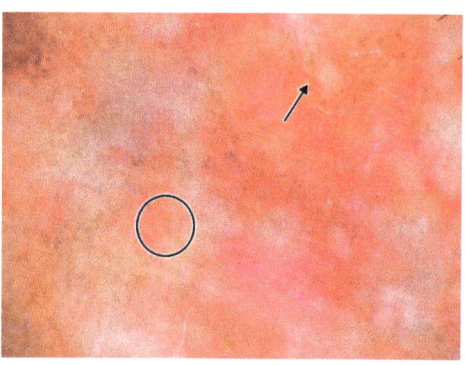

Fig. 4: Fine telangiectasias (black arrow) on a typical yellow to golden-colored background (black circle).

CHAPTER 32: Dermoscopy: Infections and Infestations

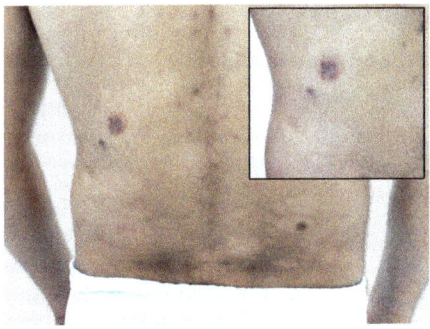

Fig. 5: Well- to ill-defined hypopigmented patch with biopsy scar mark over left flank (close up in inset).

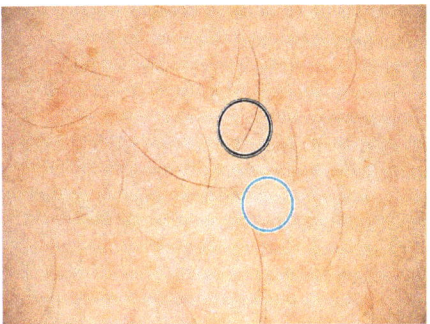

Fig. 6: Featureless white area (blue circle) with reduced hair density along with some branching vessels (black circle).

not in reaction, is characterized by featureless white area with reduced hair density along with yellow globules, decreased white dots along with some branching vessels[4] (Fig. 6).

VIRAL INFECTIONS

Hand, Foot, and Mouth Disease

Hand, foot, and mouth disease (HFMD) is generally a benign and self-limiting disease caused by *Coxsackievirus A16 (CVA16)* and *Human enterovirus 71 (HEV71)*, and rarely by some other members of the Picornaviridae family. Lesions are characterized by vesicles over the distal extremities including palms and soles as well as the mouth, where petechiae may be present as well (Figs. 7 to 9), in addition to the gluteal regions.[5] Though the diagnosis of HFMD is predominantly clinical, but sometimes, difficulty arises in early and atypical lesions where dermoscopy can be handy. Typical feature of HFMD shows appearance of vesicle in vesicle along with occasional hemorrhagic crust (Fig. 10).

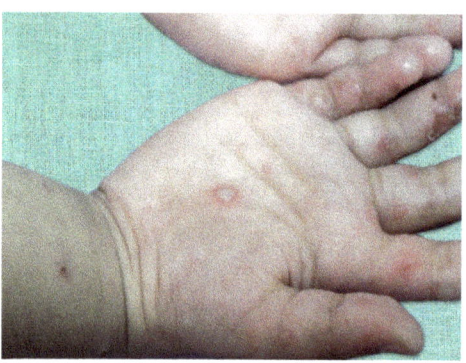

Fig. 7: Clear fluid-filled vesicles over palm.

CHAPTER 32: Dermoscopy: Infections and Infestations

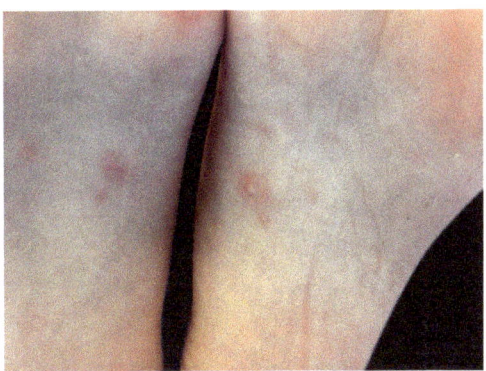

Fig. 8: Vesicles over soles.

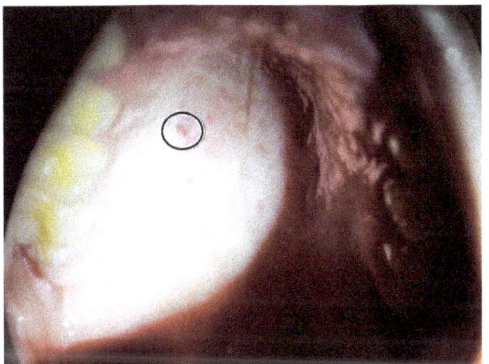

Fig. 9: Petechiae over hard palate (black circle).

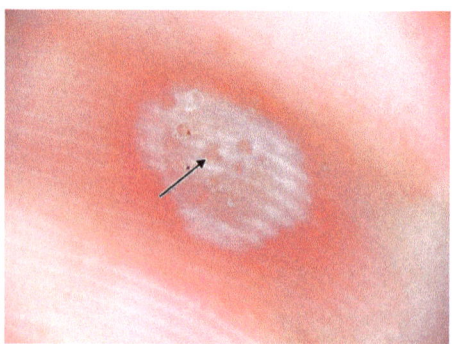

Fig. 10: Appearance of vesicle in vesicle (black arrow).

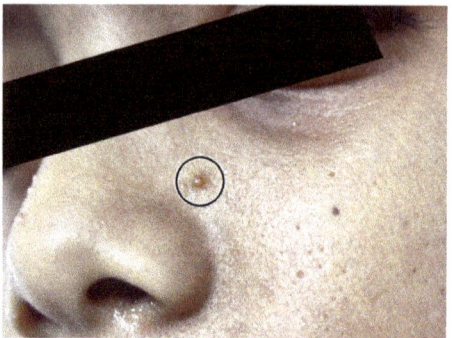

Fig. 11: Umbilicated white papule (black circle).

Molluscum Contagiosum

It is caused by a DNA poxvirus with characteristic pearly white papules with central umbilication (Fig. 11). Dermoscopy

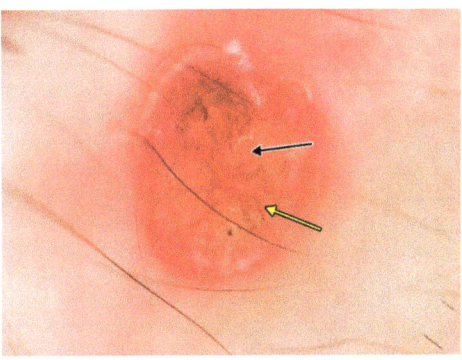

Fig. 12: Central umbilication with molluscum bodies (black arrow) is surrounded by blood vessels in a crown pattern (yellow arrow), also known as the red corona.

reveals central crater surrounded by multilobulated, yellowish white, amorphous structures (black arrow) that correlates with epidermal hyperplasia. Linear radiating vessels in crown pattern (red corona) surround the central crater[6] (Fig. 12). The pattern is produced by linear vessels originating from the periphery of the lesion and radiating toward the center but not crossing the center. The pattern is probably caused by compression and separation of the vessels by collagenous septa.[7]

Verrucae

This results from epidermal hyperplasia induced by human papilloma virus infection. Clinical differential diagnosis includes corns and calluses (Fig. 13).[8] Dermoscopy shows

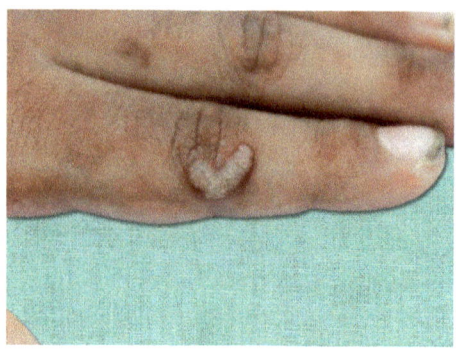

Fig. 13: Skin-colored papule with rough surface.

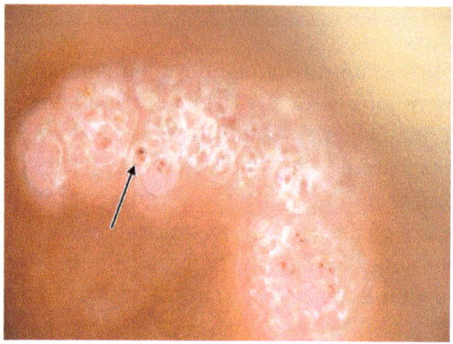

Fig. 14: Multiple densely packed papilla, each containing a central red or black dot (black arrow).

numerous closely packed papillae, each showing a central red or black dot or loop with a whitish halos (Fig. 14). While the red dots represent normal capillaries, the black dots correlate with thrombosed capillaries.[9]

FUNGAL INFECTIONS

Tinea Capitis

Tinea capitis is characterized by patchy areas of scaly hair loss (Fig. 15), sometimes with features of kerion or favus. Though potassium hydroxide (KOH) mount and fungal culture are the gold standard of diagnosis in tinea capitis, trichoscopy provides quick bedside help. Most common trichoscopic signs include comma and corkscrew hairs.[10] Comma hairs[8] (yellow arrow) (Fig. 16) are curved, C-shaped hair shafts associated with *Microsporum canis* and *Trichophyton tonsurans* infections. Corkscrew-shaped hair is described with *Trichophyton violaceum*, *Trichophyton soudanense*, and *M. langeroni*

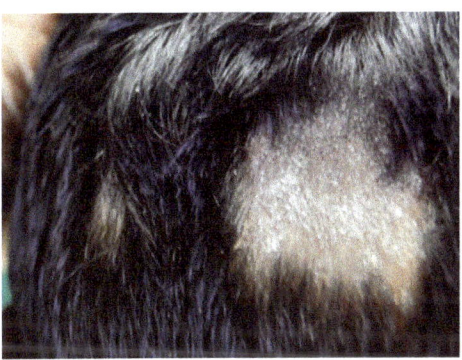

Fig. 15: Patchy area of scaly hair loss.

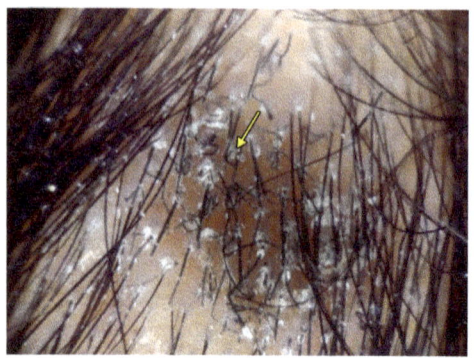

Fig. 16: Comma-shaped hair (yellow arrow).

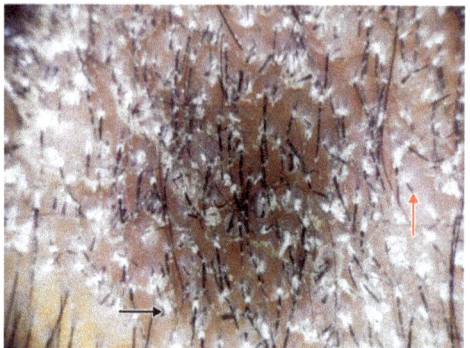

Fig. 17: Broken hair (red arrow) and black dot (black arrow).

infections. Less common signs are black dots (black arrow, Fig. 17), broken hair (red arrow), morse code hair, i-hair, and tufted folliculitis.[11-13]

Pityriasis Versicolor

It clinically presents as well defined hypopigmented/brown/black/red-colored macules over back or seborrheic distribution (Fig. 18). Dermoscopy of achromic/hypochromic lesions of *pityriasis versicolor* usually shows a fairly well demarcated white area with fine scales that are commonly localized in the skin furrows, and around hair follicles (Fig. 19).

INFESTATIONS

Pediculosis Capitis

Pediculosis capitis, caused by lice infestation, presents as itchy, scaly scalp. It needs to be differentiated from tinea capitis, seborrheic dermatitis, and atopic dermatitis. Presence of nits attached to hair shafts 1–2 mm from surface indicates

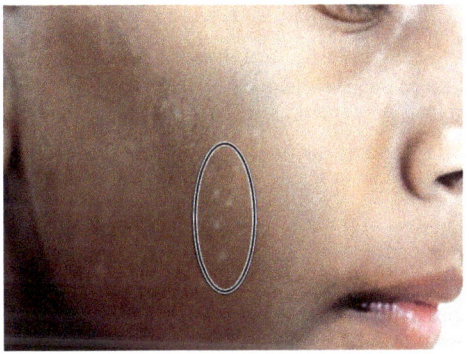

Fig. 18: Well-defined hypopigmented scaly macules (black oval).

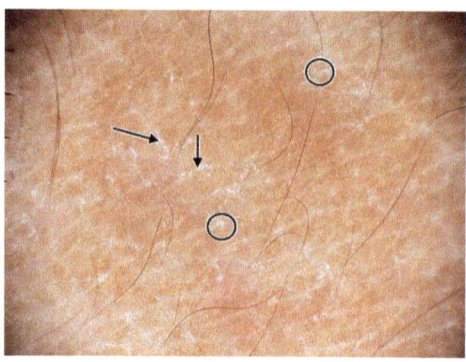

Fig. 19: Fine scale around hair follicle (black circles) and in skin furrows (black arrows).

active lice infestation. Nits can be differentiated from scales by dermoscopy. It can also help in determining whether nits are viable or dead and whether infestation is responding or not.[12] Viable nits are ovoid and brown while dead nits (empty eggs) are translucent, oval with a flat free end (Fig. 20). Dead nits may sometimes be partly brown due to collapsed nymph and partly translucent due to an air pocket.[13,14]

Scabies

Scabies is an extremely itchy condition caused by *Sarcoptes scabiei var hominis*. Scabies have characteristic lesions called burrows predominantly in flexures and multiple skin colored papules in characteristic distribution of "circle of Hebra". Nocturnal symptoms, distribution of lesions (Fig. 21) and family

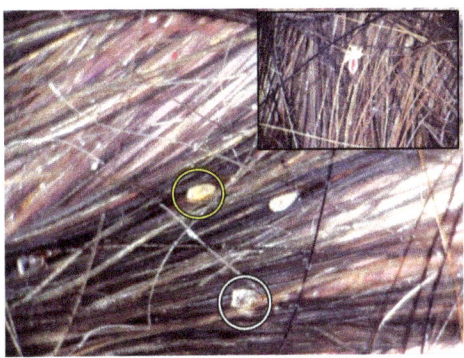

Fig. 20: Nits; viable nits (yellow circle); empty egg cases (white circle) and live lice in inset.

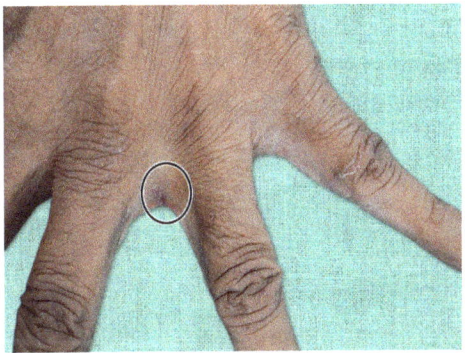

Fig. 21: Characteristic burrow visible in web space (black circle).

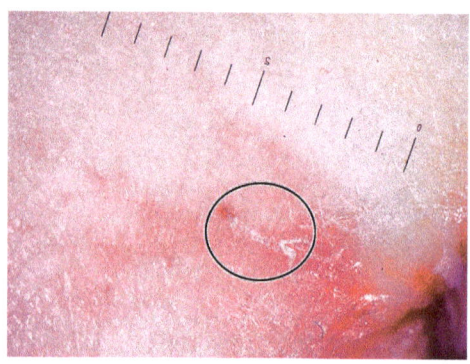

Fig. 22: "Delta wing and Jet contrail sign" with delta formed by triangular hyperpigmented area, which contains mite with jet contrail formed by burrow (black circle).

history most of the time clinches the diagnosis but difficulty arises in diagnosing atypical cases and scabies-in-clean cases. Dermoscopy reveals characteristic sign called as "delta wing with contrail" or "hanging glider sign" where contrail is burrow and delta wing is the mite seen in web spaces (Fig. 22).[15,16] Often the area near burrows shows hyperpigmented triangular solid structure, which is scybala of scabies mites also known as "mini triangle sign".[17-19]

CONCLUSION

Infections and infestations in which characteristic features in dermoscopy have been described have been mentioned here. There are a number of other infections and infestations in which dermoscopic features are not described/validated or whose dermoscopic features are not characteristic. Those have not been alluded to in this chapter.

REFERENCES

1. Weinberg JM, Tyring SK. Retapamulin: an antibacterial with a novel mode of action in an age of emerging resistance to *Staphylococcus aureus*. J Drugs Dermatol. 2010;9(10):1198-204.
2. Brasiello M, Zalaudek I, Ferrara G, et al. Lupus vulgaris: a new look at an old symptom—the lupoma observed with dermoscopy, Dermatology. 2009;218(2):172-4.
3. Lallas A, Argenziano G, Apalla Z, et al. Dermoscopic patterns of common facial inflammatory skin diseases. JEADV. 2014;28(5):609-14.
4. Balachandra S, Punit S. Dermoscopy of borderline tuberculoid leprosy. Int J Dermatol. 2018;57(1):74-6.
5. Sharma N. Hand, foot, and mouth disease: current scenario and Indian perspective. Indian J Dermatol Venereol Leprol. 2013;79:165-75.
6. Haliasos EC, Kerner M, Jaimes-Lopez N, et al. Dermoscopy for the pediatric dermatologist part I: dermoscopy of pediatric infectious and inflammatory skin lesions and hair disorders. Pediatr Dermatol. 2013;30(2)163-71.
7. Zaballos P, Ara M, Puig S, et al. Dermoscopy of molluscum contagiosum: a useful tool for clinical diagnosis in adulthood. J Eur Acad Dermatol Venereol. 2006;20:482-3.
8. Bae JM, Kang H, Kim HO, et al. Differential diagnosis of plantar wart from corn, callus and healed wart with the aid of dermoscopy. Br J Dermatol. 2009;160:220-2.
9. Fazel N, Wilczynski S, Lowe L, et al. Clinical, histopathologic, and molecular aspects of cutaneous human papillomavirus infections. Dermatol Clin. 1999;17:521-6.

10. Slowinska M, Rudnicka L, Schwartz RA, et al. Comma hairs: a dermatoscopic marker for tinea capitis: a rapid diagnostic method. J Am Acad Dermatol. 2008;59:S77-9.
11. Sandoval AB, Ortiz JA, Rodríguez JM, et al. Dermoscopic pattern in tinea capitis. Rev Iberoam Micol. 2010;27:151-2.
12. Hughes R, Chiaverini C, Bahadoran P, et al. Corkscrew hair: a new dermoscopic sign for diagnosis of tinea capitis in black children. Arch Dermatol. 2011;147:355-6.
13. Mapelli ET, Gualandri L, Cerri A, et al. Comma hairs in tinea capitis: a useful dermatoscopic sign for diagnosis of tinea capitis. Pediatr Dermatol. 2012;29:223-4.
14. Pinheiro AM, Lobato LA, Varella TC. Dermoscopy findings in tinea capitis: case report and literature review. An Bras Dermatol. 2012;87:313-4.
15. Suh KS, Han SH, Lee KH, et al. Mites and burrows are frequently found in nodular scabies by dermoscopy and histopathology. J Am Acad Dermatol. 2014;71:1022-3.
16. Criado PR. Entodermoscopy: dermoscopy for the diagnosis of pediculosis. An Bras Dermatol. 2011;86(2):370-1.
17. Di Stefani A, Hofmann-Wellenhof R, Zalaudek I. Dermoscopy for diagnosis and treatment monitoring of pediculosis capitis. J Am Acad Dermatol. 2006;54(5):909-11.
18. Grover C, Jakhar D. Dermoscopy in diagnosis of scabies. Int J Dermoscope. 2017;1(2):67-8.
19. Fox G. Diagnosis of scabies by dermoscopy. BMJ Case Rep. 2009;2009. pii: bcr06.2008.0279.

Index

Page numbers followed by, *f* refer to figure,
fc refer to flowchart, and *t* refer to table

A

Acantholytic dyskeratotic acanthoma, subungual 293
Acanthosis nigricans 95, 100, 102*f*, 104*f*
    dermatoscopy of 25*f*
    mild 101*f*
    moderate 102*f*
    severe 103*f*
    sulci pattern of 104*f*
Acanthotic epidermis 463*f*
Accentuated dark-brown pigment network 117
Achromatic lens 5
Achromic areas 173
Acne vulgaris 107*f*, 455
Acral amelanotic melanoma, dermoscopic features of 444
Acral skin 53
Acrosyringia 231
Acrotrichia 231
Actinic keratosis 71, 80, 434
    clinical variants of 435
    dermoscopy of 435
    diagnosis of 434, 435
    hypertrophic 435, 436*f*
    nonpigmented 435
    pigmented 435, 437*f*
    proliferative 435
    various grades of 436*t*
Actinic lentigo 117
Active papular lesion 399*f*
Active scleroderma pattern 328*f*
Adnexal openings, characteristic sparing of 127
Adnexal tumors 69
Alcoholic disinfectant 25
Alopecia
    areata 82, 314, 315*f*, 334, 344, 345*f*, 346*f*, 369, 370*f*, 373*f*, 374*f*
        active border of 371*f*

dermoscopic findings of 370
    stable patch of 372*f*
  chemotherapy-induced 351, 351*f*
  congenital triangular 349
  frontal fibrosing 337, 357
  patchy
    nonscarring 369
    scarring 379
  temporal triangular 349
Alopecic patch 344
Ameboid 170, 173, 179
  pattern 177, 200, 201*f*
Amyloidosis, systemic 276
Anagen
  matrix, affection of 373
  telogen ratio 387, 392
Androgenetic alopecia 335, 341, 342, 363, 364
  dermatoscopy of 82
Angiofibroma 411, 423
Angiogenesis 324
Angiokeratoma 411, 423, 425*f*
Angioma serpiginosum 154
Anisotrichosis 342
Annular granular pattern 435
Antigen 300
Antiseptic solution 2
Apocrine hidrocystoma 411, 428
Arboriform vascular pattern 349
Arciform structures 143*f*
  short 142

Argyriasis 96
Arrector muscle bundles 157
Arsenic pigmentation 96
Ashy dermatosis 246, 247*t*, 249*f*, 250*f*, 251*f*, 253
  dermoscopy of 253*f*-255*f*
Ataxia telangiectasia 158
Atopic dermatitis 104*f*, 266, 485
Atrichia 449
  focal 343
Atrophy 141, 401*f*
  epidermal 251*f*
  focal epidermal 248
Atypical pigment network 20
Atypical red vessels 262, 266, 268*f*, 354
Aurora borealis pattern 284*f*
Avascular areas 324, 325

B

Bamboo hair 361
Bannayan-Riley-Ruvalcaba syndrome 158
Basal cell
  carcinoma 18, 69, 78, 89, 90*f*, 293, 307, 428, 434, 441, 441*f*-443*f*, 459, 468*f*
    dermatoscopy of 91*f*
    dermoscopic features of 440*t*
    dermoscopy of 440
    early 467*f*

multiple 466
nodular 69
pigmented 17*f*
syndrome 466, 469
degeneration 248
Basal keratinocytes, vacuolar alterations of 231
Basal layer vacuolar change 460
Beaded hair 359
Becker's nevus 96, 156, 157*f*, 159*f*-161*f*, 165
   center of 163
   classical lesion of 160
   dermoscopic findings of 159
   diagnosis of 157
   periphery of 160
Benign acral nevi, lattice pattern of 444*f*
Benign skin tumors 410
   dermoscopy of 410
Bizarre pigmentation pattern 109
Black colloid milia 141
Black dots 335, 336*f*, 363, 364*fc*, 484
Bleomycin 295
Blood
   inclusion of 419
   vessels 57, 340, 355, 434
      macrophages around 154
Bloom syndrome 158
Blue nevi 415

Blue-gray
   blotches 114, 467, 467*f*
   dots 100, 463
   globules 109, 440, 467*f*
   ovoid nests 440, 441*f*
   pigmentation 468
Blue-white
   lacunae 423
   structures 446
   veils 20, 231
Bone and joint 294
Borderline lepromatous Hansen's disease 404
   hypopigmented patch of 405*f*
   ichthyotic patch of 404*f*
Borderline lepromatous leprosy, ichthyotic lesion of 404
Bowen's disease 80, 293, 301, 305, 306, 434, 437, 438*f*, 459
   dermoscopy of 437
Brain-like cerebriform appearance 79*f*
Breast 294
Broken hair 344, 347*f*, 349, 363, 364*fc*, 370, 371*f*, 484, 484*f*
   majority of 82
   short 347
Brown black pigment 308
Brown crusts 238

Brown dots 268, 337
Brown globules 110, 238
Brown skin, diseases of 10
Brownish granules, form of 232
Brownish orange dots 264
Brownish peripheral rim 423
Bushy capillaries 289, 325

C

Cadaverized hairs 335, 369
Café au lait macules 156-158, 158*f*, 161, 161t-163*f*
 dermoscopy of 160
Canfield VEOS DS3 30, 41, 42, 43*f*
Canfield VEOS HD1 27
Capillaroscopic microvascular morphology 322
Capillaroscopy 24
 pattern 325
Capillary architecture 325
 disorganization of 289
Capillary dilation 289
Capillary distribution 55
Capillary loop
 clusters 324
 inextricable knot of 321
Capillary loss 289, 325, 329
Carcinoma, onychodermal 294
Caviar-like papules 136, 139
Cellulitis, dissecting 335, 358
Central centrifugal alopecia 353, 358
Central linear depigmented macule 172
Central red globules 152
Central white crust 185
Central yellow-brown areas 231
Cerebriform pattern 20
Cherry angioma 73, 79*f*, 411, 416, 418*f*
Chloronychia 277, 278*f*
Chromonychia 281
Chromophores 12
Chronic granulomatous infection 404
Chrysalis 440, 442
Cicatricial alopecia 353
 causes of 379
 inflammatory 89
Cicatricial patches 383
Clark's level of invasion 309
Clear cell acanthoma 80
 characteristic of 62
Clustered glomerular vessels 438*f*
Coiled hairs 344, 348
Colloid bodies 248
Combines standard epiluminescence microscopy 392
Comb-like white structures project 210
Comedo-like openings 181, 420
Comedones 469

Comet-tail
  appearance 177
  like projection 170*f*
Comma hair 334, 347*f*, 375, 483
Comma vessels 16, 63, 66, 67*f*, 268, 354
Common benign tumors, classification of 411*t*
Compound nevus 67*f*, 415
Compulsive disorder 377
Concomitant atopy, manifestation of 453
Confetti macules 169*f*
Confetti-like depigmented dots 144
Confocal reflectance microscopy 93
Connective tissue
  disease 321, 322, 325
  papillae 51
Contact dermatoscopy, nonpolarized 54
Contact dermoscope 7
  principle of 3*f*
Contact leukoderma 33, 166
Coral vessels 71
Corkscrew 16, 347
  hairs 334, 347, 347*f*
  vessels 64, 70
Cornoid lamella 459, 459*f*
Corns 481
  pearls 231

Cosmetic dermatitis, pigmented 109
Coudability hairs 344
Coudability sign 344
Coxsackievirus 478
Crawling snake 361
Crista intermedia 444
Crista limitans 443
Crista profunda
  intermedia 53
  limitans 53
Crown
  pattern 481
  vessels 63, 68, 423
Cryosurgery 295
Cupuliform depressions 313
Curvilinear depressions 105
Curvilinear structures 144
Cutanea tarda, porphyria 96
Cutaneous horn 302
Cutaneous inflammatory diseases 84
Cutaneous lupus vulgaris, plaque of 397
Cuticle 55, 272*f*
Cyst
  malignant onycholemmal 294
  milia-like 27, 397, 412, 420, 475
  onychodermal 294
Cystic lesions 469
Cytoplasmic organelles 125

D

Darier's disease 276, 277f, 301
Dark blue lagoons 423
Dark brown macules 157
Dark lacunae and scar-like appearance 416
Deafness 449
Delta wing 488f
Demodex 338
Dendrites 125
Depigmentation, islands of 176
Depression, margins of 471
Dermabrasion 145
Dermal collagen 31
Dermal granuloma 397
   suggestive of 407
Dermal melanocytes, melanin of 173
Dermal melanocytic nevus 411
Dermal melasma 131f, 136
Dermal nevi 18
Dermal papillae 106
Dermal pigmentation 35
Dermal plexus, subpapillary 60
Dermal vascular plexuses, anatomy of 59
Dermatitis
   seborrheic 266, 268f, 353, 354t, 485
   stasis 154, 266
Dermatofibroma 18, 19, 73, 80, 411, 416
   hallmark of 416
Dermatoglyphic furrows 443
Dermatoglyphic lines 471
Dermatoglyphic ridges 444
Dermatomyositis 86f, 289, 324, 325
Dermatopathology 11
Dermatophyte infection 374
Dermatoscope 1, 30
   choice of 23, 37t
   compact 29
   history of 23
   nonpolarized 24, 26
   polarized 26
   traditional 40
   types of 24
Dermatoscopy 11, 23, 31, 32, 80, 84, 89
   application of 76, 77, 197
   expediency of 77
   green light in 34
   guided biopsies 78
   nonpolarized 27
   oral mucosal 34
   patterns 84
   role of 148
   yellow light in 34
Dermatosis
   common inflammatory 84
   inflammatory 4
   lesions, purpuric 148f
   progressive pigmentary 147f
Dermis 111
   diffuse fibrosis in 113
   reticular 96

Dermlite 3Gen DL1 41
Dermlite carbon 27
Dermlite DL1 43, 44*f*
   basic 30
Dermlite DL200 HR 27
Dermlite Hüd 30
Dermoepidermal junction 443
   damaged 111
Dermoepidermal structures 10
Dermoscope
   component of 6
   parts of 5
   role of 166
Dermoscopic analysis 156
Dermoscopic appearance varies 435
Dermoscopic criteria 89
Dermoscopic findings, basis of 434
Dermoscopic vascular patterns 63*t*
   shortlist of 62
Dermoscopy 10, 11, 60, 73, 107, 111, 123, 141, 150-153, 175, 192, 253, 259, 295, 377
   based classification 126
   basic of 1
   clinical need of 148
   findings 375
   infections 473
   infestations 473
   principles of 1, 2
   purpose of 204, 369, 374, 377, 380, 382
   specificity of 435
   techniques of 1
   use of 197, 410, 431
   value of 145
Desmin 300
Desquamative patches plaques 89
Diamond necklace 463, 464*f*
Diffuse brown pigmentation 49
Diffuse erythema, presence of 105
Diffuse structureless brownish areas 219
Digital dermatoscopes 333
Digital fibrokeratoma 293, 294, 302
   toenail, acquired 302*f*
Digital mucous cyst 293, 304, 304*f*
Direct skin contact fluid 77
Discoid lupus 89
   erythematosus 82, 82*f*, 96, 112, 334, 356, 363, 376, 381, 383*f*, 384*f*
      dermoscopic features of 382
Disseminated superficial porokeratosis 457, 458*f*

Distal end onychoscopy 285f
Distal interphalangeal joint 304
Dot pattern 51
Dotted vessels 62, 63, 183, 191
Double follicular units 56
Doucas and Kapetanakis, eczematoid-like purpura of 146, 148f
Dowling-Degos disease 469, 470f, 472f
   late macule of 471f
Dyskeratosis congenita 96
Dyskeratotic cells 460
Dystrophic hair 357

E

Eccrine
   pores 100
   sweat glands 53f
Ectodermal dysplasia 449
Eczema 259
   chronic 238
   dermoscopic features of 268t
   dermoscopy in 264
   follicular 453, 453f
   nummular 265
Eepidermal thickness, reduced 105
Electrodessication 307
Empty hair follicle 344f
   presence of 343
Entomodermatoscopy 23
Entomodermoscopy 80
Epidermal cyst 411, 426, 427f
Epidermal growth factor receptor 298
Epidermal hyperplasia, mild 250f
Epidermal melanin, loss of 176
Epidermal nevus, androgen-dependent 156
Epidermal rete ridges, types of 53
Epidermis 106, 111
   upper layer of 129, 449
Epiluminescence microscope 1, 47
Episcope 1
Erbium-doped yttrium aluminium garnet laser 295
Erosion 400
Eruptive vellus hair cyst 455
Erythema 104f, 141, 141f, 172f, 236f, 377, 397, 434
   blotchy 107
   dyschromicum perstans 96, 98, 246
   mild 187f
   peripheral 423, 425f
Erythrodermas 89
Erythronychia 276, 276f
   longitudinal 277f

Exclamation mark hairs 344, 349, 370, 371*f*, 372, 373, 378
Exogenous ochronosis 96, 98, 135, 135*f*, 136, 139, 142
    diagnosis of 145
    incidence of 135
    initial stage of 141*f*
    over malar area 140*f*
    over zygomatic process 140*f*
Exostosis, subungual 293, 294, 303

F

Face 49, 253, 255, 258
Facial
    acanthosis nigricans, early 104*f*
    hyperpigmentation 95, 96
        dermoscopy of 119
        disorders of 95
    inflammatory skin diseases 89
    melanosis, common 132*t*
    pigmentary disorders 136
    skin, dermatoscopy of 50*f*
Faint erythema 127
Fanconi anemia 158
Fern leaf pattern 209
Fibrokeratoma 301, 411, 428
Fibrous tissue tumors 294
Filaggrin 449
Filiform wart 68*f*
Fine short linear vessels 183
Fingerprint-like
    pattern 51
    structures 416
Fish scale-like pattern 51
Fissures, longitudinal 281
Fixed drug eruption 96, 111, 111*f*
Flame hairs 349
Focal hyperpigmented dots 100
Follicles 349
Follicular globules 105, 129*f*
    forming sulci pattern 105
Follicular hyperplasia 358
Follicular openings 219, 449, 451*f*
    loss of 400
    obliteration of 135
Follicular orifice 363, 363*fc*
Follicular ostia 56, 357, 359, 373, 374*f*, 435
    empty 378
    loss of 112
Follicular ostium, single 56
Follicular papules, prominent raised 454
Follicular plugs 110, 380, 397, 400, 407
Follicular red dots 356
Follicular scale-crust 377
Follicular structures 142
Follicular unit hair transplantation 82

Folliculitis 455
    bacterial 341
    decalvans 341, 353, 358
    dissecting 358
    tufted 353, 358, 484
Fotofinder dermoscopeó 31
Fotofinder handyscope 30, 41, 44, 45f
Freckles 96
Frontotemporal hairline 357
Fungal
    elements 375
    infection 483
        deep 402

G

Galaxy sign 178f, 198, 199f
Genetic hair shaft abnormalities 359
Genitourinary tract 294
Genodermatoses 466
Genus Leishmania 190
Giant capillaries 324, 325
Giant melanosomes, occasional presence of 157
Giant vessels 55
Globular yellowish brown pigmentation 237
Globules 151, 163, 209
Glomerular vessels 64, 70, 71f, 191, 262, 268, 340f, 353f, 354, 437
    presence of 154
Glomus cells 299
Glomus tumor 276, 293, 294, 299, 300, 300f, 301
    vascularity of 31
Glutaraldehyde 295
Glycerin 2
Granular layer
    absence 459
    reduced 459
Granuloma
    annulare 405
        annular plaque of 406f
    noncaseating 406
    pyogenic 411, 417, 419f
    pyogenicum 293, 294, 297, 297f
Granulomatous dermatoses, patterns of 396
Granulomatous disorders 396, 405, 407
Granulomatous skin disease
    dermoscopic hallmark of 397
    dermoscopy of 396
Gray dots 150, 337
Gray-black granules 100
Grayish white veil-like structureless WS 224
Guttate hypomelanoses 173
Guttate lichen sclerosus 166
Guttate psoriasis 262, 263f
Guttate vitiligo 179, 197, 199f
    lesions of 198

H

Hailey-Hailey disease 276
Hair
    and scalp 56
        dermatoscopy 56
        diseases 23, 80
    chromophores of 12
    clipping of 387
    density 343, 386
    diameter measurement 389
    follicle 49, 161, 373, 486*f*
        openings 334
    growth 391*f*
        rate, measurement of 394
    length of 390, 391*f*
    loss
        assessment of 386
        disorders 373
        female pattern 341
        irregular patches of 379
    monilethrix-like 344
    parameters of 386
    pulling tic 377
    regrowth 346
    shafts 56, 333, 378
        diseases 82
    short stubs of 375
    zigzag-shaped 347
Hairpin
    loops 60
    vessel 16, 63, 67, 68*f*, 191
Halo nevus 411, 413, 415*f*

Hand
    eczema, chronic 264, 265
    foot, and mouth disease 473, 478
    illuminated microscopes 8
Hanging curtain sign 233
Hanging glider sign 488
Hansen's disease 189, 404, 473, 475
    hypopigmented patch of 189, 190*f*
Hebra circle 486
Heine delta 20 plus 27
HEINE iC1 30, 41, 44, 45*f*
Hemangioma 18
Hematomas, subungual 275*f*
Hemorrhage 55, 326*f*, 328*f*
    perifollicular 378
    splinter 277*f*, 278, 279*f*, 281, 300, 313, 314, 317
Hemosiderin laden macrophages 153
Hidden hair 262, 266, 354
High-resolution ultrasonography 310
Histoplasmosis 402
    indurated plaque of 403*f*
    umbilicated papule of 403*f*
Homogeneous globular
    components 114
    pattern 114
Homogeneous purpuric patches, irregular-shaped 153

Homogeneous round achromic
    areas 164
Honeycomb-like reticular
    pigment network 57
Honeycomb pigment
  networks 112
  pattern 268
Honeycomb pigmentation 339*f*,
    343
Hori nevus 133
Human enterovirus 478
Human papillomavirus 295
Hutchinson's sign 308
Hybrid dermatoscopes 27
Hydroquinone 145
  prolonged application of 139
  use of 134
Hypergranulosis 248
  wedge-shaped 231
Hypergranulotic infundibula
    232
Hyperkeratosis 248
  subungual 285*f*, 313
Hyperkeratotic follicular
    plugging 383
Hyperkeratotic ridge, diamond
    necklace appearance
    of 464*f*
Hypermelanotic rete ridges 412
Hyperpigmentary skin 126
Hyperpigmentation 96, 141, 161,
    197, 247, 338
  blotchy areas of 159
  diseases of 198
  disorders of 95
  evaluation of 105
  honeycombed 380
  macular 163
  parafollicular 160, 160*f*, 161,
    163
  perifollicular 102, 106, 107*f*,
    171, 172*f*, 250*f*, 378, 412
  perilesional 171
  periorbital 95, 105
  peripheral reticulate 402*f*
  postinflammatory 95, 105,
    107*f*, 148, 218*f*
Hyperpigmented
  border 460
  globules 100
  lesion 157*f*
  macules, areas of 136
  maculopapular diseases 89
  margin 112, 170
  papules 224
  plaque 476*f*
  rete ridges 117
  tracks 463
  triangular solid structure 488
Hyperplasia
  epidermal 481
  focal 252*f*
    epidermal 248
  rete ridge pattern of 248
  sebaceous 68, 69*f*, 411, 423,
    424*f*

Hypertrichosis 134f, 156, 157f, 412
Hyphal pattern 51
Hypomelanosis 176
    pharmacologic 176
Hyponychium 54, 55, 280, 281f
Hypopigmentary disorders 175
Hypopigmentation 197
    central 469
    diseases of 198
    disorders of 166, 175, 176
    perifollicular 160, 160f, 453
    postinflammatory 92f, 176, 177, 187f, 188f, 191, 191f
Hypopigmented
    area 192
    halo 247
    holes 126
    lesions, differential diagnosis of 175
    macular dermatosis 89
    macules 185
    mycosis fungoides 176, 183
    patch 189, 402f, 477f
        accentuation of 31
        dermoscopic evaluation of 183
    scaly macules 485f
    vellus hairs 344
Hypovitaminosis A 455

I

Ice pick scars 106
Ichthyosis 449, 453
    follicularis 449
    vulgaris 449
Idiopathic guttate
        hypomelanosis 166, 175, 179, 197, 198, 202f
    dermoscopy of 181f
    petaloid pattern of 180f
Imiquimod, topical 307
Impetigo 474, 474f
Inbuilt illuminating system 5
Inbuilt photography systems 6
Infections 283
    bacterial 176, 474
Infectious disease
    common 80
    transmission of 80
Inflammatory disease 23, 277, 369
    dermoscopic examination of 84
Inflammatory disorders 47
Inflammatory purpura, types of 153
Inflated balloon appearance 400
Infundibulum, follicular 111, 225f, 449
Ingrown hair 454
Ink furrow test 445f

Interfollicular
    area 383
    dermis 380
    epidermis 338
Interfollicular region 110, 383
Intrapapillary capillary loops 52
Irregular brown globules 100
Irregular polycyclic margin 173
Isopropyl alcohol 25
Itchy 485
    papulonodular lesions 89
Ivory white
    areas 359
    background 428
    color 427

J

Jelly like synovial fluid 305
Jelly sign 127, 129f
Jet contrail sign 488f

K

Keratin
    filled craters 221
    plugs 112
        over follicular ostia 49
Keratinization, disorders of 449
Keratinocyte 125, 410
Keratinous plug 448, 451f
Keratitis 449
Keratoacanthoma 67, 293

Keratosis
    pilaris 448, 452f
        clinical differentials of 454
        dermoscopic features of 449
        dermoscopy of 448, 450f
        differential diagnosis of 453, 455t
        pathogenesis of 449
        reduction of 449
    subungual 281
Keratotic
    follicular papules 453
    papules, dermoscopy of 224
    ridge 458f
Koebner's phenomenon 200, 211, 242, 242f
    classical 214f
    dermoscopy of 243f
Koenen's tumor 293, 294, 302, 303, 303f
Kumkum pigment, granules of 111

L

Large blue-gray ovoid nests 443
Large brown globules 102, 105
Laser irradiation 145
Late scleroderma pattern 329f
Leaf venation pattern 209
Leishmaniasis 176, 190
    cutaneous 80, 190

Lentigines 96
Lentiginosis 164
Lentigo
- maligna 19
- simple 78
- simplex 117
  - dermoscopy of 118*f*

Leopard syndrome 158
Leprosy 176, 177
- hypopigmented patch of 189, 189*f*

Lesion
- annular 220*f*
- center of 159
- dermoscopic image of 217*f*, 218*f*, 234*f*, 235*f*, 239*f*
- dermoscopy of 236*f*
- distribution of 486
- evolution of 150
- periphery of 160, 161*f*

Leukocytoclastic vasculitis 149
Leukonychia 171, 276, 276*f*, 278, 313, 317
- longitudinal 277*f*

Lice nits 362*f*
Lichen
- planopilaris 82, 224, 335, 353, 354, 355*f*, 370, 379
  - characteristic feature of 381*f*
  - dermatoscopy of 28*f*, 35*f*
  - dermoscopic features of 380
  - dermoscopic image of 381*f*, 382*f*
  - scalp 226*f*
  - trichoscopy of 83*f*
- planus 86, 154, 204, 212*f*, 301
  - annular 219
  - classic lesion of 214*f*
  - dermoscopic evaluation of 209
  - dermoscopy in 204
  - diagnosis of 204
  - early lesion of 210*f*
  - follicular 224, 455
  - hypertrophic 221, 221*f*-223*f*
  - lesions, dermoscopy of 205
  - lesions nearing resolution 216*f*, 217*f*
  - mucosal 224
  - pigmented lesions of 219
  - pigmentosus 96, 98, 99*f*, 131, 133, 246, 247*t*, 249*f*-252*f*, 255, 257*f*
    - dermoscopy of 256*f*
    - lesions of 249*f*
  - subsided lesion of 218*f*
  - types of 205
- sclerosus et atrophicus 181, 182*f*
- scrofulosorum 397, 399*f*, 400*f*
- simplex chronicus 238, 240*f*

Lichenoid
  actinic keratosis 435
  dermatosis 146, 244
  drug eruption 232, 237f
  papules 247
Light dermoscopy, polarized 106, 460
Light-brown blot 119
Light-colored calms 161
Light-emitting diode 5
  bright illumination of 11
Linear crista cutis 100
Lip mucosa, dermatoscopy of 52f
Liquid paraffin 25
Loop pattern 51
Lung 294
Lunula 272f, 301, 313
Lupus erythematosus 232, 236f
  early lesion of 235f
Lupus vulgaris 89, 397, 398f, 473, 474
  lesion 399f
  reddish plaque of 398f
Lymphangioma circumscriptum 411, 419
Lymphocytes 250f
  less infiltration of 153
  perivascular infiltrate of 151, 154

M

Macular hypomelanosis,
  progressive 166
Macule
  border of 247
  depigmented 136, 171
  hyperpigmentated 158f
Majocchi's disease 146
Majocchi's purpura 147f
Malar 123
Malignant cutaneous tumors,
  dermoscopy of 434
Malignant melanoma 293, 294, 307
  dermoscopy of 443
  histological subtypes of 443
Maple leaf-like areas 440, 442, 442f
Marginal reticular pigmentation 171
Mastocytoma 119
Mastocytosis
  cutaneous 119
  maculopapular 119
Matrix cyst 293
Mature lesion 213f, 226
Mature melanocytic nevi,
  diagnosis of 66
Mature melanosomes 125
Mature violaceous
  papules 211
  plaques 211
McCune-Albright syndrome 158
Medulla, intermittent 360
Melanocyte 117, 125, 410
  epidermal 95, 175

follicular 95, 175
loss of 167
Melanocytic criteria 423
Melanocytic lesion 18, 59
Melanocytic nevus 24, 78, 293, 294, 411
  acquired 17*f*, 412, 414*f*, 443, 445*f*
  congenital 157, 163, 164*f*, 411, 412, 413*f*
  dermoscopy of 177
  junctional 411
Melanodermatitis toxica 109
Melanoma 18, 69, 276
  dermoscopy of 177
  metastasis 70
  ungual 308*t*
Melanonychia 273
  benign 275*f*
  longitudinal 307
Melanophages 106
  clusters of 100
  presence of 125, 144
Melasma 96, 126, 127*f*, 132, 145
  characteristic feature of 127
  classification of 126*t*
  clinical classification of 123, 124*f*
  dermoscopic
    characteristics of 128*t*
    features of 126
  dermoscopy in 122
  displays, dermoscopy of 142

epidermal 97*f*, 130*f*, 136
global feature of 128*f*
histopathological
  classification of 125*t*
lesions of 145
mixed 98*f*
patches 140*f*, 142
prognosis of 136
Methylated spirit 7
Mibelli classic porokeratosis 458*f*
Microhemorrhages 289
  local 324
Micro-Hutchinson sign 274
Micro-Koebner's phenomenon 167
Micropustules 377
Microscopic pigmentation, retention of 444
Microsporum 346
  canis 483
Microvascular involvement, different patterns of 287*t*
Microvascular loops 324
Microvessels, cutaneous 333
Mid spinous layer 460
Milia 411, 423, 426*f*
Mini triangle sign 488
Moh's micrographic surgery 307
Molescope 41, 44, 46*f*
Molluscum bodies 481*f*

Molluscum contagiosum 68, 81f, 473, 480
Monilethrix 334, 359, 359f
    hair shaft defect, trichoscopy of 83f
Morphea 96
Morse code hair 484
Moth eaten borders 420
Mucosa 50
    dermatoscopy of 50
Multilobular white-yellow amorphous structures 80
Multiple blue-gray globules 440, 443
Multiple endocrine neoplasia 158
Multiple follicular plugs 384f
Multiple lentigines syndrome 158
Multiple small erosions 442
Mycobacterium leprae 404
Mycobacterium tuberculosis 475
Mycosis fungoides 183
Myosin 299
Myxoid cyst 294

N

Nail 47, 54
    apparatus, melanoma of 443
    bed 55, 278, 281, 294
        hyperkeratosis 309
        involvement 313
        vessels 280
    chromophores of 12
    disorders 271
    dystrophy of 308
    fold
        abnormalities 23
        capillaroscopy 7, 85f, 287, 321
        lateral 272
        videocapillaroscopy pattern, normal 323f
    lichen planus 281, 282f
    matrix 278, 293, 300
        involvement 313
    melanin unit 294
    pigmentation 273
    pitting 281
    plate 55, 272f, 273, 278, 300, 309
        depression, linear band of 303f
        dermatoscopy of 55f
        greenish discoloration of 278f
    psoriasis 260, 261, 261f, 277, 281f, 283, 313
        dermoscopic features of 317t
        dermoscopy of 313
    trichrome vitiligo 166
    tumors 276
    unit
        benign tumors of 293t, 295
        different parts of 272f

malignant tumors of 293t, 305
melanoma, onychoscopic diagnosis of 274
pigmentation 274fc
trichrome vitiligo of 173
tumors, classification of 292
Naked eye
　diagnosis 78
　examination 244
Nebula-like appearance 190
Nebular pattern 198
Nebulous pattern 171, 199f
Necrobiosis lipoidica 406, 407
　dermoscopic examination of 407
　lesions of 407
Neodymium-doped yttrium aluminum garnet 134, 295
Neoplastic nail unit disorders 292
Netherton syndrome 361
Neurofibroma 302, 411, 416, 417f
Neurofibromatosis 158, 158f
Nevoid basal cell carcinoma 468f, 469f
　syndrome 466
Nevus depigmentosus 166, 192, 193f
　dermoscopy of 192f

Nevus depigmentosus
　hypopigmented macules of 192
　irregular border of 193
Nevus of Ota 114
　dermoscopy of 113f, 114
Nevus spilus 114, 115f, 164, 411, 414
　dermoscopy of 114, 164
Nevus types 415
Noncicatricial alopecia 341
Noninfectious balanitis 89
Noninflammatory purpura 153
Noninflammatory tinea capitis 377
Noninvasive alternative method 158
Nonmelanocytic round structure 455
Nonscarring alopecia 89
Normal pigmentary network lines 160
Normal scalp, trichoscopy of 341
Normal skin 48
　and appendages, dermatoscopy of 47
　dermatoscopy of 48f
　dermoscopy of 127f
Numerous brown pigment globules 142
Numerous cutaneous diseases 76

O

Occipital scalp 57
Ochronosis 131, 132, 139
  diagnosis of 144
Oil-drop patches 313
Onychocytic matricoma 293
Onychodermal band 272*f*, 314
Onycholemmal cyst, proliferating 294
Onycholemmal horn 294
Onycholysis 261, 261*f*, 278, 280*f*, 281, 285*f*, 307, 313, 317
  dermoscopy of 318*t*
  traumatic 318
Onycholytic bands 284*f*
Onychomatricoma 276, 293, 300
Onychomycosis 283, 283*f*-285*f*, 301, 306, 313, 318, 319*f*
  distal lateral 318, 318*t*
  proximal subungual 284*f*, 318
  total dystrophic 318
Onychopapilloma 276, 293, 301
Onychoscopy 23, 278, 310
  indications of 273*fc*
  overview of 271
Optilia digital capillaroscopy system 31
Orange-yellowish patchy areas 183, 185
Orthohyperkeratosis 243
Orthokeratosis 232
Osteochondroma 294

P

Pale cytoplasm 299
Palmar
  pits 469*f*
    dermoscopic image of 472*f*
  psoriasis 264, 264*f*
  skin, dermatoscopy of 53*f*
Palmoplantar
  lesions 224
  skin 53
Palms 47
Papillary dermal structures 10
Papillary dermis 96, 100
Papillomatosis 157
Papular lesions 449
Papule
  dermoscopy of 242*f*
  early 209
  erythematous 236*f*
  numerous skin-colored 402
Papulonodules 141
Papulosquamous disorders 204
Parallel pattern 51
Parasitic infection 176
Paronychia, chronic 306
Patch
  dermoscopy of 142*f*
  histopathology of 144*f*
Patchy alopecia 369
  trichoscopy of 369
Pediculosis capitis 362, 485

Periappendageal pigment loss 187f
Perifollicular cellular infiltrate 252f
Perifollicular depigmentation 167, 169f
Perifollicular discoloration 343
Perifollicular epidermis 333, 338
Perifollicular erosion, dermoscopy of 398f
Perifollicular erythema 378, 382f
    varying degrees of 448
Perifollicular halo
    diffuse telangiectasia 110
    typical 112
Perifollicular lymphocytic infiltrate 248
Perifollicular openings, sparing of 129
Perifollicular pigmentation 173, 199f, 202f, 262, 263f, 268, 354, 380
Perifollicular region, sparing of 111
Perifollicular scale 221, 352
Perifollicular white scale 266, 268f
Perifolliculitis capitis 358
Periorbital melanosis 105
    evaluation of 105
Peripheral brown rim 428
Peripheral globules 412
Peripheral microscales 239f
Peripheral pigment network 416
Peripheral reticular network 412
Peripheral vessels, prominent 215
Peripilar cast 380
Peripilar gray-white halo 358
Peripilar sign 339f, 343
Periungual tissue 294
Periungual warts 286, 286f, 296f
    fingerlike projections of 296f
    multiple coalescing 286f
Perpendicular axes 446
Petaloid 179
    pattern 177, 200f
Petechiae over hard palate 479f
Phototrichogram 386, 387, 392, 395
    automated 392
    classical 394
    contrast-enhanced 391
Pig tail 344
Pigment
    around hair follicle, retention of 178f
    brown granules of 180f
    brownish 221
    clusters, granules of 100
    diffuse network of 164
    incontinence 248
    loss, perifollicular accentuation of 188f

network
- distribution of 200
- gradual loss of 185
- like structures 420
- loss of 167f, 382
- perifollicular sparing of 106
- presence of 200
- reduction of 167f
- reticular pattern of 50, 100
- reversed 167, 177
- pattern, accentuated 119

Pigmentary demarcation lines 96, 116f, 117, 131, 133
Pigmentary dermatoses 8
Pigmentary disorders, primary 84
Pigmentary network 161
- absent 177
- interrupted 164

Pigmentary purpuric dermatosis 84
Pigmentation 49
- black dotted 338f
- blotchy 159, 376
  - homogeneous 164
- bluish gray 135
- depth of 96
- disorders of 197
- distribution of 249f
- enhancement of 125
- intense 471
- pattern of 105, 119
- perifollicular retention of 166, 167, 168f
- postinflammatory 164, 244
- pseudoreticular pattern of 153f
- reservoirs of 171
- structures 397, 407
- tends 209
- visualized 205
- well-defined 173

Pigmented contact dermatitis 109, 109f, 110, 110f
- pathology of 110

Pigmented lesions 13
- hallmark of 49

Pigmented macules 469
- dermoscopy of 470f

Pigmented purpuric dermatoses 146, 150f, 151f
- types of 155

Pigmented rings 469
Pigtail hairs 334, 346
Pili annulati 334, 360, 361
Pili torti 334, 360
Pilosebaceous units, presence of 49
Pits 278
- over nail plate 317

Pityriasis alba 166
Pityriasis lichenoides 185, 192

chronica 176, 187*f*
    active lesion of 186*f*
Pityriasis rosea 88*f*, 233, 238*f*, 239*f*
Pityriasis rubra pilaris 455
Pityriasis versicolor 185, 187*f*, 188*f*, 474, 485
    hypochromic lesions of 485
    white light image 185
Plane warts 242
Plantar lesions 227*f*
Plaque psoriasis 260, 260*f*
Plexus, subpapillary 59, 60
Pohle-Pinkus constrictions 344
Poikiloderma of Civatte 123
Polka dot 167, 168*f*
Polygonal globules 20
Polymyositis 289
Pompholyx 265, 266*f*
Porokeratosis 457, 460, 464*f*
    hallmark of 458*f*
    histopathology of 459*f*
    of Mibelli 457
    superficial 31
Post-kala-azar dermal leishmaniasis 191, 400, 401*f*
    plaque of 401*f*
Potassium hydroxide 319, 483
Prephotodynamic therapy 91*f*
Proximal erythematous band 280*f*

Proximal nail fold 54, 280, 295, 296*f*
    capillaries 283
    dermatoscopy of 54*f*
Prurigo nodularis 241, 241*f*
Pruritus 247
Pseudofolliculitis 454*f*
Pseudomonas aeruginosa 277
Pseudopelade 370
    of Brocq 353, 357
Pseudopods 20
Pseudoreticular pattern 106
Psoriasis 233*f*, 259, 279*f*, 285*f*, 314, 314*f*-317*f*, 353, 354*t*
    chronic plaque of 232, 234*f*
    dermatoscopy of 27*f*, 87*f*
    dermatoscopic features of 268*t*
    dermatoscopy in 260
    follicular 455
    scales 353*f*
    vulgaris 84
Purpura
    annularis telangiectodes 146, 147*f*
    steroid-induced 153
Purpuric clothing dermatitis 148
Purpuric dermatosis, progressive pigmented 146
Pustules, follicular 358

Q

Q-switched neodymium-doped yttrium aluminum garnet laser 134

R

Ramirez ashy dermatosis 98
Raynaud's phenomenon 287, 321, 322
Recurrent nevi 13
Red blood cells, extravasation of 151
Red dots 149, 151, 230, 262, 337, 337f, 354
   presence of 154
Red globules 230, 231, 262, 354
Red spots 313
Reddish brown crust 241
Reddish homogeneous areas, presence of 417
Reddish tinge reduces 152
Reflectance confocal microscopy 77
Regrowing hair 344, 346
Residual perifollicular pigmentation, presence of 171
Reticular pattern 164, 412
Reticular pigmentation, lesional 171
Reticular streaks 397, 407
Reticuloglobular network, irregular accentuation of 109
Reticuloglobular pattern 95, 97f, 98f, 107, 114, 117
Reverse skin pigmentary network 404
Riehl's melanosis 109, 131, 133
Ring-like pattern 51
Rolling scars 106
Rosacea 89
Round corneal structures 221
Round-to-oval red lacunas 154
Russell-Silver syndrome 158

S

Sagrada Familia sign 301
Salicylic acid 295
Salmon 313
   colored ovoid structures 400
   patch 278, 279f
Sarcoid granulomas 406
Sarcoidosis 89, 406, 407
Sarcoptes scabiei var hominis 486
Scabies 486
   scybala of 488
Scale
   color 268
   distribution 268
   peripheral collarette of 233
Scaling 377, 467, 468
   scalp disorders 89

Scalp 47
dermatoscopy of 56*f*, 57*f*
dissecting cellulitis of 358
psoriasis 66*f*, 262, 263*f*, 352, 353
Scaly hair loss, patchy area of 483*f*
Scanty white crusts 266
Scarring alopecia, multiple patches of 381
Scars, pitted 469
Schamberg's disease 146, 147*f*, 148, 149*f*, 153*f*
Scleroderma 288*f*, 289*f*
pattern 325
early 326*f*
Sclerosis
systemic 287, 321, 324, 325
tuberous 158
Scurvy 455
Sebaceous glands, absence of 449
Seborrhea 352*f*
Seborrheic alopecia 352
Seborrheic distribution 485
Seborrheic keratosis 13, 14*f*, 18, 67, 73, 411, 420, 422*f*
dermatoscopy of 79*f*
Semicircular hair 451*f*, 452*f*
Senile purpura 153
Siderophages 153
Sieve-like pattern 260

Signet ring vessels 262, 268, 340, 354
Silvery-white scaling 259
Single-lens reflex 27
Skin
biopsy 77
cancers, keratinizing 434
chromophores of 12
colored papule 242*f*, 482*f*
diseases, infectious 396
disorders, inflammatory 87*f*
furrows 485
interfollicular 57
lesions
nonpigmented 396
pigmented 396
lightening agents 135
perifollicular 57
sun-damaged 435
surface microscope 1, 332
tumors, evaluation of 396
Smartphone
dermatoscopes 29, 40, 44
dermoscopy 41
Snail-track appearance 162*f*
Solar lentigo 78, 117
Sparkle pattern 114
Sparse hair 378
Spitz nevus 411, 416
Spoke wheel
appearance 17*f*
area 20, 440, 442, 443
Spongiosis, follicular 110

Sprinkled hair 349
Squamous cell carcinoma 19, 67, 69, 80, 293, 295, 306, 434, 439*f*
   dermoscopy of 438
   types of 437
Starburst pattern 20, 397
Starry sky pattern 209, 355
Stasis pigmentation 148
Steatocystoma 411, 428, 429*f*
Steroid
   abuse, treatment assessment of 131
   application 117
   topical 136
Stratum malpighii 12
Strawberry pattern 20
Subtle leukotrichia, unmasking of 176
Subtle sulci pattern 100
Subungual warts, fingerlike projections of 296*f*
Sulcus cutis 100
Superficial papillary dermal vessels, hemorrhage of 146
Superficial perivascular infiltrate 250*f*
Superficial small blood vessels, macrophages around 151
Supernumerary digits 302
Sweat gland openings 49
Syringoma 411, 430, 430*f*
Systemic lupus erythematosus 329

T

Tapering hairs 351, 372
Tapioca sago 170
T-cell lymphoma, common primary cutaneous 183
Telangiectasia 172*f*, 182, 302, 337, 402, 407, 468, 476*f*
   arborizing 191, 397, 443
   deeper 183*f*
   fine focused 397
   globular 404
   linear 110, 402
   macularis eruptiva perstans 119
   presence of 171
   reticular 119
   short 112
   superficial 440, 441*f*
Telogen
   effluvium 343, 344*f*
   hairs 391*f*
Terminal hair 56*f*
   pilosebaceous unit of 449
Thick honey color crust-scale 475*f*
Thyroid diseases 122

Tinea capitis 341, 346, 347*f*, 374, 375, 375*f*, 474, 483, 485
  dermoscopic image of 376*f*
Tiny lichenoid papules 397
Traction alopecia 349, 350*f*
  hair cast 350*f*
Tranexamic acid 134
Triangular pigmentary band 274
Trichoanalysis 30
Trichoepithelioma 411, 428
Trichophyton 346
  soudanense 483
  tonsurans 483
  violaceum 483
Trichoptilosis 344, 347, 378
Trichorrhexis
  invaginata 334, 361
  nodosa 334, 344, 361
Trichoscan 386, 392, 395
Trichoscopy 23, 82*f*, 332, 333, 359
  equipment 333
  overview of 332
  patterns 333
  structures 333
  terminologies 333
Trichothiodystrophy 360
Trichotillomania 82, 334, 347, 348*f*, 377, 378
  dermoscopic
    findings in 378
    image of 379*f*
Trichrome
  pattern 177
  sign 168*f*
Tuberculosis
  cutis lichenoides 397
  cutaneous 397
Tuberculous foci 475
Tubular casts 354
Tubular perifollicular scales 354, 355*f*, 356*f*
Tulip hair 349
Tumors
  benign
    melanocytic 411*t*
    nonmelanocytic 411, 411*t*
  metastatic 293
  nail specific 294*f*
  subungual filamentous 293

U

Ulcer 400
Ulceration 89, 309, 440, 441*f*, 442, 443, 467
Ultraviolet 31
  light 31, 175
    dermoscopy 463, 464*f*
  radiation 122
  use of 377
Upper epidermis appears 96
Urticarial vasculitis 154

V

Vascular endothelial growth factor 122
Vascular lacunae 79f
Vellus follicle 450f
Vellus hair 56, 56f, 346, 370
  follicles 402
  nonpigmented 159
  short 344, 372
Verruca 293, 481
  plana 14f, 242f, 243f
  vulgaris 302
Vessels
  arborizing 69, 70f, 89, 356, 440
  coral pattern of 72f
  crown of 80
  cutaneous 13
  linear 14, 16t, 224, 427, 428
    irregular 64, 71, 191, 460
  onychodermal 317
  pattern of 268
  polymorphous 73
  thrombosed 295
  tortuous 224
  types of 268
  variable dermoscopic pattern of 183
Videodermoscope 5, 8f
  principle of 3f
Videodermoscopy
  principles of 1
  techniques of 1
Violaceous brown pigmentation 356f
Viral infections 473, 478
Visceral leishmaniasis 191, 400
Vitiligo 176, 177t, 178f, 179, 179f, 203
  active lesion of 169f
  dermatoscopy of 32f, 33f
  dermoscopic signs of 189
  dermoscopy in 166
  diagnosis of 166
  evolving lesions of 179
  histopathology of 198
  hypopigmented
    macules of 176
    patch of 190
  lesions of 202
  like perifollicular
    pigmentation, dermoscopic features of 200
  localized 197
  macule 176
  perifollicular pigmentation hallmark of 202f
  progressive 170f
  repigmenting 171
  stable 171, 171f
    repigmenting 172f

Volcanic crater 460
V-pattern 51
V-sign 349

W

Wart 294
    viral 295, 301
White chrysalis-like areas 182
White discoloration 343
White dots 335, 336*f*, 349
White light dermoscopy 460
White rail line 417
White starburst pattern 242
White track 460
Whitish irregular blotches 106
Whitish papules 224
Whitish-blue areas, structureless 428
Wickham striae 204, 205, 211*f*, 212*f*, 221, 230, 235*f*
    annular 211
    demonstration of 244
    linear 205
    patterns of 206*f*-208*f*
    rapid recognition of 204
    reticular 211
    ring-shaped 219
    round 205
    whitish globular 224
Wood's lamp 123, 125, 126*t*, 198
Woolly hair syndrome 361

Y

Yellow clods 49
Yellow dots 268, 334, 335*f*, 349, 371*f*
Yellow orange blot 119
Yellow scales 183
Yellowish brown hyperkeratotic plug 86
Yellowish scales 266
Yellowish tubular scaling 358

Z

Zygoma 123
Zygomatic region 141*f*

EU GSPR Authorised Reprsentative
Logos Europe, 9 rue Nicolas Poussin
1700, La Rochelle, France
Phone: +33 (0) 6 67 93 73 78
E-mail: contact@logoseurope.eu

www.ingramcontent.com/pod-product-compliance
Ingram Content Group UK Ltd.
Pitfield, Milton Keynes, MK11 3LW, UK
UKHW021826140426
5217IPUK00016B/1229